3rd EDITION
THE KID-FRIENDLY
ADHD& AUTISM
C⊙⊙KBOOK

THE ULTIMATE GUIDE
TO THE MOST EFFECTIVE DIETS
WHAT THEY ARE • WHY THEY WORK • HOW TO DO THEM

Pamela J. Compart, MD and Dana Laake, RD, MS, LDN

FAIR WINDS

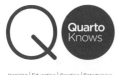

Brimming with creative inspiration, how-to projects, and useful information to enrich your everyday life, Quarto Knows is a favorite destination for those pursuing their interests and passions. Visit our site and dig deeper with our books into your area of interest: Quarto Creates, Quarto Cooks, Quarto Homes, Quarto Lives, Quarto Drives, Quarto Explores, Quarto Gifts, or Quarto Kids.

© 2006, 2009, 2020 Quarto Publishing Group USA Inc.
Text © 2006, 2009, 2020 by Pamela J. Compart and Dana Godbout Laake

First Published in 2006 by Fair Winds Press, an imprint of The Quarto Group, 100 Cummings Center, Suite 265-D, Beverly, MA 01915, USA.
T (978) 282-9590 F (978) 283-2742 QuartoKnows.com

Second edition published in 2009

Fair Winds Press titles are also available at discount for retail, wholesale, promotional, and bulk purchase. For details, contact the Special Sales Manager by email at specialsales@quarto.com or by mail at The Quarto Group, Attn: Special Sales Manager, 100 Cummings Center, Suite 265-D, Beverly, MA 01915, USA.

24 23 22 21 20   1 2 3 4 5

ISBN: 978-1-59233-850-4

Digital edition published in 2020

Library of Congress Cataloging-in-Publication Data available

Design: Danny Yee, Yee Design
Cover Images: Shutterstock.com
Page Layout: Claire MacMaster, barefoot art graphic design

Printed in China

The information in this book is for educational purposes only. It is not intended to replace the advice of a physician or medical practitioner. Please see your health-care provider before beginning any new health program.

This book is dedicated to all the courageous children and to all who love and serve them. We are humbled in your presence.

With gratitude, we also dedicate this edition to our distinguished colleagues in functional medicine and nutrition whose contributions have helped advance treatments and improve recovery rates for children with ADHD and autism.

With special appreciation, we also recognize the Autism Research Institute for its unwavering commitment to supporting research, educating professionals, families and patients, and providing opportunities for practitioners from diverse fields to convene and share their knowledge and expertise.

Our hope is to continue to educate ourselves, our patients, and their families as we share their journeys. Our goal is to help those with ADHD and autism achieve their best individual potential.

And finally, we honor the three pioneers whose foresight and brilliance changed the trajectory of evaluation, research, and treatment, achieving a far-reaching paradigm shift: Bernard Rimland, Sidney MacDonald Baker, and Jon Pangborn.

Contents

Preface

When I went to medical school over twenty years ago, nutrition was given very little attention. Although I attended a very open-minded, cutting-edge school, my nutrition training consisted of one week of lectures. This left my colleagues and me with the impression that, at the time, nutrition was not felt to be very relevant to the practice of medicine. As I proceeded through my traditional training, not much happened to dispel that notion. It was only after I completed my formal training and began practicing in the "real world" of developmental pediatrics that I realized how critically important nutrition is to overall health and, in particular, to brain functioning.

Early on in my training, when parents would ask me if they should try special diets or nutritional supplements for their special-needs children, I distinctly remember advising them not to waste their time, as there was no evidence to show that they helped. I wish now that I could find all those parents and tell them they were right to be thinking outside the box. Parents have always been motivated to look at all options to help their children, especially those with special needs. It is only now that science is catching up with what those parents asked many years ago. Part of the role of this book is to explain the science behind the diets and why these diets may be worth trying with your child.

I am grateful that I came to an understanding of nutrition via a traditional medical route. I was not at all predisposed to believing that diets would help

change behavior, development, and brain function. So when I saw diets working, I knew it was not a placebo effect. Still, I wanted to know *why* they worked and have now devoted my medical practice to understanding these less traditional approaches. My traditional training also reminds me that there is no one way to treat children with special needs. Many people in both camps (traditional and nontraditional) assume that the type of intervention they favor is the right one. I believe strongly in using all the tools I have at my disposal to help children reach their potential, whether those tools are traditional (therapy, school placement, medications, etc.) or less traditional (diet change, nutritional supplements, digestive support, etc.). This book addresses some of these less traditional tools, specifically diet and nutrition.

Dr. Sidney Baker, in his book *Detoxification and Healing*, outlines a helpful context for thinking about the role of diet in brain function. In essence, he asks two basic questions that, for me, form the basic foundation of my approach to caring for children with special needs. Paraphrased here, these two questions are:

1. Is this child's body and brain getting all that is needed to perform optimally?

2. Is there something getting to this child's brain that interferes with its ability to perform optimally?

Diet and nutrition are clearly involved in answering both of these questions. An optimized diet, along with nutritional supplements, provides nutrients that are essential for body and brain functioning. In addition, breakdown products from certain foods (particularly dairy and glutens) can interfere with brain functioning. These concepts will be explained further in the chapters that follow. The recipes in this book are designed to give the body and brain what is needed and to eliminate those substances that are most likely to interfere with function.

In medicine, there is a saying that you don't have to remember everything, you just have to remember where you filed the article. In the same way, I don't have to know everything about nutrition; I have to know who my good resources are to complement my medical knowledge of health and nutrition; Dana Laake, my coauthor, is such a resource.

Pamela J. Compart, MD

My introduction to nutrition began through a career in dental hygiene. I learned the powerful effects of food on the body and mind from Emanuel Cheraskin, a physician and dentist, who was an internationally renowned researcher and expert in the field of nutritional medicine. While attending a course led by this pioneer, whose influence would guide me for decades, I fell in love with the fields of nutrition and preventive medicine. Cheraskin opened the first of many doors in this challenging and steadily evolving field. His legacy was great, but I remember him most for the simplicity of his favorite statement, "Man is a food-dependent creature; if you don't feed him he will die. If you feed him improperly, a part of him will die."

In 1979, George Mitchell, our family physician, invited me to join him in opening a preventive medicine practice in Washington, D.C. He introduced me to the innovators and visionaries in nutrition and alternative medicine. Though criticized in their new ideas, most prevailed and received the recognition they deserved.

Early on in the practice, I experienced a challenge when a seven-year-old boy was brought in by his distraught mother. She said that he was a conundrum to his family, teachers, and pediatrician. Beginning at two years of age, he was physically violent toward others, including routinely striking his father, and was unable to function in school because of poor attention span, impulsivity, acting out, and aggression.

He had chronic bowel problems, wet his bed nightly, and was in a constant state of agitation and unhappiness. Showing the reports from his teachers, his mother cried as she confessed, "each teacher tells me that he is the worst child they have ever encountered."

A review of his diet revealed that milk products and glutens (wheat) were his most common and favorite foods. This occurred in the era when there was little acceptance of the connection between food and behavior. I had read about the connections in newsletters from Bernard Rimland, PhD, founder of the organization that became the Autism Research Institute. Although we did not have the quality and accuracy of testing so prevalent today, the anecdotal evidence was growing. Since a trial of food avoidance fits the medical dictum, "do no harm," I recommended a trial avoidance of milk products and gluten.

The results stunned me as much as the parents. After the first few days without milk products and gluten, the boy became worse, which was what we understood to be withdrawal. But within a week of avoidance, he began to improve; he cooperated at school, began to progress in achievements, received outstanding behavior reports, and stopped aggressive and impulsive behaviors. His bowels improved, and he no longer wet the bed at night. Most importantly, he stopped hitting his father and began hugging again. Thinking he was "cured," his parents allowed him to have cake and ice cream at a birthday party, only to have him relapse into the full spectrum of aggressive symptoms and bed-wetting. They returned to the diet, and his symptoms resolved once again. I am eternally grateful for what this child taught me; he sparked the beginning of my journey into a new and expanding territory that continues to enlighten me every day.

Dana Godbout Laake, RDH, MS, LDN

Introduction

"There is one thing stronger than all the armies in the world, and that is an idea whose time has come."

—Victor Hugo

Why Buy This Book?

Although written for children with Attention Deficit Hyperactivity Disorder (ADHD) or autism spectrum disorders (ASD), it can be helpful for any child with a variety of behavioral or developmental challenges. Because it may be easier to change the entire household's diet at the same time, this book is also written for the families. Other family members are often surprised by improvements in their own health and behavior.

You may wonder how this book is different from other elimination diet recipe books. We believe this book is different in several ways:

- When implementing a special diet, it is hard to take "on faith" that it may help. This book explains the reasons why diet changes may help your child's brain and body function better.

- We recognize that it is much easier to recommend a specialized diet than to actually implement it. This book includes helpful suggestions on how to begin and how to maintain a specialized diet.

- We are aware that changing diets in children, especially children who are picky, can be a challenging undertaking. This book includes many helpful hints for dealing with the picky eater.

- Not everyone likes or has time to cook. We have included "Quick N Easy" versions of recipes for parents on the go. For those who prefer more complex recipes, we have included those as well.

- Children with ASD often have additional challenges, in both behavior and biochemistry, which can make feeding an even more difficult task. This book includes ways to hide or disguise nutritious and healthy foods in ways children will accept.

- Many books about specialized diets focus only on the elimination of gluten and casein. There are subsets of children who may also react to other common offending foods such as soy, egg, corn, and nuts; yeast-promoting foods; and food components such as phenols (including salicylates), double sugars (disaccharides), and oxalates. This book includes recipes that are free of multiple offending foods.

- This edition includes more of the diets currently being used for children with autism, ADHD, and other challenges. It also includes new recipes or modifications to previous recipes, appropriate to the additional diets.

- This book focuses not only on what is being taken out of a diet, but also on what is put back in. The goal of elimination diets is not just removing unhealthy or potentially harmful foods, but also providing nutritious, appealing foods in their place.

What Is Attention Deficit Hyperactivity Disorder?

ADHD is a collection of symptoms including inattention, hyperactivity, and impulsivity. There is no blood test that can diagnose ADHD. It is diagnosed by a certain number of symptoms presenting in a particular combination. A paraphrasing of these symptoms from the manual that provides the current definition of ADHD, the *Diagnostic and Statistical Manual of Mental Disorders, 5th edition*, or *DSM-5*, follows:

- **INATTENTION SYMPTOMS:** Failure to pay close attention to details or making careless mistakes in schoolwork or other activities, difficulty sustaining attention, often not seeming to listen when spoken to directly, often not following through on instructions or failure to complete tasks, difficulty organizing tasks and activities, avoiding tasks that require sustained mental effort (such as homework), losing things necessary for tasks and activities, easy distractibility, and frequent forgetfulness in daily activities (tying shoes, zipping up pants, etc.)

- **HYPERACTIVITY SYMPTOMS:** Fidgeting or squirming, difficulty staying seated when expected to, running or climbing in situations in which it is inappropriate, difficulty playing quietly, often acting as if driven by a motor, and talking excessively

- **IMPULSIVITY SYMPTOMS:** Blurting out answers before questions are finished, difficulty awaiting his/her turn, and often interrupting conversations or intruding

Children who have at least six symptoms of inattention are described as having ADHD, Predominantly inattentive presentation. Children who have at least six symptoms in some combination of hyperactivity and impulsivity are described as having ADHD, Predominantly hyperactive-impulsive presentation. Children who meet both of these requirements are described as ADHD, combined presentation.

There are some important things to keep in mind regarding the diagnosis of ADHD:

- Everyone can experience periods of difficulty with attention or hyperactivity. An ADHD diagnosis requires that symptoms be present for at least six months.

- By definition, ADHD symptoms begin before age twelve. This does not mean symptoms were significantly impairing before twelve because symptoms may not become a problem until demands exceed the child's abilities.

- To have ADHD, symptoms must be impairing to social or academic functioning. ADHD symptoms are not always a problem; it is a matter of degree. They must also occur in more than one setting, such as at home and at school.

- Symptoms must be inappropriate for the child's developmental age, not chronological age. If a four-year-old child has developmental delays and is functioning at a two-year-old level, his ADHD symptoms must be out of the norm for a two-year-old, not a four-year-old.

- Most important, not every child who presents with ADHD symptoms has ADHD. Part of the definition is that these symptoms must not be better explained by some other diagnosis. Children who are anxious or depressed or who have learning disabilities or allergies and food intolerances will also not pay attention well.

There are many approaches to treating ADHD. This book is not meant to diagnose ADHD or take the place of advice from your child's medical professional. Rather, it provides ideas for how to optimize your child's nutrition so that his or her brain can work at its best. For some children, diet changes alone may be sufficient to treat symptoms. For others, some combination of diet, nutritional supplements, school accommodations, therapies, tutoring, and/or medication results in the best outcome. When the brain is working at its best, a child can be more responsive to these other treatments.

What Is Autism? Why Is It Called Autism Spectrum Disorder?

Autism is a developmental disorder that is also defined according to the *DSM-5, The Diagnostic and Statistical Manual of Mental Disorders, 5th Edition*. It is a much more complex disorder than ADHD, but like ADHD, it has no specific blood test or brain scan that can make the diagnosis. It is also a collection of symptoms. In May 2013, when the *DSM* was revised to its *5th* edition, there were some significant changes made to the diagnostic criteria for autism. Previously, autism was characterized by symptoms in 3 different areas: social interaction, communication, and restricted interests/repetitive behaviors, with a combination of some, but not all, symptoms required for a diagnosis. In the *DSM-5* criteria, social interaction and communication were combined into a single category. Individuals must now have all 3 criteria in the social interaction and communication category along with at least 2 out of 4 criteria in the restricted interests and repetitive behaviors domain. In addition, for the first time, sensory symptoms were included in the diagnostic criteria. The diagnostic categories are:

■ **PERSISTENT DEFICITS IN SOCIAL COMMUNI-CATION AND SOCIAL INTERACTION:**

1. Deficits in social-emotional reciprocity: Ranging from abnormal social approach and failure of normal back-and-forth conversation; to reduced sharing of interests, emotions, or affect; to failure to initiate or respond to social interactions

2. Deficits in nonverbal communicative behaviors used for social interaction: Ranging from poorly integrated verbal and nonverbal communication; to abnormalities in eye contact or body language or deficits in understanding and use of gestures; to a total lack of facial expressions and nonverbal communication

3. Deficits in developing, maintaining, and understanding relationships: Ranging from difficulties adjusting behavior to fit various social contexts; to difficulties in sharing imaginative play or in making friends; to absence of interest in peers

■ **RESTRICTED, REPETITIVE PATTERNS OF BEHAVIOR, INTERESTS, OR ACTIVITIES:**

1. Stereotyped or repetitive motor movements, use of objects or speech (e.g., simple motor stereotypes, lining up toys or flipping objects, echolalia, idiosyncratic phrases)

2. Insistence on sameness, inflexible adherence to routines, or ritualized patterns of verbal and nonverbal behavior (e.g., extreme distress at small changes, difficulties with transitions, rigid thinking patterns, greeting rituals, need to take same route or eat same food every day)

3. Highly restricted, fixated interests that are abnormal in intensity or focus (e.g., strong attachment to or preoccupation with unusual objects, excessively circumscribed or perseverative interests)

4. Hyper- or hypo-reactivity to sensory input or unusual interest in sensory aspects of the environment (e.g., apparent indifference to pain/temperature, adverse response to specific sounds or textures, excessive smelling or touching of objects, visual fascination with lights or movement)

Another significant change within the *DSM-5* was the elimination of previous diagnostic categories such as Pervasive Developmental Disorder (PDD) and Asperger's Disorder; they are now all included under the broad label of Autism Spectrum Disorder (ASD). The term ASD encompasses the wide range of combinations of symptoms and levels of severity that can be seen within an autism diagnosis. From a functional medicine perspective, the distinctions are less critical, since the goal of treatments such as elimination diets is to improve *function* regardless of the "label" applied to the symptoms.

DSM-5 also changed the age of onset criteria. The previous criteria required that symptoms be present before age 3 years. In the *DSM-5*, symptoms must be present in the early developmental period, but the criteria allow for the fact that these may not become fully evident until social demands exceed the child's limited capacities.

An important feature of ASD is that the diagnosis is not just about delayed development or lack of certain skills. Much of it is about the quality of a skill or interaction. A child can amass a great deal of language, but if it is not used to communicate, that is unusual. For example, a child may be able to recite an entire book from memory but not be able to have a conversation. His language may seem advanced, but his ability to communicate is not typical.

Regardless of the label given to a particular child's symptoms, many children with ADHD or ASD respond very well to changes in diet and nutrition. The purpose of optimizing nutrition is to also optimize brain and body function, so that children can respond to all the other treatments provided and have the best possible outcome. Other chapters in this book will describe some of the unique biochemical problems children with ASD have that are different from those seen in children with ADHD.

What If I'm Not Sure If My Child Has ADHD or Autism? Can This Book Still Help?

Your child does not need to have a specific diagnosis in order to benefit from this book. As you read about the symptoms and the dietary connections, you may find that some of the advice resonates with your child's symptoms. Again, this book provides help in giving the brain and body what is needed and taking away what is not needed in order to achieve optimum results.

Will Diet Alone Be Enough to Treat My Child's Symptoms?

Children with ADHD or ASD often require a comprehensive set of treatments. There is no one cause of ADHD or autism and, therefore, no single treatment. Particularly for the child with autism, he or she may have genetic predispositions, inborn errors of metabolism, immune dysfunction, maldigestion, malabsorption syndromes, and food reactions. These differences are then modified by a wide range of environmental factors that can potentially increase susceptibility to autism: birth trauma, pathogen exposure, toxins, heavy metal exposures, unusual vaccination reactions, allergens, pesticides, poor diet, nutritional deficiencies, and other stressors. Typically, it is not any single factor that is the cause, but the cumulative effect known as the "total load" that tilts the balance in these children. The current research focus is aimed toward identifying the many potential risk factors, establishing more preventive measures, improving early diagnosis, establishing early interventions, and expanding the effectiveness of therapies and treatments.

We visualize our approach as three "legs" on the treatment "table," all of which are important for keeping the table steady and balanced.

- **THERAPIES.** These can include behavioral therapies or organizational strategies and educational interventions (special education, speech or occupational therapy, etc.).

- **MEDICATIONS.** Depending on the need, medications are used as appropriate to each child.

- **BIOMEDICAL COMPONENT.** Diet and nutrition are critical components of the overall treatment plan because they address underlying core problems affecting the body and the brain. We are much more than what we eat—we are what we eat, digest, absorb, and utilize. Unfortunately, diet and nutrition are often overlooked or dismissed, when, in fact, many of the symptom presentations in ADHD or autism are directly related to nutritional deficiencies, disturbances in nutrient metabolism, poor diet, the negative effects of specific foods, and problems in digestion and absorption.

For optimum results, all three legs need to be considered. This book focuses on one part of the biomedical leg of that table—the diet.

What Are the Diets?

There is no one diet that is right for all people, and this is especially true in those with ADHD or autism who can benefit from one or more elimination diets. Based upon each individual's unique biochemistry, digestive status, and reactions to foods and food components, there are many types of elimination diets that are helpful. It is important to understand that these diets or combination of diets are specific to the individual's sensitivities and are not necessarily applicable to all children diagnosed with ADHD or autism. The most common, and frequently most effective, elimination diet for autism and ADHD is a regimen of eating and drinking that focuses on the elimination of gluten and casein. Although other foods may also be bothersome, these two proteins are by far the most common offenders. Casein is the main protein found in milk products, but don't confuse "milk-free" with "casein-free," as casein is found in products other than milk. It is found in other dairy products such as yogurt and ice cream and also in many baked goods and other unexpected places such as certain canned tuna.

Gluten is a protein found in wheat and other grains. Again, "wheat-free" is not the same as "gluten-free." A more in-depth discussion of these proteins, their sources, and substitutes can be found in Chapter 4.

For many children, the elimination of casein and gluten is enough. There are increasing numbers of children who react to other foods such as soy or corn. Others may react to chemicals in foods (such as phenols or salicylates) or to artificial preservatives and dyes. Still others may have difficulty tolerating certain types of carbohydrates. A subset may need to adjust diet to address bacterial overgrowth of the intestine. This edition includes more in-depth discussions of diets beyond the gluten-free casein-free diet, including the Feingold/low phenol/low salicylate diet, the Specific Carbohydrate Diet (SCD), GAPS diet, low oxalate diet (LOD), FODMAP, and diets focused on targeting yeast overgrowth and inflammation. Most of the recipes in this book are gluten- and casein-free; others are also free of soy, corn, and other potentially bothersome foods. We have also adapted the recipes, where possible, to be compatible with the other diets discussed. In Chapter 2, we provide a concise overview of the diets and support strategies, followed by individual chapters on each of the diets beginning with specifics on a healthy diet. In Chapters 12 and 13, we provide tips on getting started and solutions for common concerns. In Part II, we provide some guidelines and recipes by categories. Our goal is to provide guidance and recipes for the broadest group of children on specialized diets.

Are There Tests to Help Determine If My Child Needs a Specialized Diet?

This question will be discussed in detail in later chapters. In general, nutritional and dietary treatment approaches should be based on determining the specific reactions, underlying biochemical, metabolic, immune, digestive, and nutritional imbalances present for each child. Fortunately, the science of nutrition has caught up with the decades of clinical and anecdotal observations. Now, there is an abundance of

sophisticated testing that has improved our diagnostic abilities. Tests include analysis for maldigestion and malabsorption syndromes; food allergies, sensitivities, and intolerances; bowel pathogens; inflammation; immune disorders; exposure to toxic metals and other harmful substances; poor nutrient levels; and defects in the metabolism of amino acids, fatty acids, carbohydrates, vitamins, and minerals. Many of the children with ADHD or autism have problems with digestion of foods and absorption of nutrients. Some have accumulation of toxic metals. Almost all of the children have nutritional deficits, and those with the most severe presentations have multiple significant nutrient deficits and metabolic disturbances.

Most of these specialized tests are not always part of the routine work-up for people with ADHD and autism. Without these tests, significant problems can be missed, rendering treatment plans incomplete.

How Will This Book Help?

This book includes chapters that address the following issues:

- Identifying sources and substitutes for the main culprits—gluten and casein—as well as soy, corn, eggs, salicylates, phenols, disaccharides, oxalates, and inflammatory foods

- What makes a food "good" or "bad" for you

- How to determine if your child is sensitive to particular foods

- How to change your child's diet

- How to get your picky eater to accept new foods

- Suggestions for dealing with common problems encountered when changing diets

In Their Own Words

No one tells the story better than the parents who have tenaciously sought and found the right treatment path for their children—and the children who have courageously walked it! The stories we've included throughout the book may differ because each child's response is unique. While some respond dramatically to a single intervention, others respond best when a combination of treatments is utilized. It is important for parents not to give up when the results are not immediate and dramatic. Remember to be persistent and patient. We'll start with Anne Evans's poignant dedication in her book, *Autism Treated and Cured*.

"Dedicated to my loving Sarah who put up with the sickness, the suffering, and the agony of recovery to forge a path toward healing for other children on the spectrum."

PREVALENCE OF ADHD AND AUTISM SPECTRUM DISORDER (ASD) IN THE UNITED STATES

ADHD

According to the CDC, approximately 11% of children ages 4–17 have ever been diagnosed with ADHD, according to a parent report from 2011–2013.

Based on data from the National Survey of Children's Health, conducted in 2011–2012, a history of an ADHD diagnosis by a health care provider increased by 42% between 2003 and 2011.

AUTISM

The prevalence of autism as reported by the CDC, based on data acquired through the ADDM (Autism and Developmental Disabilities Monitoring) Network:

Year	Prevalence per 1,000 children	Number of children
2000	6.7	1 in 150
2006	9.0	1 in 110
2008	11.3	1 in 88
2010	14.7	1 in 68
2012	14.6	1 in 68
2014	16.8	1 in 59*

The report of April 2018 is based on data from 2014. ASD is about 4 times more common among boys (1 in 37) than among girls (1 in 151).

Studies in Asia, Europe, and North America have identified individuals with ASD with an average prevalence of 1–2%.

The number of children who have autism symptoms from early infancy has not changed significantly over time. What has escalated exponentially is regressive autism, which occurs between 12 and 24 months, after a period of normal development and behavior.

Since autistic behaviors are usually present prior to the age of 3 years, early diagnosis is critical. The best success results from early intervention treatments.

CHAPTER 1

Food Reactions:
What They Are and How to Test for Them

"The important thing in science is not so much to obtain new facts as to discover new ways of thinking about them."

—William Bragg

Food Allergies versus Food Sensitivities and Intolerances

Many people use the term "food allergies" to describe all reactions to food, but this is not accurate. Allergy is one type of reaction to food. There are also numerous sensitivities and intolerances to foods that are not classified as allergic reactions. Many children with ADHD or ASD have multiple types of reactions to foods, ranging from allergies to a variety of types of sensitivities and intolerances. The type of reaction least likely to cause behavioral symptoms is the traditional type of food allergy with obvious symptoms such as sneezing, hives, and wheezing. Children with ADHD or ASD tend to have food reactions best labeled as "sensitivities" or "intolerances." Some of the most common foods that cause food intolerances and sensitivities are similar to those that cause allergies— milk, wheat, and soy. Corn is also a frequent offending food, but almost any food can trigger reactions due to sensitivity and intolerance.

There are many types of food sensitivities and intolerances that result from poor digestion and/or poor absorption of specific food substances. For the purposes of this chapter, when we refer to food sensitivities, we are referring to the delayed (immunoglobulin G, or IgG) type of food reactions. Food intolerances can include a wider range of reactions, such as intolerances to lactose, fructose, other carbohydrate sugars, phenols, salicylates, and gluten (in celiac disease) and intolerance to byproducts of abnormal digestion, such as opiate peptides from milk/casein, gluten, and soy. More recent research suggests that gluten may also be problematic by causing inflammation in the body and the brain.

Food Allergies

The antibodies (immune cells) in the body that result in traditional allergies are called immunoglobulin E (IgE) antibodies, which trigger the release of histamine. The antibodies that result in one type of food sensitivity are immunoglobulin G (IgG) antibodies. The reactions are different and the testing is different. This distinction will be important when we discuss types of blood tests commonly available to test for food reactions later in this chapter. The most confusion comes from testing for traditional (IgE) allergy reactions versus delayed (IgG) reactions.

IgE reactions are obvious and fast. We are all familiar with traditional allergic reactions in some fashion. A person eats a food and develops hives or wheezing. A person with a severe peanut allergy can develop a life-threatening allergic reaction after eating peanuts. The immune pathway in the body that results in these reactions is very fast-acting. Cause and effect is usually easy to figure out because the reaction happens so quickly. These reactions do not have a direct negative effect on the brain. While people may become irritable from the discomfort of the allergy symptom, such as itching or wheezing, they are not irritable due to a specific effect of the food on the brain. The most common foods that provoke allergic reactions are milk, eggs, peanuts, tree nuts (almonds, cashews, pecans, and walnuts), fish, shellfish, soy, and wheat.

Food Sensitivities

Most types of food reactions, however, are not IgE reactions; most fall into the other categories. IgG food sensitivities can result in physical symptoms similar to allergies. However, they may also result in a much broader array of symptoms, including behavioral or developmental symptoms. A striking difference between food allergies and food sensitivities is the time it takes for the reaction to occur. Whereas food allergy symptoms occur quickly, symptoms of food sensitivities can occur at any time within three days of eating the food. Most commonly, these reactions occur within one to two days. This often makes it very difficult to figure out which food caused which behavioral reaction. With food allergies, keeping a food diary can be very helpful. Because of the delayed nature of food sensitivities, food diaries are less helpful.

For those with compromised systems, the number of IgG sensitivities may be high and include most of what the person eats. For that reason, rotation diets are frequently recommended to limit the damaging effect on the immune system. The concept behind a rotation diet is to limit the exposure to the same food and, more specifically, the same family of foods. By not repeating the suspect or reactive foods daily, the body's reactions to the foods will be more limited. The most common food rotation programs suggest not eating the same foods more often than once per day in four or more days. Food rotation diets are discussed in Chapter 9.

Food Intolerances

These reactions are not immunoglobulin (IgE or IgG) reactions. Intolerances include problems with digestion of foods due to the lack of specific enzymes including maldigestion of lactose, carbohydrate double sugars (disaccharides), and proteins from gluten and milk (casein). Celiac gluten intolerance is not due to maldigestion but to an autoimmune response that damages the intestinal villi in response to gluten exposure.

Intolerances also include inability to metabolize a component of a food such as fructose, phenylalanine, phenols, and salicylates. Food intolerances may result in immediate and also delayed reactions, depending on the situation. With lactose intolerance, the effects (diarrhea, cramps) may be notable within hours. Gluten celiac type reactions may also be immediate (stomach pain, cramps, diarrhea) and long-term (growth delay, skin conditions, fatigue, and neurological or behavioral/developmental symptoms). For intolerance to phenols and salicylates (a type of phenol), some reactions may be more immediate (stomachache, red face or ears, hyperactivity, hives, and headaches) whereas others are more delayed (dark circles under the eyes, short attention span, sleep disorders, speech difficulties, tics, behavioral problems, and head banging).

Symptoms of Food Sensitivities and Intolerances

Symptoms of food sensitivities and food intolerances can be broad:

- **GENERAL SYMPTOMS:** Fatigue, food cravings
- **SKIN:** Eczema, unexplained rashes, allergic shiners (dark circles under the eyes), red face/ears
- **DIGESTION:** Stomachaches, loose stools or diarrhea, constipation, alternating diarrhea and constipation
- **RESPIRATORY:** Mucus production, congestion
- **IMMUNE, INFLAMMATORY, AND AUTOIMMUNE REACTIONS**
- **CARDIOVASCULAR:** Abnormal pulse, elevated blood pressure
- **NEUROLOGIC:** Headaches (e.g., migraines), ringing in the ears, tingling, dizziness, tics
- **PSYCHOLOGICAL:** Depression, mood disorders, anxiety, panic attacks, aggression, sleep disorder
- **BEHAVIOR/DEVELOPMENT:** ADHD symptoms (decreased attention, hyperactivity, impulsivity), mood swings, irritability, anxiety, autism symptoms (poor eye contact, social withdrawal, decreased language, obsessions, repetitive behaviors)

Causes of Food Reactions: The Digestive Connection

Normally, when foods are digested in the small intestine (the upper part of the intestine), they break down into their smallest components: proteins to amino acids, fats to fatty acids, and carbohydrates to simple sugars. Along with nutrients, these are allowed to cross the intestinal lining into the bloodstream, where they travel to other parts of the body, including the brain.

A critical part of this healthy system is the lining of the intestine. This lining needs to be a good barrier so that foods cannot enter the blood until they have been fully digested. It functions like a window screen, letting in good air but not larger items like pesky flies or harmful bugs. When the intestinal lining is damaged, potentially harmful large food molecules can enter the bloodstream—like holes in the window screen letting in bugs. This condition is commonly referred to as a "leaky gut," since food molecules leak through the microscopic holes in the intestinal lining.

Many children with ADHD or autism have problems with their intestinal lining. Children with autism also may not have enough digestive enzymes, or the body may not release them at the right times or in sufficient amounts. The type of food that causes the most problems for children with ADHD or autism is protein, specifically proteins from milk, wheat, and soy. Dietary proteins (fish, fowl, meat, eggs, dairy, beans, nuts, seeds, and grains) consist of many chains of amino acids and are not useful until they are broken down into individual amino acids by digestive enzymes. The foods themselves are like dollar bills that will not work in a coin machine. They must be broken down first into individual coins (amino acids). Visualize these proteins as long metal chains, with each link being an amino acid; digestive enzymes break the connection between links and free the amino acids (links) for further use. The amino acids are very small and are absorbed through the intestinal lining into the body. The amino acids can then be put back together in different combinations to make peptides and proteins again. These can be used to build important structures in the body, such as muscle, or to send messages in the body, for example, as hormones or transmitters in the brain.

During digestion, not all of the amino acid chains are completely digested. What results are residues of short chains of amino acids called peptides. The peptides, however, are large and should not be absorbed unless the gut is damaged and, therefore, too permeable or leaky. Think of amino acids like Scrabble letters. Peptides are the "words" made from those letters. Depending on how the letters (amino acids) are arranged, different "words" (peptides) are formed. The body recognizes these "words." If, however, the letter arrangement does not spell a "word," the body considers it to be foreign. Likewise, if the intestinal lining is damaged, the body may consider the peptides that leak into the bloodstream to be foreign. If they are not recognized because they are foreign, the body sends specialized cells to get rid of them. When the peptides are "words" the body recognizes, the body allows them to remain. If the "words" have receptors in the brain, they may cross the brain and send a signal. If the signal is not one that should normally occur in the brain, there can be a short circuit in brain functioning. This can contribute to many of the symptoms seen in children with ADHD or autism.

> "I used to lie down and cry and hold my stomach. I had continuous stomachaches. No one knew how bad it hurt. No one believed me. They thought that I was telling stories. I did not pay attention in school. I was in the bathroom all of the time. The teachers used to complain. I wasn't good at reading. I had bad grades. I think I was failing. I didn't really like school. Learning wasn't fun. I used to be in a daze."
>
> —**Ashley Stilson**,
> *age fourteen, originally diagnosed with*
> *pervasive developmental disorder*

The Dope on Opiates

While short-circuiting of the brain from "misspelled words" can occur in a variety of conditions, a feature that is more common in autism but occasionally found in ADHD is the creation of "words" or peptides that have an opiate-like effect on the brain. If the amino acid "letters" in the peptide "word" are arranged in a specific order, the peptide looks like an opiate and acts like an opiate—similar to morphine. "Opiates" refers to the narcotic alkaloids found in opium such as morphine and heroin. An "opioid" has an opiate-like reaction. Casein and gluten are the most common foods that result in these opiate-like substances. Soy is also likely a source of these opiates. Casein and gluten contain a similar sequence of amino acids. They have, embedded within their long chains of amino acids, sequences of these short opiate-like peptides. These peptides are not available or active unless the proteins are incompletely broken down due to digestive enzyme deficiencies such as lack of dipeptidyl peptidase IV (DPP-IV). The resulting opiate-like endorphins have very specific amino acid sequences. For gluten the result is gliadorphin (tyr-pro-gln-pro-gln-pro-phe) and for milk casein, the result is casomorphin (tyr-pro-phe-pro-gly-pro-ile). These opiate-like peptides are generally large and unable to pass through the intestinal lining. When the lining is leaky, these peptides can enter the bloodstream and travel to the brain, having an opiate-like effect there. These opiate peptides have been found in the spinal fluid and the urine of children with autism. The effect of opiates on the brain can certainly explain some of the symptoms seen in autism.

Many children crave dairy and wheat products. There are some children whose parents describe them as "milk-aholics" because of the intensity of their craving for milk. These cravings may be similar to drug-seeking types of behaviors. A child may not want other foods because they don't give the brain the same "high" as the opiate-producing foods. Food "hunger strikes" and refusal to eat can occur. This may also account for the behaviors—from irritability to rage—seen in many children when dairy and wheat are initially removed from the diet. They are, in effect, having drug-withdrawal symptoms.

These opiate-like peptides mimic the effects of drugs like morphine and have been shown to react with areas of the brain that are involved in speech and auditory processing. Opiate-like effects on the brain could also result in social withdrawal. A child may "zone out" or "be in his/her own world." He/she may laugh or giggle for no apparent reason. In addition, a child may have a high pain tolerance since opiates, like morphine, are excellent painkillers. We are aware that there are likely other psychoactive and neuroactive peptide possibilities. It is not unusual

---

Support for the Opioid Theory

According to the research of Kalle Reichelt, MD:

- Food-source opioids have been reported in the cerebrospinal fluid, breast milk, blood, and urine, particularly in patients with autism, depression, and schizophrenia.

- Addictive behaviors are present when on glutens and casein, and withdrawal symptoms can occur with removal.

- Opioids decrease in the urine of those on a GFCF diet.

- For those with autism, as with morphine users, their pupils are small while "under the influence" and large when going through a period of abstinence.

- Constipation, self-absorption, and insensitivity to pain are markers for opioid effect in autism.

Source: http://www.gluten-free.org/reichelt.html

---

for the casomorphin and gliadorphin tests to be negative, yet the child shows a significant improvement in behavior and focus when either milk casein and/or glutens are removed from the diet. It is certainly likely that there are other types of reactions occurring. For these reasons, when a child presents with an extremely limited diet and/or an addictive focus to the classical problem foods (e.g., milk products, glutens, and possibly soy), these are signs that an avoidance trial may be helpful.

Lab Tests: What They Tell Us and What They Don't

In medical practice, where possible, we like to have information about whether certain treatments are indicated. Sometimes we can tell this simply based on examining a child. Other times, lab tests are ordered. So it seems logical that testing for food reactions (allergies, sensitivities/intolerances) would be a reasonable thing to do. However, this is actually a source of some debate among practitioners. Some believe food testing should always be done before starting an elimination diet; others believe it is not necessary or can be deferred to a later date. Regardless of when food testing is done, it is important to understand what the tests tell us and, equally important, what they do not reveal.

Like the misunderstanding of the difference between food allergies and food sensitivities, many people use the words "allergy testing" to describe testing for all types of food sensitivities or intolerances. Testing for food allergies is different from testing for food sensitivities. If you take your child to a traditional allergist, testing will be done for food allergies, the immediate, fast-acting immune response (IgE). This is done by either skin testing or blood testing. The blood testing, or radioallergosorbent testing (RAST), can be ordered through a traditional laboratory. This type of testing provides reliable information about the immediate types of allergy reactions, the types that can cause hives, wheezing, and a host of other physical symptoms. Neither the skin nor the IgE blood testing gives any information about food IgG sensitivities, which is the type of reaction related to ADHD, autism, and other behavioral symptoms. Therefore, if you want to have your child tested for food sensitivities, a referral to a traditional allergist may not provide the answers you are looking for.

There is another type of testing, for those delayed food reactions, called IgG testing. This type of blood testing is offered only through specialized labora-

tories and is often not covered by insurance plans. While some traditional laboratories may offer it for casein and/or gluten, traditional laboratories typically do not offer a full panel that includes a variety of foods and food groups. These tests are expensive, and cost needs to be considered as one factor in determining whether or when to test your child.

Reactions that indicate a problem with foods are called positive reactions. They are reported in various degrees, based on the strength of the reaction. There are a number of points to keep in mind when interpreting food IgG test results:

- Finding a positive reaction in blood testing does not guarantee that removal of the food will result in improvement. It is revealing that molecules from that food "leaked" into the bloodstream, triggering a response from the body's immune system, resulting in an increase in these IgG antibodies. Removal of the offending foods and/or rotation does reduce the total load and hence can potentially reduce symptoms. The IgG reaction is common in many with autism. IgG reactions contribute to overall body burden.

- The absence of a food reaction does not guarantee your child is not reactive to that food in another category of reactions, sensitivities, or intolerances.

- Reactions may be positive to foods your child has never eaten. This is because certain food groups can cross-react, causing false positive reactions.

- Some children have positive reactions, of varying degrees, to a large number of foods. If fifteen or more reactions are present, this is thought to be more of an indicator that the intestinal lining is leaky (too permeable to large molecules) rather than each individual food being a problem. In other words, this shows that the intestinal barrier is unable to keep out a variety of food molecules and the immune system has responded by making antibodies against all of those foods. It does not necessarily mean that all fifteen foods need to be eliminated from the diet. Also, when the number is large, the foods are usually those most commonly consumed.

So what to make of these tests? How best to use them to help guide treatment? It is our opinion that food testing generally does not need to be done initially. Again, removing foods based solely on food IgG results does not guarantee improvement in symptoms.

Given these caveats, why and when should you consider food IgG testing? Food testing may be more helpful if conducted after other treatments have already been completed, such as those that help heal the "leakiness" of the intestinal lining. When the intestinal lining is a better barrier, it will be harder for food molecules to enter the bloodstream. The food molecules that do enter and still trigger immune reactions might then have more significance. Food testing may also be helpful in a situation in which the most common offending foods have been removed from the diet and other treatments (such as nutritional supplements) have been started and the child is still not showing adequate improvement. In that case, food testing may then provide guidance on which of all the foods in a child's diet might still be causing problems. This would help guide further dietary elimination trials.

"Be not astonished at new ideas; for it is well known to you that a thing does not therefore cease to be true because it is not accepted by many."

—**Spinoza** *(1632–1677)*

Are There Any Helpful Tests to Do Before Starting a Special Diet?

Two types of tests are helpful to have at the beginning of this process:

- For children with ADHD or autism: Blood testing for celiac disease
- For children with autism: Urine testing for opiate peptide residues caused by gluten, casein, and soy

Food allergy and sensitivity testing may be considered, with the caveats discussed above.

As mentioned in the introduction, the physician treating your child may expand testing to include assessments based upon previous test results and symptom presentation. Tests to consider discussing with your child's physician include:

- CBC to check for possible anemia
- Vitamin A and D levels to check for deficiency
- Metabolic profile

Specialty lab testing may also be considered:

- Organic acid urine analysis for cellular nutrient and enzyme functions (the gold standard in nutrient function testing)
- Amino acid analysis (plasma and urine)
- Stool analysis may include pathogens, parasites, gut microbiota, and markers for digestion, occult blood, and inflammation.
- There are many other kinds of tests that may be considered including genetic, mitochondrial, immune/autoimmune panels, and markers for toxic exposures.

CELIAC DISEASE

Celiac disease is a medical disorder in which gluten is not tolerated. In this disease, intake of gluten results in what is called an autoimmune reaction; the result is that the body recognizes the cells in the lining of the small intestine as foreign and reacts against them. This changes the anatomy of the intestinal lining and makes it "leaky."

The traditional view of celiac disease was that it had to cause diarrhea or affect a child's growth. However, recent studies reveal that bowel movements and growth may be normal, and a child may instead exhibit behavioral, developmental, or neurological effects from this disease. Celiac disease may also be present in a small percentage of children with ADHD or ASD. Celiac disease also occurs in 10–15% of children with Down Syndrome. The reason for testing for celiac disease before starting a gluten-free diet is that the only current treatment for celiac disease is 100 percent strict, lifelong elimination of gluten. Even 99 percent elimination of gluten will not cure the disease. In children, with 100 percent strict elimination of gluten, this disease is virtually completely reversible, and the intestinal lining will return to normal. This often results in improvement in behavioral and developmental symptoms. In addition, if celiac disease is present and not treated for years, the risk of other autoimmune disorders (such as rheumatoid arthritis or lupus) and certain cancers is increased. It is felt that treating celiac disease lowers the future risk of these disorders.

While some children with ADHD or autism require 100 percent strict elimination of gluten in order to see benefit, there is not a medical consequence to only partial elimination. With celiac disease, partial treatment may result in medical problems in the future. Testing for celiac disease includes two kinds of tests: one that identifies specific antibodies to gluten (anti-endomysial, anti-gliadin, tissue transglutaminase, reticulin) and one that identifies genetic markers (HLA DR by PCR, specifically HLA DQ2 and/or HLA DQ8). The antibody tests must be accomplished while gluten is still in the diet. For the genetic test, exposure to gluten is not required. Genetic testing is generally done if there is a family history or if the screening antibody tests are abnormal. Therefore, it may be worth asking your child's physician to order blood testing for celiac disease before you start eliminating gluten.

"Travis underwent the stool, urine, and blood tests this summer. The doctors found abnormal yeast overgrowth, inefficient production of digestive enzymes, deficiency in vitamin A, and food sensitivities to many more foods, the foods he ate the most—including eggs, soy, tomatoes, yeast, canola, cantaloupe, and coconut. He has been off these foods for four weeks now. There was a regression for the first two weeks, but now Travis is much better and more energetic."

—Letter from
Michele Pacifico in 2000, regarding son Travis

According to the experts in celiac disease, there can also be gluten intolerance that is not celiac disease (i.e., specific celiac testing will be negative). As with gluten, individuals can also react in more than one way to milk products and to soy. Testing for food sensitivities or intolerances can produce a false negative result. It is our experience that avoiding suspect foods is the most reliable means of determining the culprits and their effects.

URINE OPIATE PEPTIDES

Urine testing is available to measure the opiate-like peptides made from casein, gluten, and soy. This testing is available only in specialized laboratories and is often not covered by insurance. It must be ordered by a physician or other practitioner such as a nutritionist. Testing directly measures opiate-like peptides from casein and gluten. Soy peptides cannot yet be directly measured and may be included in the measurements of casein and gluten peptides. The degree of elevation of peptides can provide helpful information regarding the amount of withdrawal symptoms to expect. When a child has high levels of opiates, it may be more difficult to remove the foods due to the intensity of the "addiction" and subsequent withdrawal symptoms. Finding opiates in the urine also provides good motivation for following the diet, as it provides evidence that the foods are creating substances that can have a negative effect on brain functioning.

The Body Doesn't Lie: The Wisdom of Trial and Response

The best test is the child's own body. We know the most common offending foods are casein, gluten, and soy. Removing these foods gives "the biggest bang for the buck" for the largest number of children.

The gold standard for food reactions is the child's response to elimination of a food. It is better than any blood test. The goal of treatments is not to make the blood tests better; the goal is to make the child better. Some children will show obvious improvement when offending foods are removed from their diet. For other children, the response is less clear. The standard way of doing a food test is to do what is called an "elimination and challenge." An offending food is removed for a period of time. If improvement is not obvious, the body is then challenged by reintroduction of that food. Often, after an offending food is removed, there will be a more obvious and stronger reaction when the food is reintroduced. This method identifies offending foods and the symptoms they cause. A complicating issue is that children may be reactive to more than one food. Even if they react to a food that is removed, other stronger food reactions may mask any improvement from removal of that single food. Sometimes, improvements are not seen until more than one food is removed from the diet. Paraphrasing Dr. Sidney Baker, if you are sitting on multiple tacks, removing only one will not make much of a difference in your comfort level.

CHAPTER 2

Contemplating the Right Elimination Diet and Support Strategies

One Size Does Not Fit All

When it comes to diet, one size does not fit all. There is no diet that is suitable for all people. Anthropological evidence indicates that the diets of the earliest humans were diverse depending upon where they lived, the season of the year, weather, and availability of food.

This is still true today. The three categories for human food have consistently included protein, fat, and carbohydrate; what has always varied are the specific choices within these categories and the relative percentages of proteins, fats, and carbohydrates.

Natural, Healthy Diets Around the World Are Diverse

There is no "standard" or "ideal" diet that is suitable for all people because natural populations throughout the world differ significantly in diet patterns, food sources, and food choices. The diet styles are based upon geographical location; availability of land and seafood sources; agriculture and aquaculture techniques; genetics and metabolism; cultural and religious customs; and individual food preferences. The outcome includes a wide variation in healthy natural diets with regard to relative intakes of proteins, fats, and carbohydrates. The range varies from carnivorous/paleo style (high animal protein and fat with low carbohydrate and fiber content) to vegetarian (no animal protein and low fat with higher carbohydrate and fiber content). There are numerous versions within this broad range in natural diets.

For all of these reasons, diets need to be flexible and suited to the individual.

The following are examples of how wide the diversity is with regard to diet categories among natural cultures throughout the world:

- The intake and type of healthy fats that meet the needs of various cultures can range from 10% in some African countries to 50% to 75% in Inuit populations and in Uruguay, Poland, Finland, and Denmark, all of which have significantly lower cardiovascular death rates.

  - Low fat diets do not necessarily reduce cardiovascular risk, and healthy fat diets can prevent cardiovascular death rates. France and Italy have a relatively high intake of healthy fats and cholesterol, yet cardiovascular death rates are among the lowest in the world and life expectancy is among the highest.

  - The type of fat makes the difference. Instead of hydrogenated oils, deep-fried foods, and high intake of vegetable oils, the healthy fat diets tend to be higher in good fats such as omega-9-rich olive and avocado oils plus coconut oil and animal fats, omega-9, and a higher intake of omega-3 oils from seafood, algae, nuts, and seeds. For these reasons, there is no one standard for all populations with regard to the type of good fat to be consumed.

- Carbohydrate intake throughout the world also varies significantly with regard to amount and type. The healthier carbohydrates in legumes (beans, peas, lentils, and peanuts), nuts, seeds, vegetables, fruits, and whole grains tend to be higher in vegetarian style diets and lower in paleo style diets. They keep blood glucose stable as compared to glycemic (sugar-raising) sweets, juices, and refined processed foods and grains—the intakes of which have significantly increased the rates of diabetes and obesity in contemporary populations.

- Relative fiber intakes and sources of fiber (legumes, beans, nuts, seeds, vegetables, fruits, and whole grains) also vary throughout the world from 10 to 40 grams/day, the lowest intake being among the more carnivorous/paleo diets. Hence, there is little validity in establishing a dietary fiber intake recommendation for all individuals.

- Protein intakes may include a range from paleo style (animal protein) diets to vegetarian style (plant protein) diets. Vegetarian diets may also include varied animal protein choices such as eggs (ovo-vegetarian), milk products (lacto-vegetarian), seafood (pesca-vegetarian), and combinations. The actual adult protein intake may vary from 40 grams/day to 70 to 130 grams/day.

There is no one diet that is suitable for every individual, given the diversity in relative intakes of protein, fat, carbohydrate, and fiber prevalent in ancestral and natural diets throughout the world. The previous USDA pyramids and the current USDA "My Plate" give the impression that grains and cow milk products are essential for humans, but this is not accurate. Although animal milk is one way to obtain protein and fat, and grains are one way to obtain carbohydrates, they are not essential to the diet. They are choices within the categories of protein, fat, and carbohydrate. Legumes, nuts, and seeds provide good protein, fat, carbohydrate, and fiber.

Elimination Diet Choices: How Do I Know Which Diet to Try for My Child?

Diets need to be individualized to the particular child. The underlying causes for reactions to specific foods are related to that child's unique biochemistry and metabolism, imbalances, nutritional status, digestive ability, gut health, enzyme function, genetic variants, and more. Additional concerns include the common problem of limited food choices due to picky appetites, sensory issues around eating, and the impact of certain medications on appetite.

In selecting an elimination diet, it is important to focus on an organic, healthy, nutrient-dense diet described in detail in Chapter 3. It is glucose stable, and includes pastured animal source foods, while avoiding foods that are refined, processed, genetically modified, reaction provoking and foods that contain

artificial additives, preservatives, coloring, flavoring, and contaminants. This "artificial stuff" places a significant burden on the individual's immunity, metabolism, energy, behavior, and nutritional status. The healthy organic diet includes proteins, fats, and carbohydrates based upon the individual's uniqueness and reactions to specific foods and food components. Removing the artificial burdens, improving the environment, and cleaning up the diet can result in noticeable improvements and allow for the appropriate elimination diet or diets to succeed.

A diet that works well for your child's classmate or next-door neighbor may not show any benefits in your child, even if both children have the same outward symptoms or diagnoses. For example, two children with ADHD may have hyperactivity and silliness. The first child does not have sufficient amounts of nutrients to support the clearance of natural phenol chemicals found in a number of fruits and some vegetables. The second child has had frequent ear infections and has taken numerous antibiotics and now has imbalanced bacteria and yeast in his intestine. Both of these conditions can result in hyperactivity and silliness, but the reasons are different and the treatments, including the choice of specific diets and/or supplements, will also be different.

The key to identifying which elimination diet is most likely going to work for an individual is to identify the symptoms that can be addressed by each potential diet. If there are no underlying symptoms suggesting that a given diet will work, then that diet is less likely to be effective. In our experience, the diet that has been helpful for the largest percentage of children, particularly those with autism, is the gluten-free casein-free (GFCF) diet. Soy elimination is also recommended during a GFCF trial. There are numerous other potentially helpful diets, summarized at the end of this chapter.

Diets low in natural salicylates, phenols, and/or chemical additives are also helpful for another significant subset of children who may have behavioral symptoms, red cheeks and ears, and/or irritability. Other diets, such as the Specific Carbohydrate Diet (SCD) focus on avoiding double sugar (disaccharide) foods, with the GAPS version being more restrictive. The anti-yeast diet addresses overgrowth of candida, which can cause rectal and/or vaginal itching and focus and attention problems. The low oxalate diet is helpful in addressing pain and inflammation associated with oxalate foods. The anti-inflammatory diet may be used individually or in combination with other diets. The FODMAP diet is highly restrictive and helpful for those who have symptoms associated with many of the diets. The rotation diet provides more flexibility when there are multiple foods to be limited. For each diet described in this book, we provide symptoms or conditions that suggest that a particular diet may be worth considering for your child in addition to what to avoid and include.

Most of the special diets tend to limit many of the plant-based foods (nuts, seeds, beans/legumes, vegetables, fruits, and grains) because plants contain components that may be irritating, improving the plant's resilience against pests and reducing the chances of being consumed. Examples include lectins, phytic acids, alkaloids, salicylates, phenols, oxalates, polyols, glutamates, purines, and amines. It is important to note that high-fiber foods can be difficult to digest, especially for those with digestive problems.

- Vegetables and fruits may be better tolerated and more easily digested when peeled, steamed, cooked, puréed, juiced, or included in soups and stews.
- Nuts, seeds, grains, and legumes/beans are more easily digested when soaked. A pressure cooker is useful in reducing some of the problems produced by legumes/beans.
- Grains can be soaked and fermented.
- Nuts and seeds can be better digested when made into nuts/seed butters.

These strategies certainly improve digestibility; however, they do not render all the components that trigger reactions less problematic. Meats, poultry, seafood, eggs, and milk products (if tolerated) do not have these natural defense mechanisms and are usually better tolerated. For this reason, most of the elimination diets lean toward animal sources.

Other Potential Culprits

As is the case with all the foods and food components we cover, not every individual reacts poorly to each of the following substances. Although there may be similar patterns in the symptoms from these foods, not all who react to a given category will have the same symptoms.

LECTINS are natural toxins found in high levels in legumes (beans, peas, lentils), grains, peanuts, corn, tomatoes, potatoes, and A1 milk. Plants with seeds also contain lectins (squash, nightshades, and some fruits). Lectins are natural toxins for protecting the plant but are like barnacles to the human gut mucosal lining. They interfere with the gut micro-biota, gut cell junctions and functions, and increase inflammation, thus contributing to a leaky gut. They can also attach to insulin receptors, impeding receptor functions and leading to insulin resistance. Lectin effects can be reduced by fermenting and pressure cooking grains and beans and peeling and de-seeding fruits and vegetables.

PHYTIC ACID is a natural substance found in plant seeds, grains, legumes, and nuts. Referred to as an anti-nutrient, it impairs the absorption of zinc, calcium, and iron. Its effects are minimized by the consumption of more anti-inflammatory foods.

SOLANINE, TOMATINE, AND NICOTINE are inflammatory alkaloids found in nightshade foods: tomato, white potato, peppers, eggplant, tobacco, okra, Goji berries, tomatillos, sorrel, gooseberries, ground cherries, pepino melons, paprika, cayenne pepper, and capsicum. They are potential culprits in increased inflammatory and autoimmune conditions

Overview of Elimination Diets: What They Are, Why They Are Needed, and Recommendations

Each of the diets has been summarized in the following grids. Each diet is explained in detail in the corresponding chapters. The following recommendations apply to all of the diets:

- Consult with a nutritionist/dietitian or physician with expertise in special diets and nutritional supplementation.

- Review the following resources for information on supplements used in ADHD and autism:
  - *The ADHD and Autism Nutritional Supplement Handbook* by Dana Laake and Pamela Compart
  - *Nutritional Supplement Use for Autistic Spectrum Disorder* by Jon Pangborn
  - *Cure Your Child with Food* by Kelly Dorfman
  - *Cooking to Heal* by Julie Matthews
  - *Nourishing Traditions* by Sally Fallon
  - *The Blood Sugar Solution* by Mark Hyman

"Hippocrates said, 'Let thy food be thy medicine and thy medicine be thy food.' Good advice, surely, but it was probably a lot easier to follow in 400 B.C., when he didn't have to contend with three McDonald's, two Starbucks, and a Cinnabon within a five-mile radius of the Parthenon. Overwhelming temptation is one reason it's hard to stay on a restricted diet, but there are plenty of others."

—Kathryn Scott,

in her article "Flirting with Disaster," from Living Without, *Spring 2006*

Overview of Elimination Diets

HEALTHY ENVIRONMENT, LIFESTYLE, AND ORGANIC NUTRIENT-DENSE DIET
Chapter 3

Why Is the Diet Needed? Contaminants, pollutants, toxins, GMO foods, and artificial additives are burdens to the body and deplete nutrients needed for growth and development.

Symptoms the Diet May Help: Generalized fatigue; headaches; "brain fog"; mood issues; inflammation; immune problems; and reactions to artificial additives and manufactured chemicals

Avoid:

- Environmental, manufactured, and natural toxic chemicals, pesticides, and pollutants
- Artificial additives, preservatives, sweeteners, coloring, flavoring, excitotoxins (MSG), and commercially processed foods
- Genetically modified organisms (GMOs); non-organic foods; contaminated food and water
- Sugars and sugar-raising foods. Trans-fatty acids, deep fried foods, canola, and corn oils.
- Any problem food or beverage that causes a reaction!

GFCFSF: GLUTEN-FREE, CASEIN-FREE, AND SOY-FREE
Chapter 4

Why Is the Diet Needed?

- Incomplete protein digestion leading to partially digested food peptides including opiate-like peptides from DPP IV enzyme deficiency.
- Leaky gut allows partially digested food peptides to cross into the bloodstream and enter the brain, causing behavior symptoms and cravings for the food sources.

Symptoms the Diet May Help: Cravings for opioid food sources (gluten, milk/casein, and/or soy); silly, "dopey" behavior; repetitive behaviors; OCD; self-injury; high pain tolerance; poor eye contact; and digestive symptoms

Avoid:

- **Gluten:** wheat, barley, rye, spelt, kamut, triticale, groats, and commercial oat
- **Milk:** animal milk products including casein
- **Soy:** edamame, miso, natto, sprouts, tamari, tempeh, tempura, tofu, yuba, lecithin, HVP, MSG, vitamin E

FEINGOLD/LOW SALICYLATE DIET
Chapter 5

What Are Salicylates and Where Are They Found? Salicylates are a type of phenol found in plants, fruits, vegetables, artificial additives, and in aspirin and other pain-relievers.

Why Is the Diet Needed? Insufficient sulfation and detoxification; inadequate gut flora

Symptoms the Diet May Help: Hyperactivity; behavior outbursts; irritability; oppositional/defiant behavior; anxiety; and learning problems

Avoid: Environmental toxins and manufactured chemicals; artificial additives and preservatives; specific fruits and vegetables (especially brightly colored), and most spices.

FAILSAFE/LOW SALICYLATE DIET   Chapter 5

What Is FAILSAFE? (**F**ree of **A**dditives, **L**ow in **S**alicylates, **A**mines and **F**lavor **E**nhancers)
Most rigid diet. Expansion of Feingold Diet by excluding glutamates and biogenic amines.

Why Is the Diet Needed? Insufficient sulfation, detoxification, and inadequate gut flora (microbiota); and chemical sensitivity

Symptoms the Diet May Help: Red cheeks/ears; hyperactivity; silliness; aggression; regressions; poor sleep; night sweats; headaches; dark circles under eyes; behavior problems (oppositional/defiant); and mood swings.

Avoid: Environmental toxins; manufactured chemicals; artificial additives and preservatives (sulfites, nitrates, benzoates, sorbates, and parabens); aromatic chemicals

- Aspirin, NSAIDs, COX II inhibitors, and salicylate-containing medications
- Glutamates: MSG additives and glutamate foods
- Neurotransmitter amines found in aged proteins and fermented foods
- All processed foods; many fruits and vegetables with a few exceptions

LOW PHENOL DIET   Chapter 5

What Are Phenols? Phenols have antioxidant qualities and are beneficial for most, but not for those who are intolerant. Phenols include phenolic salicylates, amines, and glutamates.

Why Is The Diet Needed? Defective phenol sulfotransferase (PST) enzyme necessary for sulfation and detoxification; inadequate gut flora; and high sulfur food sources

Symptoms the Diet May Help: Red cheeks/ears; hyperactivity; silliness; aggression; regressions; poor sleep; night sweats; headaches; dark circles under eyes; behavior and learning problems; and mood swings.

Avoid:

- Environmental toxins, manufactured chemicals, artificial additives and preservatives.
- Aspirin and salicylate-containing medications
- **Main Food Avoids:** Apples; bananas; berries; chocolate; milk products; oranges; orange juice; raisins; red grapes; soy; tomato; and vanillin
- **Other avoids:** Beans (black, white); cherries; cloves; globe artichoke heads; honey; nuts (almonds, hazelnuts, pecans, walnuts); olives; plums; spinach
- If improvement is insufficient, try avoiding more phenolic salicylates, amines, and glutamates.

SCD (SPECIFIC CARBOHYDRATE DIET) AND GAPS (GUT AND PSYCHOLOGY SYNDROME) Chapter 6

Why Are the Diets Needed?

- **SCD:** Deficiencies of disaccharidase enzymes which digest double sugars (lactase, sucrase, maltase, isomaltose); leaky gut; digestive and intestinal conditions; and small intestinal bacterial overgrowth (SIBO)
- **GAPS:** Persistence of inflammatory bowel disease (IBD); irritable bowel syndrome (IBS); and digestive problems

Symptoms the Diets May Help:

- **SCD:** Persistent belching; gas; cramping; constipation; diarrhea; yeast issues; celiac disease; diverticulitis; inflammatory bowel disease (IBD); small intestinal bacterial overgrowth (SIBO); and other digestive problems
- **GAPS:** When the SCD has not been fully effective. GAPS is more strict

Avoid:

- **SCD:** All disaccharides (lactose, sucrose, maltose, and isomaltose) found in sugars; grains; pseudo grains (amaranth, buckwheat, and quinoa); some beans; dried fruit, starchy vegetables; and some milk products
- **GAPS:** Expansion of SCD: additional removal of milk products and casein

ANTI-YEAST (ANTI-CANDIDA) DIETS Chapter 7

What Is Yeast/Candida? Yeast is a normal fungus in the intestine, and *Candida albicans* is the most common yeast. The problem is the overgrowth of yeast, which produces toxins that cause damage.

Why Is the Diet Needed? Yeast overgrowth from intestinal microbiota imbalance, known as dysbiosis. Antibiotics and/or poor fiber increase yeast overgrowth, which damages the intestinal lining.

Symptoms the Diet May Help:

- Abdominal bloating; loose or smelly stools; sugar cravings; rashes; thrush; rectal and vaginal itching
- Silly or inappropriate laughing; inattention; brain fog; and mood and behavior changes

Avoid: Consider the SCD diet first. If not sufficient, add this anti-yeast diet.

- All sugars and sweeteners; high sugar fruits (bananas, dates, grapes, mangoes, raisins, ripe fruit); and sweet juices
- Starchy veggies (most beans, beets, corn, parsnips, peas, potatoes, yams); processed foods; deli meats; grains; most dairy; moldy cheeses; and moldy nuts

LOW OXALATE DIET (LOD) Chapter 8

What Are Oxalates? Oxalates are in foods, in fungi and yeast, and made by the body. Plants make oxalates to protect against infection and consumption.

Why Is the Diet Needed? The problems are caused by insufficient good flora to metabolize oxalates and prevent yeast overgrowth. Inadequate fecal calcium impairs oxalate elimination. Oxalate crystals can damage the GI tract, cross into the bloodstream, and damage tissues, causing inflammation and pain.

Symptoms the Diet May Help:
- Kidney stones; inflammation and pain—urinary, genital, joint, muscle, and eyes
- Headaches; digestive tract inflammation; and self-injurious behavior (common in autism)
- Oxidative stress; glutathione depletion; poor energy metabolism; and poor detoxification

Avoid:
- Nuts, seeds; grains; beans (black, navy, pinto, soy)
- Fruits: berries; citrus; dates; kiwi
- Vegetables: beets; Brussels sprouts; carrots; celery; green olives; potatoes; sorrel; sweet potatoes; tomatoes; zucchini
- Spices/herbs: black pepper; cinnamon; oregano; turmeric
- Other: chocolate; date sugar; stevia; tea

ANTI-INFLAMMATORY DIET Chapter 9

What Is Inflammation? Chronic inflammation begins slowly and can last for months to years. Contributors: pathogens; toxins; problem foods and food components; GMO foods; trans-fatty acids and autoimmune antibodies. Nightshades, alkaloids, and lectins are among the most inflammatory components and are the focus in this diet. Other problem foods include oxalates, phenols, salicylates, phytases, FODMAPs and purines.

Why Is the Diet Needed? Chronic inflammation of the gut and brain is a hallmark in autism and issues in ADHD. Maternal-fetal antibodies may contribute to autism. An anti-inflammatory diet allows for healing.

Symptoms the Diet May Help: Digestive problems including "leaky gut"; brain inflammation; behavior changes; irritability; self-injury; mood disorders; joint and muscle aches/pain; and poor cognition and function

Avoid:
- Nightshade/solanine/tomatine and alkaloid foods: white potatoes, tomatoes, eggplant, okra, peppers, tomatillos, sorrel and other related foods, gooseberries, ground cherries, pepino melons, paprika, cayenne pepper, capsicum, and tobacco (nicotine) exposure
- Lectins (legumes, corn, nuts, seeds, squash, grains, caraway, nutmeg, peppermint, marjoram), phytates, and alkaloid containing foods: blueberries, Goji berries, and huckleberries
- Commercially processed foods, artificial additives, GMO foods, trans-fatty acids, sugars, gluten and possibly other grains and grain substitutes, cow milk products, soy, corn, nuts, and legumes

What Are FODMAPs? Fermentable Oligosaccharides, Disaccharides, Monosaccharides, And Polyols. If poorly digested, these short-chain carbohydrates can ferment in the gut to cause digestive distress. FODMAPs are found in many natural foods and food additives.

Why Is the Diet Needed? For those sensitive to many foods noted to be culprits in many of the elimination diets. The more reactions and symptoms, the more likely the FODMAPs diet will help.

Symptoms the Diet May Help: Multiple digestive conditions and symptoms: irritable bowel syndrome (IBS); inflammatory bowel disease (IBD); and small intestinal bacterial overgrowth (SIBO)

Avoid:

- Processed and deli meats
- Oligosaccharides: fructo-oligosaccharides (FOS), inulin, grains, onions, leeks, and garlic; Jerusalem artichokes; legumes, beans, nuts, and seeds
- Disaccharides: soft cheeses, yogurt, milk products
- Monosaccharides: high fructose corn syrup, watermelons, pears, mangoes, apples, and honey
- Polyols: sorbitol, xylitol, isomalt, and mannitol; mushrooms, apples, apricots, nectarines, peaches, pears, plums, prunes
- Commercially processed foods, artificial additives, GMO foods, trans-fatty acids, sugars, gluten and possibly other grains and grain substitutes, cow milk products, soy, and corn

What Is a Rotation Diet? The diet avoids repetition of foods based upon a four- to seven-day rotation by food families. Families are how biologically related foods are grouped. Rotating by food families provides more options. The diet can reduce reactions to mildly reactive foods and help identify problem foods.

Why Is the Diet Needed? When there are multiple food reactions and very limited choices, rotation expands nutrient diversity and allows inclusion of mildly reactive foods and other nonreactive foods.

Symptoms the Diet May Help: Persistent digestive problems; autoimmunity; inflammation; skin problems; depression; anxiety; behavioral problems; and inattention

Avoid:

- Artificial additives, processed foods, GMO foods, trans-fatty acids, sugars, contaminated food and water
- Foods identified as highly reactive by lab testing, observation, or elimination diet responses
- Food families where many foods are reaction-provoking

CHAPTER 3

Beginning Your Journey:

What to Leave Behind and What to Take with You

"The doctor of the future will give no medicine, but will interest . . . patients in the care of the human frame, in diet, and in the cause and prevention of disease."

—Thomas Edison

THE HEALTHFUL RECOMMENDATIONS IN THIS CHAPTER apply to all individuals and particularly to those with ADHD, autism, and similar disorders. This is the core diet for those with ADHD or autism.

Beyond the challenges of developmental delays and disorders of sensory, language, processing, and motor functions, many children with ADHD, and more so autism, have additional burdens to their already overchallenged systems. Environmental deterioration exposes them to indoor and outdoor manufactured, nutrient-depleting chemicals; pesticides; and toxic metals; in addition to inhalant allergens and rapidly expanding electromagnetic fields and radiofrequency radiation. Through food, children take in a wide range of artificial additives, endure food reactions and frequent infections, and have restricted appetites and poor nutrition. For children who are biochemically less resilient, any one of these issues may be tolerated, however the total load and complexity have become overwhelming.

Any effort to reduce the burden on children's systems can help them improve. Any positive change is helpful. A healthier environment and diet along with optimum nutritional status are cornerstones, not options. This holds true for all adults and children, especially those with ADHD and autism.

Environmental Considerations: Outdoors and Indoors

In the last 100 to 200 years, we have created and allowed an exponentially increasing number of manufactured chemicals into our indoor and outdoor environments and the addition of artificial additives and contaminants into the food supply. Regulation by the 1976 Toxic Substances Control Act (TSCA) has been disastrous for the environment. Currently, there are more than 90,000 manufactured chemicals, 62,000 of which were grandfathered in without testing. There are 700 new chemicals per year and testing is voluntary. If tested, the results must still be revealed. Over 16,000 are permitted to be kept secret from the public. The EPA acknowledges that only 200 manufactured chemicals have been tested for safety. The bottom line is that for more than 99% of environmental chemicals, there is a scarcity of research, woefully inadequate testing, and lenient, inadequate regulations. Grassroots efforts to improve this act continue.

As of June 2016, the TSCA has been amended to mandate EPA evaluation of existing chemicals and increase public transparency. As of 2019, there are EPA strategies to prevent pollution, and there is greater transparency in tracking active new chemical cases.

Indoor pollution sources that release gases or particles into the air are the primary cause of indoor air quality problems. Inadequate ventilation can increase indoor pollutant levels by not bringing in enough outdoor air to dilute emissions from indoor sources and by not carrying indoor air pollutants out of the area.

Note that when these manufactured chemicals, toxicants, and naturally occurring toxins (such as lead, arsenic, cadmium, mercury, and aluminum) come into our bodies, the impact can be devastating.

TOXINS ARE NUTRIENT ANTAGONISTS AND DEPLETE HEALTHY NUTRIENTS, which are "spent" trying to rid the body of these culprits. For those with autism and, to a lesser degree, those with ADHD, it is not uncommon to find defects in glutathione and other detoxification "disposal" systems. The challenges are far beyond the diet's ability to compensate.

Even if some of the 90,000 manufactured chemicals are banned, and there is a reversal of the TSCA section that permits 16,000 to be kept secret, we will not eliminate those already present long-term in our environment and deep within our bodies. We will pass them on to the next generations.

The position paper on pesticides from the American Academy of Pediatrics (*Pediatrics* 2012;130e1757–e1763) concluded: Epidemiological evidence demonstrates associations between early life exposure to pesticides and pediatric cancers, decreased cognitive function, and behavioral problems. Related animal toxicology studies provide supportive biological plausibility for these findings. Recognizing and reducing problematic exposures will require attention to current inadequacies in medical training, public health tracking, and to regulatory action on pesticides.

How Problematic Is the Environmental Toxic Load?

Beyond exposure to natural toxins, the toxic load now includes manufactured chemical components in plastics, pesticides, fire retardants, nonstick cookware, herbicides, artificial turf, building products, cosmetics, personal care products, household cleaning agents, disinfectants, air fresheners, fabric softeners, dental implants and restorative materials, and more.

They can cause behavioral, cognitive, and learning problems and respiratory conditions, and also increase cancer risk, immune dysfunction, and, as endocrine disrupters, they negatively affect hormone metabolism, reproduction, and fetal development. In the cord blood of newborn babies, there are more than 200 industrial pollutants, some of which are known carcinogens and endocrine disrupting hormonal agents. This has been termed "born pre-polluted."

Important and increasing is our exposure to electromagnetic fields (EMFs) and radiofrequency radiation (RFRs) from our technological devices, appliances, and meters, which are now ubiquitous in our indoor and outdoor environments. The deleterious effects on the nervous system are well known. There is increasing concern about the safety of these lifetime exposures and the lack of regulations regarding human exposures.

The evidence of harm is already known; action is what is needed.

Most Contaminated Produce:

Buy organic.

- Apples
- Bananas
- Celery
- Cherries
- Grapes
- Lettuce
- Nectarines
- Peaches
- Pears
- Peppers: sweet bell and hot peppers
- Potatoes
- Red raspberries
- Spinach
- Strawberries
- Tomatoes

Least Contaminated Produce:

If you buy it, wash it well. Organic is still best.

- Asparagus
- Avocados
- Broccoli
- Cabbages
- Cantaloupes
- Carrots (peeled)
- Cauliflower
- Citrus fruits
- Corn (sweet)
- Eggplant
- Honeydew melons
- Kiwis
- Mangoes
- Onions
- Papaya
- Peas (sweet) frozen
- Pineapples
- Sweet potatoes

Source: Environmental Working Group's 2018 Shopper's Guide to Pesticides in Produce at https://www.ewg.org/foodnews/

GLYPHOSATE, an herbicide linked to cancer by California state scientists and the World Health Association, is the active ingredient in the most heavily used pesticide in the US. It is used on grain crops, especially genetically engineered soy and corn as well as wheat and oat products. It is also sprayed on non-GMO crops prior to harvesting. It is found in more than 95% of conventionally grown oat products. See the Environmental Working Group site for more detailed information: www.ewg.org/childrenshealth/glyphosateincereal/

Excellent Nutrition Is Not Optional . . . It Is Vital

In the 1960s, nutritionist Adelle Davis wisely said "you are what you eat." We have modified that to "you are what you eat, digest, absorb, transport, uptake, and utilize based upon your healthy or unhealthy exposures and your own unique genes and biochemistry."

To have excellent nutrition, it's important to understand what nutrition is. Your diet is what you eat. Nutrition is what the cells derive from what you eat. When you consume poor-quality food, your nutritional status will be poor. However, a healthy diet may still result in poor nutrition if there are problems in one or more of the following: food digestion, nutrient absorption, transportation to the tissues, uptake and utilization of nutrients by the tissues as impacted by helpful nutrients, and/or interfering substances, such as environmental and dietary toxins, herbs, and medications (e.g., antacids, diuretics).

In the past 100 to 150 years and with the evolution of the "modern" diet, healthy fats were replaced with damaging commercially hydrogenated fats (trans-fatty acids) and artificial fats (Olestra). Meanwhile, genetically modified foods, imitation foods, refined foods, and copious amounts of artificial additives, sweeteners, coloring, flavoring, preservatives, and sugars have become part of the modern diet. In addition to chemicals in cookware, many food containers have harmful chemicals that can seep into the food. There are more than 3,000 FDA additives included in food in the US, which includes the GRAS (Generally Recognized As Safe) list. Our advice: go organic. (See page 48.)

Health Enemies: Leave These Behind

1. SAY NO TO NATURAL TOXINS AND ARTIFICIAL INGREDIENTS, INCLUDING ARTIFICIAL FOOD ADDITIVES, PRESERVATIVES, SWEETENERS, TASTE ENHANCERS, ARTIFICIAL FLAVORING AND COLORING AGENTS, EXCITOTOXINS, GMO FOODS, TRANS-FATTY ACIDS, AND COMMERCIALLY PROCESSED FOODS.

The FDA oversight and regulation of food additives, which are so abundant in non-organic, processed foods, is not consistent with the increasing scientific findings about the detrimental health impact of singular and combined chemical additives in our foods. Even if a single additive has a mild negative effect, there are combinations of mild-effect additives that can have potent synergistic negative effects. When consuming many processed foods, consumers have no way of knowing what those combinations do to their immunity, brain health, neurological system, hormonal functions, and more.

The Environmental Working Group (ewg.org) provides information important to consumers with regard to scientific concerns on the safety of already approved and new food additives. Use EWG's Food Scores to find foods without the problematic additives. See the following for more information:

- EWG's Food Scores at www.ewg.org/foodscores/
- EWG's Dirty Dozen Guide to Food Additives at www.ewg.org/research/ewg-s-dirty-dozen-guide-food-additives

Generally Recognized as Safe?

The **FDA** classifies approximately 3,000 additives as Generally Recognized as Safe (GRAS), though studies can indicate otherwise. Beyond this are more questionable GRAS additives that come into contact with food through food containers and packaging. For new ingredients, the law recommends safety evaluation through the FDA approval process. In 1997, the FDA established a voluntary system for manufacturers, which allows them to establish their own GRAS determination, sharing the information with the FDA. Because it is voluntary, many additives are being used in foods and are not known to the FDA.

The Following GRAS Items Are of Significant Health Concern:

Genetically modified organisms (GMOs) are living organisms whose genetic material has been artificially manipulated in a laboratory through genetic engineering creating combinations of plant, animal, bacteria, and virus genes that do not occur in nature or through traditional crossbreeding methods. More than 80% of all GMO crops worldwide have been engineered for herbicide tolerance (pesticide "ready"). GMO crops have caused the emergence of "super weeds" and "superbugs" that can only be killed with evermore toxic poisons. According to animal studies and human observation, GMO exposures can have a negative effect on digestion, immunity, food tolerances, reproduction, and development. They do not increase crop yield and can cross-pollinate in crops, contaminating them long-term, harming the land and sea ecosystems. When the US failed to require GMO labeling, the Non-

GMO project was created to give consumers the informed choices they deserve. See the following for more information:

- EWG's 2014 Shopper's Guide to Avoiding GMO Food at www.ewg.org/shoppers-guide-to-avoiding-gmos
- The Non-GMO Project at www.nongmoproject.org

The following are examples of more of the GRAS items that are of significant health concern based on current scientific data: aluminum (a known neurotoxin); artificial colors (behavioral and attention problems); artificial sweeteners (weight gain and diabetes risk); Bisphenol A/BPA (hormonal effects); BHA and BHT (potential carcinogens); nitrates and nitrites (cancer causing); natural flavors (permitted to contain numerous synthetic chemicals); GMO foods (endocrine disruption, herbicide tolerance, and immune dysregulation); sulfites (allergenic); animal growth promoting hormones, antibiotics, and steroids; and "excitotoxins" including MSG (monosodium glutamate), which causes problems in development, behavior and neurological function.

Abundant in processed foods, there are more than 70 types of dietary excitotoxin sources which include artificial additives, preservatives, artificial sweeteners, taste enhancers, and artificial flavoring and coloring agents. Glutamate (and glutamic acid), especially MSG, are the most notable excitotoxins; however, there are others such as aspartame, aspartate, cysteine, and casein. They are able to cross the blood-brain barrier and affect brain function by overstimulating the natural body neurotransmitter known as glutamate, which is balanced by the naturally occurring, calming neurotransmitter, GABA (gamma–aminobutyric acid). Glutamate and GABA occupy the two ends of a teeter-totter that is thrown out of balance by excessive glutamate overexciting the neurons, thereby reducing the calming neurotransmitter, GABA.

Monosodium Glutamate (MSG)

MSG deserves special mention, due to its prevalence and its potential for causing significant symptoms. It is common in processed foods, especially Asian foods, and canned foods. Incorrectly termed a "flavor enhancer." it actually alters the brain's perception of taste, increases hunger, and overstimulates the excitatory neurotransmitters. It can cause headaches, flushing, sweating, behavioral problems, neurological symptoms, arrhythmias, chest pain, nausea, and weakness. In the US, if MSG is used directly in the food, it must be listed on the label. However, if an ingredient contains MSG, only the ingredient must be listed. The following items contain MSG: hydrolyzed protein, autolyzed yeast and yeast extracts, glutamic acid, and more. For those who are highly sensitive to glutamate and MSG, naturally occurring sources may need to be avoided: potatoes, peas, tomatoes, tomato juice, mushrooms, grapes, grape juice, and Parmesan and Roquefort cheeses.

2. SAY NO TO DRINKING WATER CONTAMINANTS.

The contamination of tap water is a concern in almost every community. Most of the problems are from pesticides, manufactured environmental chemicals, and toxic metals.

■ **CONTAMINANTS** that increase risks for cancer, fetal development, and cognition problems include: solvents, arsenic, herbicides, chromium-6 (not nutritional chromium), copper from copper plumbing, lead, manganese (excessive), nitrates (fertilizer), nitrosamines from the use of chloramine disinfectants, perchlorate, and radiological contaminants that leach into water from minerals and mining.

● The EPA reports that more than 1,000 communities have water tainted with lead, which impairs cognition in children and increases cardiovascular risk in adults.

● **SULFURYL FLUORIDE** (pesticide) increases fluoride exposure exponentially, adding significantly to total fluoride exposure.

■ **DISINFECTION BYPRODUCTS (DBPS).** There are more than 600 byproducts in chlorinated drinking water, the main groups of which are potentially harmful to fetal development and can increase cancer risk: trihalomethanes (THMs), haloacetic acids (HAAs), chlorate, and bromate. For more information, read www.ewg.org/tapwater/reviewed-disinfection-byproducts.php#

■ **FLUORIDE** has been added to public water supplies in order to reduce dental decay. The CDC, National Research Council of the National Academy of Medicine (formerly the Institute of Medicine), the American Public Health Association, and the US Department of Health and Human Services have been concerned about the lack of safety testing of **SILICOFLUORIDE (SIF)** used in 92% of the public water supplies. Fluoride has been identified as a chemical of significant concern with regard to health issues, including recent research (2019, *JAMA Pediatrics*) validating previous findings that higher water fluoride levels correspond to lower IQ scores, most strongly in boys. The US Department of Health and Human Services already proposed lowering fluoride in public water supplies. This has been accomplished in many communities attempting to reduce harm from excess fluoride exposure.

There are a variety of filter options that vary significantly in terms of cost. For more information, check with the Environmental Working Group's Tap Water Database: www.ewg.org/tapwater

3. SAY NO TO SUGARS AND SUGAR-RAISING FOODS.

Understanding the Glycemic Impact on ADHD and Autism

Glycemic means "sugar raising." The glycemic index (GI) is a measure of how a food triggers a rise in blood glucose. The range is zero (fats, oils, cheese, and seafood) to 100 (glucose). Glycemic foods include all sugars, caffeine, refined carbohydrates (including breads, pasta, crackers, pretzels, bagels, and white rice), sweets, caffeine, sodas (diet and regular), fruit juices, juice drinks, dried fruits, potatoes, and corn.

When a glycemic food is consumed alone, the sugar enters the bloodstream quickly, raising blood glucose. The more of the glycemic food consumed, the higher and faster the glucose rises. This triggers an excess release of insulin, which drives the glucose into the cells and converts some of it to fat (triglycerides, which store as "belly fat"). Also, as the glucose drops, there is "brain fog," irritability, hunger headaches, visual disturbances, fatigue, muscle weakness, and/or cravings for a "quick fix"—more of the sugar sources.

Most children with ADHD or autism eat sugar-raising, low-protein, and low-fiber diets. They crave "white foods," refined grains and processed carbohydrates—pasta, breads, crackers, pretzels, bagels, and sugars. They also crave sugary sweets, sodas, and juices. Besides wearing out the body's ability to handle sugar and setting up children for early diabetes, glycemic foods have a serious negative effect on mood stability, focus, and attention. Because children with ADHD or autism already suffer from these problems, it is important to not reward good behavior and attention with sugar treats and candies. Many parents describe "hangry" (a combination of *hungry* and *angry*) behaviors in their children from the blood glucose drop after a high glycemic meal or snack or when not eating sufficient protein, good fats, and fiber to keep blood sugar regulated between meals.

The key is to slow down the entry and quick rise of glucose by including healthy **fats**, **proteins** (nuts, seeds, beans, meats, poultry, seafood, tolerated milk products), and **fiber** (vegetables, beans/legumes, nuts, seeds, limited grains, and some fruits). These choices will blunt the glucose-raising effect of food that is more glycemic. When hungry, there is a tendency to consume more of the first food served. Avoid serving breads or any glycemic food first. Instead, serve the healthy, low glycemic foods first.

- **HIGH FRUCTOSE CORN SYRUP (HFCS)**, manufactured primarily from genetically modified corn, has replaced sugar in most processed foods and drinks. It is high in fructose (42 to 50%). It has double the sucrose (sugar) effect and increases weight gain, diabetes risk, triglyceride, LDL, high blood pressure, and risk for kidney damage. The high content of fructose can increase pancreatic cancer risk. Reports indicate the presence of mercury in 50% of the HFCS.

- **SUGAR BLUES:** white table sugar (cane sugar), sugar in the raw, brown sugar, and corn syrupIn 1820, in the US, sugar consumption was less than 10 pounds (4.5 kg) per year per person. By 1900, it was 50 pounds (23 kg) per year. In 2000, it was 100 pounds (45.5 kg) per year. Currently, the average US sugar consumption is 130 to 170 pounds (59 to 77 kg) per year. Sugar increases blood glucose, which increases risk for diabetes, which has increased 90% in the last decade. For more information, see Sugar Consumption in the US

Diet between 1822 and 2005: http://onlinestatbook.com/2/case_studies/sugar.html

- **AGAVE SYRUP** is high in fructose, which increases diabetes risk more than pure glucose and also increases nonalcoholic fatty acid liver disease.
- **SUGAR DRINKS AND JUNK ELECTROLYTE DRINKS:** Juice drinks are juices with sugar and/or HFCS added. These are highly glycemic and must be avoided. The most popular electrolyte drink is primarily sugar in various forms with artificial coloring. For a better electrolyte drink, consider organic coconut water plain or with some organic fruit juice added. Organic vegetable juices are nutrient dense. Drink water and organic vegetable juice.
- **SODAS (DIET AND REGULAR):** Sodas, both diet and regular, are a problem, and not just because they take the place of drinking more water and nutritional beverages. They provide a combination of artificial coloring and flavoring in addition to artificial sweeteners. They are high in phosphorus, a nutrient abundant in any diet. Excess phosphorus via sodas can bind with minerals, making them unavailable for use by the body. Phosphorus depletes calcium, magnesium, zinc, and vitamins C and B. Sodas are the opposite of electrolyte drinks; they are electrolyte thieves. They take nutrients out of the nutrient stores. The body cannot easily compensate for the depletion.

Both diet and regular sodas significantly increase risk for obesity, diabetes, and metabolic syndrome, and confer a 48% increased risk for cardiovascular disease including strokes. Diet sodas are worse because they contain artificial sweeteners. Human and animal studies have demonstrated that artificial sweeteners slow metabolism down and impair regulation of calorie intake—leading to overeating and the long-term health consequences of overeating. All sodas and artificial sweeteners must be avoided.

- Children with ADHD or autism characteristically

have low levels of minerals and vitamins. Especially in autism, the nutrient deficiencies are significant, and the nutrient needs are well above what is standard due to metabolic inefficiencies. What these children do not need is a drink that deprives them further and increases their risk for mood swings, diabetes, obesity, and behavior problems.

- **REFINED GRAINS:** Because a product says "whole grain" does not mean that it is nutrient-dense and fiber-rich. All grain products come from "whole grains," including refined white breads, so don't be fooled. Grains that are less glycemic include barley, bulgur, and rye (if gluten is tolerated), gluten-free oats (steel cut), oat bran, wild rice, and pseudo-grains such as quinoa, buckwheat, and amaranth. The more refined the grain, the higher the glycemic (sugar-raising) effect. This includes bagels, white breads, pretzels, pizza dough, and brown and white rice.

Unless a bread is high in fiber or includes nuts and vegetables, the glycemic effect can be almost as high as that of sugar. Almost all cold cereals are glycemic; we like to think of them as "desserts," and not necessarily healthy. So just as you would not start dinner with dessert, we suggest starting breakfast with good protein, healthy fat, and good fiber. If transitioning from a typical high sugar, non-organic cold cereal to a healthier version, after the healthier foods are consumed, offer a small serving of the organic, low glycemic cold cereal. This will blunt the blood sugar raising effect of the glycemic cereal alone.

- **CAFFEINE:** The quick wake-up jolt from caffeine (no matter the source) is ultimately glycemic. Caffeine stimulates the adrenals to put out adrenaline, the hormone responsible for the "fight or flight" response that occurs under stress and dangers. Adrenaline directs the liver to break down glycogen and release glucose into the bloodstream, which initiates the glycemic response. Children with ADHD or autism are more sensitive to the effects of caffeine and more at risk for excitability and anxiety.

4. SAY NO TO PROBLEM FATS.

- **PARTIALLY HYDROGENATED OILS/TRANS-FATTY ACIDS:** When healthy oils are hydrogenated to become unhealthy mutant, plastic, saturated fatty acids, it is analogous to good Dr. Jekyll becoming evil Mr. Hyde. Hydrogenation is the industrial processing of vegetable oils (corn, sunflower, safflower, canola, peanut, cottonseed, or soy) to form unhealthy, highly saturated, trans-fatty acids. The process involves bubbling hydrogen through the oil at high temperatures using toxic metal catalysts such as nickel and cadmium. Partially hydrogenated oils (PHOs) contain the unnatural, harmful "trans-fatty acids," which are far worse than any naturally occurring saturated fatty acid. In fact, trans-fatty acids from commercial hydrogenation do not occur in nature at all and do not belong in the human body.

Commercial trans-fatty acids from commercial hydrogenation are found in numerous processed foods. They are nutritionally inferior, have absolutely no health benefit, and are severely detrimental to health in ways that affect all people. They are antagonists to omega-3 fatty acids.

So how bad can trans-fatty acids be, and why are they important when it comes to children with ADHD or autism? In the body, trans-fatty acids look like and take the place of the natural and essential fatty acids within the cell membrane. They are similar to a key that looks like your door key, fits in the lock, and becomes stuck, blocking the right key from fitting in. Trans-fatty acids become part of the cell membranes, hardening them. This interferes with the ability to transport nutrients into the cell and remove metabolic waste (garbage) from the cells. Mitochondrial function is impeded, resulting in increased cell death in hippocampus brain cells. Children

US Bans Trans-Fatty Acids

Since the 1970s, researchers have reported mounting concerns about the safety of trans-fatty acid consumption. In 2000, after five decades of recommending partially hydrogenated oil trans-fatty acids, the US government began questioning their safety and by 2013 stated that PHO trans-fatty acids were no longer Generally Recognized as Safe (GRAS), establishing a ban that took effect in 2018. Some natural trans-fatty acids are present in small amounts in meat and dairy products, but the structure is not the same as the harmful commercial PHO trans-fatty acids. By banning PHOs, the US government expects to reduce cardiovascular-related deaths by 7,000 per year. This is consistent with findings in local communities and other countries around the world.

with ADHD or autism already have problems with cell function and toxic accumulation without adding trans-fatty acids from partially hydrogenated oils to the diet.

Trans-fatty acids interfere with cell function, reproduction (male and female), fetal development, brain structure and development, breast milk quality, immunity, and metabolic enzymes. They increase the risk for poor-quality lipids, diabetes, obesity, inflammation, immune disorders, cancers, and autism.

Studies in pregnant women indicate increased risk for autism in children whose mothers consumed PHO trans-fatty acids. Trans-fatty acid levels in the cord blood matched serum levels in the mothers. Breast-fed infants' intake of trans-fatty acids is directly affected by the mother's dietary intake of trans-fatty acids. Based on the importance of omega-3 fatty acids in neural development, it is understandable that trans-fatty acid consumption could affect developmental issues including autism. When it comes to spreads, butter is better, but not for those with casein/milk problems. The alternative is ghee, which is clarified butter, also called drawn butter.

- **DEEP FAT FRIED FOODS** are high in calories and lack nutrient density (empty calories). The most common oils for deep frying are canola, cottonseed, and soybean. The high temperature cooking increases the rancidity of the oil. Some of the oils contain a possible carcinogen, acrylamide, which is a byproduct of deep fat frying. Roasting and stir frying are healthier options.

- **CANOLA OIL:** The canola plant was bred from the rapeseed plant, which has large amounts of erucic acid, known to contribute to health problems including cardiovascular diseases. In 1995, Monsanto produced a genetically modified version of canola (named for Canada—oil). Canola oil is partially hydrogenated, and currently over 90% of canola oil comes from genetically modified canola.

- **GMO SOY OIL AND CORN OIL,** like canola oil, are not the best choices. More than 90% of soy crops and corn crops are genetically modified and engineered to survive being doused with large amounts of herbicides. If soy is the only option as a milk substitute, it must be 100% organic (USDA Organic).

- **PALM KERNEL OIL:** Derived from the seed of the palm fruit, this oil is less beneficial and less nutritional as compared to the unrefined palm fruit oil (red palm oil).

5. SAY NO TO NON-ORGANIC DELI MEATS, PROCESSED FOODS, AND CONTAMINATED SEAFOOD.

- **NON-ORGANIC DELI MEATS** are preserved with nitrites, which, in significant enough amounts, can deactivate hemoglobin, impeding the carrying of oxygen by red blood cells. Nitrites also can convert to nitrosamines, which are carcinogenic.

- **PROCESSED FOODS** are calorie high, nutrient low, fiber low foods that increase blood glucose levels and the risk for obesity, diabetes, immune disorders, and developmental delays. They are usually high in artificial ingredients, preservatives, glutamates, and excitotoxins.

- **CONTAMINATED SEAFOOD:** Seafood is abundant in healthy nutrients, especially protein, zinc, omega-3 fatty acids, and iodine. Seafood is generally much easier to digest than animal protein (meats, poultry). Some of the concerns lie in environmental issues, such as inadequate conservation efforts to avoid depletion of certain species of fish and the increasing contamination from industrial pollutants. The species most likely to have higher levels of toxins and pesticides include the large steak fish that feed on smaller fish and bottom-feeders. The toxins move up the food chain, becoming more concentrated and detrimental. Farming techniques contribute to the toxic content of farm-raised fish, depending on what they are fed. The location of the seafood determines the type and level of toxins present. Currently in the United States, there is no USDA organic certification for seafood or aquaculture production. Problems associated with contaminated seafood:

  - Chemicals and contaminants: mercury, polychlorinated biphenyls (PCBs), chlordane, dioxins, DDT, cadmium

  - Toxins are higher in the organs and fatty tissues (shellfish "mustard" or "tamale").

  - Government monitoring is poor. There is no USDA organic certification for seafood.

  - The more contaminants, the higher the risk.

  - Fetuses, young children, and those with immune problems are at increased risk for cancers, neurological problems, learning disorders, cognitive decline, and developmental delays.

SEAFOOD TO AVOID

(The highest risk is during pregnancy and to fetuses, infants, children, and those with immune disorders.)

Mercury (found in big, old fish)

Blue fish

Halibut

Kingfish

Lobster

Mackerel (King)

Mahi

Marlin

Sea bass

Shark

Swordfish

Tilefish

Tuna (Bigeye)

Tuna (canned light and albacore)

High in PCBs (polychlorinated biphenyls)

Catfish

Carp

Lake trout

Muskellunge

Northern pike

Shark

Striped bass

Walleyes

Higher in Other Contaminants

Carp

Catfish

Flounder

Grouper

Orange roughy

Shellfish

Farm-raised fish—*raised in crowded pens with processed feed*

The mustard in blue crabs or tamale in lobsters

Raw fish (sushi, sashimi)—*risk of parasite exposure*

Resource for seafood safety: Calculate your safe intake of seafood using EWG's Seafood Calculator

https://www.ewg.org/research/ewg-s-consumer-guide-seafood/seafood-calculator#

6. SAY NO TO ANY FOOD OR BEVERAGE THAT CAUSES A NEGATIVE REACTION.

Make certain the reaction is due to the food or beverage and not to artificial additives, preservatives, coloring, and flavoring. If a food or beverage causes a reaction (for example hyperactivity, aggression, or irritability), make sure that food is organic and does not have artificial additives before eliminating the food. For example, if your child is reacting to a fruit punch that has red dye, switch to an organic fruit juice that does not have additives and observe the reaction. If the reaction persists in an organic juice, then that fruit and its juice may be the problem.

We have described the negative effects from numerous single environmental and dietary culprits discussed in this chapter. As exposure to combinations of these culprits increases, the effects are not additive, they are compounded exponentially, and the consequences gravely endanger health at every stage from conception to death. All of these are considered health, neurological, and behavioral risk factors to humans, and especially to the more susceptible individuals with immune, metabolic, or developmental issues.

Many families observe significant improvements in behavior and learning by making adjustments to diet (including going organic), household environment, and toxic outdoor environmental exposures. If the total load of culprits remains in the diet and environment, success with an elimination diet or diets may be blunted. Having said this, we believe that any effort you make is a positive step.

Healthy Foods for Your Journey

The right diet depends upon genetics, family history, ethnicity, culture, age, gender, stage of life, health status, lifestyle, stress, food reactions, and food aversions. A healthy diet is an organic, nutrient-dense diet appropriate to the uniqueness of the individual's digestion, biochemistry, and nutrient needs.

1. DON'T TRY TO FOOL MOTHER NATURE—GO ORGANIC.

This is not fluff or a trendy concept. The US Department of Agriculture (USDA) Organic seal is a certification that mandates specific standards. Organic foods *may not* be irradiated or produced with genetically modified organisms (GMOs). All organic farmers and processors are required to meet the standards of the USDA and the National Organic Standards Board (NOSB). Organic foods are grown without relying on synthetic chemical pesticides. Techniques must help protect the air, soil, water, and food supply from potentially toxic chemicals and other pollutants. Organic farming conserves natural resources by recycling natural materials, protecting ecosystems, and preventing contamination of crops, soil, and water by plant and animal pathogenic organisms, heavy metals, or toxic residues.

The definitions are strict and easy to understand:

- *100% ORGANIC:* This means that 100% of all the ingredients are organic, and animals are fed 100% organic feed. Labeling may include the **USDA ORGANIC SEAL** and/or **100% ORGANIC** claim. Labeling must identify organic ingredients.

Organic meat regulations require that animals are raised in living conditions accommodating their natural behaviors (e.g., pastured), fed 100% organic feed and forage, and not administered antibiotics or hormones.

- *ORGANIC:* This means that 95% are organic ingredients, free of synthetic additives like pesticides, chemical fertilizers, and dyes, and must not be processed using industrial solvents, irradiation, or genetic engineering. The remaining 5% may only be foods with additives on an approved list. Labeling may include the **USDA ORGANIC SEAL** and/or **ORGANIC** claim. Labeling must identify organic ingredients.

- *MADE WITH ORGANIC:* This means that the product does not qualify for the USDA Organic seal. It indicates that the product contains 70% or more organic ingredients, and the remaining 30% of the ingredients are produced without using prohibited practices (e.g., genetic engineering) but can include substances that would not otherwise be allowed in 100% organic products.

Reading the Food Labels:

- *Organic.* The following USDA certifications qualify for the "Organic" Seal:
  - USDA Organic
  - 100% Organic
  - Organic (95% organic ingredients)
- *Made with organic ingredients*—does not qualify for the USDA Organic seal.
- *Pastured* indicates the animal was raised on grassy land (includes chickens, pigs, goats, cows, beef cattle, and sheep).
- *Grass-fed* applies to beef, indicating that the animals have continuous access to grass during the growing season and it is their sole source of food after weaning. Cattle tend to be herbivores.
- *Natural* is a meaningless and an unregulated term. Natural does not mean "nontoxic" (arsenic is natural).
- *Fresh* means never frozen, but not indicative of when slaughtered. Use fresh or frozen organic foods.
- *Cage-free* applies only to birds raised for eggs, not those raised for the poultry meat.
- *Free-range* suggests that the animals had some access to the outdoors, but does not indicate how long and what they were fed.
- *Hormone-free* is mandated in poultry and hogs; however, hormones are permitted in beef cattle, sheep, and other animals unless certified hormone-free.
- *Antibiotic-free* indicates birds were given no unnecessary antibiotics for fattening, but does not address the living conditions or what they ate.
- *Arsenic-free.* Arsenic, used to fatten, is important to avoid. Being free of arsenic does not address quality of the feed and living conditions.

Resources:
- USDA Organic 101
  https://www.ams.usda.gov/sites/default/files/media/Organic%20101%20Training%20Final%20June%202015.pdf
- *Food: What the Heck Should I Eat?* by Mark Hyman, 2018, pp 65–75.
- 2017 EPA-FDA Advice about Eating Fish and Shellfish
  https://www.epa.gov/fish-tech/2017-epa-fda-advice-about-eating-fish-and-shellfish

As a rule, we recommend using organic foods whenever possible, primarily because it avoids so many of the aggravating effects from artificial additives. Some children with ADHD and many children with autism already have inefficiencies in metabolizing and eliminating their own toxins, placing a burden on their systems. Ingesting harmful pesticides, additives, contaminants, and toxins can increase that burden. USDA organic products are therefore safer to consume. When buying organic produce is not possible, focus on the less contaminated "clean 15" foods and wash them thoroughly. (See page 39.)

2. BE IN CONTROL OF YOUR BLOOD SUGAR (GLUCOSE) LEVELS.

Guidelines for Maintaining a Stable Blood Sugar (Glucose):

- Never consume a glycemic (sugar-raising) food on an empty stomach: sugars, sweets, sodas, caffeine, fruit juices, and refined grains (bread, pasta, crackers, pretzels, bagels, most cold cereals, and white rice).

- Good protein, fats, and fiber help keep blood glucose stable. They also reduce the problems with glycemic foods.

- The first food or beverage of the day sets the glucose standard for the day. It must be low in sugars and refined carbohydrates. This helps maintain healthy glucose levels throughout the day.

- Consume healthy, organic sources appropriate to the diet:

  - **PROTEIN:** seafood; pastured poultry, meat, and eggs; and legumes, beans, nuts and seeds
    If tolerated/allowed: pastured source organic cheese, Greek yogurt, and cottage cheese (included in some elimination diets)

  - **FATS AND OILS:** coconut, butter, lard, seafood, fish oils, algae, and oils of olives, almonds,

avocados, pumpkin seeds, walnuts, macadamias, flaxseeds, perilla, peanuts, and vegetable oils

- **FIBER FOODS:** beans, nuts, seeds, grains, non-starchy vegetables, and low glycemic fruits (cherries, grapefruit, prunes, apples, pears, strawberries, and peaches)

- **NATURAL SWEETENER OPTIONS (USE SPARINGLY):** organic stevia, coconut sugar, raw honey, maple syrup (grade B), blackstrap molasses, banana purée, real fruit jam/spread, and Sucanat

3. JACK SPRAT WAS WRONG: GOOD FATS TO THE RESCUE.

A common diet myth is that animal fats are all saturated and vegetable fats are all unsaturated. Dietary fats and oils are combinations of saturated and unsaturated fatty acids, both of which occur naturally in animal and plant sources. Cholesterol is found only in animal food sources. Fat is important in energy production, providing part of the structure of the cell membranes; absorption and carrier of fat soluble vitamins A, D, E, and K; and functioning as a precursor source to the essential omega-6 (linoleic acid LA) and omega-3 (linolenic acid ALA) fatty acids.

Polyunsaturated Fatty Acids

POLYUNSATURATED FATTY ACIDS include the best-known essential fatty acids, omega-6 and omega-3.

- **OMEGA-3 AS ALPHA-LINOLENIC ACID (ALA)** is a precursor to the omega-3 EPA and DHA. ALA is found in plant sources only, such as flaxseeds, walnuts, pumpkin seeds, and hemp and perilla seed oils.

- **OMEGA-6, LINOLEIC ACID (LA)**, is found in vegetables, nuts, seeds, and their oils and is more abundant in the Western diet.

- **OMEGA-3 EPA AND DHA** sources include seafood, fish oils, and algae. EPA and DHA are critical to brain structure and function, vision, cognition, skin health, immunity, hormones, reproduction, development, and more. Not all people thoroughly convert the precursor plant source omega-3s to EPA and DHA.

- **RATIO OMEGA-6 TO OMEGA-3.** The ratio of 1 to 1 is ideal with a healthy range up to 4 to 1. Omega-6 and omega-3 fatty acids are both important in human health. In Western cultures, the ratio of omega-6 to omega-3 fatty acids is skewed toward omega-6, which can promote inflammation. Based on inadequate intakes or individual biochemical uniqueness, those with ADHD or autism tend to have higher needs for omega-3 fatty acids. This can be determined by dietary history and documented via testing.

Monounsaturated Fatty Acids

OLEIC ACID is an **OMEGA-9** monounsaturated fatty acid, found in olive oils, avocados and avocado oil, macadamia nuts and macadamia oil, and peanuts and peanut oils. Oleic acid is also abundant in animal fats such as lard and tallow.

Saturated Fatty Acids

SATURATED FATTY ACIDS are found in coconut oil and red palm oil, poultry, meats, seafood, milk fats, and butter. The short-chain fatty acids are found in butter, coconut oil, and palm oil and have lower melting points than longer-chain saturated fatty acids. Medium-chain saturated fatty acids are found in foods as medium-chain triglycerides (MCT) and are used in special medical formulas for those who cannot absorb the longer-chain fatty acids. These are especially important in infant formulas where they duplicate the medium-chain saturated fatty acids found in human milk. The longer-chain saturated fatty acids are the most common fatty acid found in foods. The long-chain fatty acids are important in membranes, especially in the brain.

Coconut Oil and Unrefined Red Palm Oil

are not the enemies. These healthy natural fats and oils were abandoned with the saturated-fat scare and replaced with partially hydrogenated oils, which consist of highly damaging trans-fatty acids, more harmful to human health than any naturally occurring fatty acid. The lauric acid found in coconut oil and mother's milk has antifungal and antimicrobial properties and is especially beneficial to infants and children. Tropical oils have been demonstrated to raise good cholesterol (HDL) levels.

Good News about Cholesterol!

Cholesterol is found only in animal sources: meats, poultry, animal milk fats, egg yolks, seafood, lard, tallow, and butter. One pervasive myth is that if high cholesterol is bad, the lower the cholesterol, the better. This is not true. Without cholesterol, the body cannot function. Cholesterol is so important to human health that the liver makes approximately 1,000 milligrams per day. Scientific studies have documented that dietary cholesterol has little effect on blood cholesterol levels. The body regulates the amount of cholesterol so that when more is consumed, the body makes less, and when less is consumed, the body makes more.

Why would the body make a substance purported to be so dangerous? Why would mother's milk be so rich in cholesterol? Cholesterol is vital to the structure of all cells. It is a major precursor of reproductive and natural steroid hormones, vitamin D, and digestive bile acids. It forms the "bricks" of the cell membranes and the covering of nerves. In fact, 25% of total body cholesterol is in the brain, critical to brain structure and function. It is important in the serotonin neurotransmitter receptor in the brain, which affects mood, social behavior, sleep, memory, and appetite. Cholesterol maintains the health of the intestinal wall, preventing leaky membranes.

Cholesterol does not attach to or attack healthy vessels. When there is injury to vessels, the body sends out more cholesterol as a repair substance or band aid for the injury. The cholesterol becomes part of the injured area of the vessel. So yes, the elevated cholesterol in the blood is associated with heart disease—but it is not the direct cause. The cholesterol plaques that form within the wall are part of the problem. The causes of vessel injury are the main source of the problem, and they include genetics, aging, high blood pressure, high blood glucose, inflammation, infections, viruses, stress hormones, deep-fried foods, hydrogenated oils, oxidized fats, lack of antioxidants, excess free radicals, lack of B vitamins, elevated C-reactive protein (CRP), methylation defects, and elevated homocysteine.

The previous and outdated limit on cholesterol intake at 300 milligrams per day was based on the faulty premise that consuming cholesterol is harmful to health. Studies show that at four times the so-called "limit," there is little impact on blood cholesterol. Cholesterol is an important nutrient for the body and is regulated by the body. If intake is low, the liver makes more, and if intake is high, the liver makes less. The Institute of Medicine has declared that cholesterol is no longer a nutrient of concern.

The Good Egg

Eggs, another item wrongly maligned over time, are not the enemy either, as confirmed by numerous current scientific studies. The egg is a high-protein, nutrient-rich food so beneficial to health that it is considered one of the leading nutrient-dense foods. The white includes amino acids; however, it is the yolk that is loaded with vitamins, minerals, antioxidants, and choline, a brain nutrient. Healthy choices include pastured sources and omega-3 enriched eggs. Because cholesterol production is regulated by the liver, egg intake contributes little to total blood cholesterol levels. In fact, egg intake is associated with increased good HDL cholesterol levels and improved cholesterol ratios.

As long as there are not allergies, eggs are, indeed, incredible. They are an excellent way of increasing good-quality protein.

Low Cholesterol Levels and Autism

Studies have found that a subset of children with autism spectrum disorders have a cholesterol level that is too low. Some of these children have low cholesterol as part of a defined genetic disorder, Smith-Lemli-Opitz Syndrome (SLOS), while others have low cholesterol that is not due to an apparent genetic disorder. In SLOS, there is a deficiency of 7-dehydrocholesterol reductase, the enzyme responsible for the final step in making cholesterol. The severity of the symptoms in this syndrome appear to correlate with the degree of deficiency in cholesterol. The cause of low cholesterol in autism is not yet known.

The use of high doses of cholesterol supplementation in individuals with SLOS and autistic symptoms can result in a decrease in autistic behaviors, irritability, hyperactivity, aggression, self-injury, temper outbursts, and improvements in physical growth, language, sleep, and social interactions. It is possible that increasing cholesterol in individuals with autism who do not have SLOS may also be helpful.

4. FISH FACTS

Seafood is abundant in healthy nutrients, especially protein, zinc, omega-3 fatty acids, and iodine. Seafood is generally much easier to digest than animal protein (meats, poultry).

Nonpolluted Seafood—Recirculating Aquaculture System (RAS) Technologies

These are gigantic land-based, closed-containment, eco-friendly aquariums. The water is 99% recycled and filtered to remove residual waste, which can be used as fertilizer. Currently, RAS facilities are commercially producing food-size Atlantic salmon, rainbow trout, sturgeon and their caviar, pike, perch, catfish, barramundi, tilapia, and other species. This allows for more variety in fish choices without the usual toxins.

For more information, see Fish 2.0: http://fish20.org/images/Fish2.0MarketReport_Aquaculture.pdf See also the Aquaculture Research at the Conservation Fund Freshwater Institute www.conservationfund.org/our-work/freshwater-institute/our-projects

Suggestions:

- Choose seafood from **RAS land-based**, **closed-containment**, **eco-friendly** sources that avoid contamination. Note that open containment exposes seafood to toxins. If you're not sure of the source, ask.
- If seafood from RAS sources is not available, follow these recommendations:
  - Avoid farm-raised fish.
  - Eat seafood caught away from major cities.
  - Avoid fish sticks; (less healthy fish are used in processed fish production.)
- When purchasing fish, notice the following:
  - Flesh should look moist and shiny.
  - Gills should be red; eyes should be bright, not dull.
  - Buy the whole fish and ask to have it filleted.

Preparing:

- Store in the refrigerator; cook and eat or freeze immediately.
- Keep mussels, clams, oysters, and shellfish alive. If they are dead, do not cook or eat them.
- Remove the skin. Trim off the dark meat and fat. Cook fish so that the fat drips away.
- Broil, bake, or grill and avoid the drippings. Poaching removes some contaminants.

The safest sources are seafood from RAS (Recirculating Aquaculture System) technologies. If not available, choose from these safer choices:

Anchovy	Herring	Scallop
Atlantic Croaker	Lobster	Sculpin
Atlantic Mackerel	Mackerel (Atlantic)	Shad
Black Sea Bass	Monkfish	Shrimp
Blue Crab (Atlantic)	Mullet	Skate
Burbot	Oysters	Smelt
Butterfish	Pacific Club Mackerel	Snapper
Catfish	Perch	Sole
Clam	Pike	Squid
Cod	Pollock	Tilapia
Crawfish	Porgie	Trout (rainbow)
Croaker	Rockfish	Tuna (canned light has less mercury than albacore, which is highest)
Haddock	Sablefish	
Hake	Salmon (wild)	Whitefish
	Sardine	

Resource for seafood safety:

• *Calculate your safe intake of seafood using EWG's Seafood Calculator*
  https://www.ewg.org/research/ewg-s-consumer-guide-seafood/seafood-calculator#

• *EWG's Consumer Guide to Seafood at https://www.ewg.org/research/ewg-s-consumer-guide-seafood/why-eat-seafood-and-how-much#*

5. FERMENTED FOODS—FRIENDS OF THE GUT MICROBIOTA

Fermentation of foods is one of the oldest forms of food preservation. The fermentation process results in the production of **probiotics**, nutrients, and enzymes. Probiotics support healthy microbiota. There are 10 trillion human cells and 100 trillion microbe cells, which renders us 1 part human and 10 part microbes. They are responsible for more than 70% of our entire immune system, and they produce short-chain fatty acids that, in balance with each other, are necessary for a healthy gut. The gut flora participate in improving digestion and nutrient absorption, neurotransmitter production, reducing inflammation, improving resistance, and reducing eczema, allergies, and asthma. Those in Western cultures have about 25% of the diversity of microbiota species, rendering us vulnerable to a wide range of problems with digestion and immunity. **Prebiotics** are indigestible carbohydrates that are "food" for probiotics. Prebiotic foods include Jerusalem artichokes, chicory root, dandelion greens, garlic, onions, leeks, asparagus, bananas, flaxseeds, seaweed, and more. Fermented foods are important and provide more diversity to the gut microbiota than you would have by merely supplementing with probiotics and prebiotics.

- **DAIRY FERMENTATION** (Note that cow milk sources are avoided in milk/casein-free diets.)

  - **YOGURT** can be made using a dairy or nondairy milk and milk or non-milk starter. The process is easy using a yogurt maker.

  - **KEFIR** is usually made from milk with kefir powder or grains as a starter.

  - **CULTURED BUTTERMILK**

  - **CHEESE**

  - **SOUR CREAM**

- **VINEGARS** have a starter (mother) that is a slimy film-like substance made of cellulose and acetic acid bacteria.

  - **APPLE CIDER VINEGAR** is the most common of the fruit vinegars.

  - **WHITE VINEGAR** is made from a vodka-like spirit distilled from grain, and the final product is comprised of acetic acid (5 to 10%) and water.

  - **WINE VINEGAR** and **GRAPE VINEGAR** are made from a two-fold fermentation of grape juice.

  - **KOMBUCHA VINEGAR** is made from kombucha.

- **YOUNG GREEN COCONUT KEFIR*** is made with the liquid of the young coconut (coconut water) and the starter.

- **VEGETABLE FERMENTATION** occurs when the natural bacteria in the vegetables break down the vegetables into forms easier to digest and more nutritious than the raw vegetable. The following are the most popular vegetables to ferment: sauerkraut, pickles, kimchi (from cabbage and other vegetables), daikon radishes, turnips, and parsnips.

- **KOMBUCHA** is a tangy fermented beverage of black tea and sugar (cane, fruit, and honey) and a slimy disc-shaped layer starter culture known as SCOBY (Symbiotic Colony of Bacteria and Yeast), mother or mushroom. The SCOBY metabolizes sugar and caffeine to create probiotics, vitamins, and enzymes.

- **MISO** can be made from soybean or brown rice.

- **TEMPEH** is made from cooked and slightly fermented soybeans and formed into a patty.

  * Young Green Coconut Kefir can be purchased at www.bodyecology.com/articles/coconutkefir.php.

  See the probiotic discussion on the previous page and the Fermented Beverages sidebar on page 68 for more in-depth information.

6. USE SALT, NOT SODIUM PRESERVATIVES.

A subset of children with ADHD or autism have constant physiologic challenges due in part to genetic predispositions, inefficiencies in energy metabolism (mitochondria), nutritional deficiencies, inability to rid toxins, and poor diet, including glycemic (high sugar) diets and low protein intake. They can experience a cluster of symptoms, including generalized physical weakness, low muscle tone, cold extremities, lower body temperatures, digestive symptoms, and extremely pale skin. There are often cravings for sweet foods and salty foods. Commonly, there is lower blood pressure, poor balance, and dizziness upon standing up too quickly. The symptoms can be signs of an imbalance in the autonomic nervous system, termed *dysautonomia*, which can also include inefficient adrenal function (not adrenal disease). Adrenals respond well to good protein intake, excellent glucose control, and optimum salt intake. Remember, the body regulates sodium levels, absorbing and retaining more when needed and less when not. For these children, salt is important. Parents often notice improved alertness and less fatigue and pallor after salt consumption, improved protein intake, and reduction of sugars.

Chloride is necessary for cell function, balance, and distribution of body fluids, and a necessary part of digestive acid (hydrochloric acid). It is depleted through sweat, vomit, and diarrhea.

The sodium preservatives (nitrites, benzoates, and MSG) are generally not well handled by children with ADHD and even less well by those on the autism spectrum. MSG-glutamate is an excitotoxin.

Do not restrict salt for your child, unless your health care provider has instructed you to do so because of specific medical conditions. Allow salt intake to be determined by taste. If your child has the symptoms described on page 55, observe to see if there is improvement in your child after salt consumption.

AVOID

- **Environmental indoor and outdoor toxins:** pesticides, glyphosate, artificial turf, and VOC chemicals in paints, building products, and furnishings; nonstick cookware; harmful ingredients in cleaning products, fabric softeners, air fresheners, personal care products (cosmetics, shampoos, fragrances, and oral care); and electromagnetic fields (EMFs) and radio frequency radiation (RFR).
- **Artificial:** additives, preservatives, sweeteners, taste enhancers, flavoring, coloring; and excitotoxins, GMOs, MSG, amines; and growth promoters in meat and milk products
- **Contaminated drinking water:** pesticides, agricultural runoff, industrial chemicals, nitrates, toxic metals, and byproducts of chlorination. Also, avoid use of plastic water bottles and food containers.
- **Sugars and sugar-raising foods:** high fructose corn syrup, sugars, agave syrup, sugar drinks, junk electrolyte drinks, all sodas (diet and regular), refined grains, and caffeine.
- **Problem fats:** trans-fatty acids, deep-fried foods, canola oil, palm kernel oil, and GMO soy and corn oils.
- **Non-organic** deli meats, processed foods, and contaminated seafood.
- **Any food or beverage that causes a negative reaction.**

INCLUDE

- **Organic foods:** USDA Organic seal, Non-GMO Project Verification, pastured animals, poultry, eggs, and milk products. Clean, contaminant-free drinking water.
- **Blood sugar control:** The first food or drink of the day sets the glucose standard for the day; it must be stabilizing and include low glycemic foods. Have protein, fiber, and good fat at meals and snacks.
- **Protein:** seafood, poultry, meat, eggs, tolerated milk products, legumes, beans, nuts, and seeds
- **Fats and oils:** coconut, butter, lard, seafood, fish oils, algae, and oils of olives, avocados, nuts
- **Fiber foods:** non-starchy vegetables, legumes, beans, nuts, seeds, and low glycemic fruits
- **Natural sweetener options:** organic stevia, coconut sugar, raw honey, maple syrup (grade B), blackstrap molasses, banana purée, real fruit jam/spread, sucanat, splash of organic fruit juice
- **Healthy fats:**
  - Omega-3: (essential) seafood sources, algae, legumes, beans, nuts, seeds, and fish oils
  - Omega-6: vegetables, nuts, seeds and their oils
  - Omega-9: plant source oils (olive, avocado, macadamia, peanut) and some animal sources
  - Saturated fatty acids: found in plants and animals
  - Cholesterol: healing substance produced by the body and found only in fats from animals and seafood
  - Eggs: nutrient-dense natural food: high protein (white), nutrients and choline (yolk)
- **Seafood:** Select the least toxic sources, and, ideally, seafood from RAS (Recirculating Aquaculture System) technologies that are land-based, closed-containment, eco-friendly aquariums producing healthy, nontoxic fish
- **Fermented foods:**
  - Probiotics from milk products, vinegars, coconut kefir, vegetables, kombucha, miso, and tempeh
  - Prebiotic fuel for microbiota growth: Jerusalem artichokes, dandelion greens, garlic, onions, leeks, asparagus
- **Salt (not sodium preservatives):** Salt is a nutrient, regulated by homeostasis and especially beneficial to those who experience generalized weakness, dizziness, salt cravings, poor endurance, and/or low blood pressure

The following charts give basic information applicable to all of the diets. All of the diets will include proteins, fats, and carbohydrates. The specific foods to include will differ among the various elimination diets.

PROTEIN	FAT	CARBOHYDRATE
Animal Source Seafood Meats Poultry Eggs Milk products **Plant Source** *Fiber sources* Beans/Legumes Nuts Seeds	**Saturated Fatty Acids** **Unsaturated Fatty Acids** Monounsaturated Omega-9 olive, avocado, almond Polyunsaturated Omega-6 *Essential* vegetables and their oils *excess depletes omega-3s* Omega-3 *Essential* *seafood fish oils, algae,* *beans, legumes, nuts, seeds*	*Fiber sources* Vegetables Fruits Grains Beans Nuts Seeds

Dietary Guidelines by Age

The following chart provides the general recommended intake by age. These guidelines are relevant to most individuals and not necessarily specific to ADHD and autism only. In the various elimination diets, there will be food restrictions. It is still important to maintain a healthy balance with any of the diets.

Daily Intake	Age 2 to 3	Age 4 to 6	Age 7 to 11	Age 12 to 17	Adult Female	Adult Male
Calories	1,000–1,400	1,200–1,800	1,200–2,000	1,600–2,400	2,000–2,400	2,400–3,000
Protein Grams	20-25	25-35	35-45	45-60	60-75	75-90
Veggies Cups	1	1.5-2	2	2-3	3-3.5	3-3.5
Fruit Cups	1	1-1.5	1.5-2	2-2.5	2-2.5	2-2.5
Grains* Ounces	0-3	0-4	0-5	0-6	0-7	0-8
Fiber Grams	5	15-19	15-20	20-25	25-30	30-35
Water Ounces	30-35	40-45	45-60	55-60	60-70	70-90

*Grains - 1 ounce equivalents = ½ cup cooked rice, cereal, pasta
1 slice bread or 1 small muffin
1 cup cold cereal flakes (organic)

Serving Size

The protein serving sizes are provided to help readers understand how much protein is in a given amount of food. The serving size equivalents provide a visual means of estimating food amounts.

PROTEIN SERVING SIZE

Each person's animal-protein serving size is equal to his or her own palm (minus fingers and thumb).

The following amounts of protein foods contain approximately 7 to 8 grams.

- 1 ounce (30 g) meat, fish, or poultry
- 1 extra large egg or 2 small eggs
- ½ cup (90 g) baked beans, (50 g) cooked dried peas, (100 g) cooked lentils
- 2 tablespoons (32 g) nut butter
- ⅓ cup (1.5 ounces, or 42 g) nuts/seeds
- 1 cup (235 ml) milk
- ½ cup (115 g) Greek yogurt or cottage cheese

VEGETABLE, FRUIT, AND GRAIN SERVING SIZES

- Raw leafy vegetables	1 cup = 1 baseball
- Fruit	1 medium = 1 baseball
- Pasta, rice, cooked cereal	½ cup = ½ baseball
- Potato	1 medium = computer mouse

SERVING SIZE EQUIVALENTS

- 2 tablespoons	table tennis ball
- ¼ cup	golf ball
- ⅔ cup	baseball
- 1 cup	tennis ball
- 3-4 ounces	deck of cards
- 3-4 ounces	1 adult palm
- 2 ounces	1 child palm
- 1 teaspoon	tip of thumb
- 1 tablespoon	whole thumb

CHAPTER 4

The Main Culprits:

Glutens, Casein, Soy, and Others

"I WAS BLESSED TO HAVE A CHILD who was an immediate and dramatically positive responder to dietary intervention. Within thirty-six hours after we stopped casein, his incessant screaming and head banging were almost gone, and we had some eye contact back. Within five days after we stopped gluten, his life-long rash was gone, and his stools improved. Dietary infractions have produced equally dramatic results, so we have been very motivated to continue the diet. Maintaining his special diet is very difficult, but not nearly as hard as living with a severely autistic child. For us, diet has been one of the top three interventions that have aided in his recovery from autism."

—MOTHER OF JOHN, *a five-year-old recovering from autism*

"It's not the food you avoid that makes you sick. It's the food you crave and eat every day!"

—*George H. Mitchell, MD*

What They Are

Glutens, animal milk casein, and soy are complex foods, which may explain why so many people have problems with one or more of them. They are listed among the most common food allergens—but the reactions (intolerances) we discuss are not classical allergic responses like hives, rashes, and itching.

Glutens are plant proteins in the subclass Monocotyledonae, found in wheat, semolina, bulgur, couscous, wheat berries, graham flour, whole meal flour, groats, malt, oats, barley, rye, triticale, spelt, and kamut. Gluten is elastic and provides the stretchiness necessary in making yeast and non-yeast breads.

Where They Are

Gluten-containing grains are the most common ingredient in breads, pastas, crackers, cookies, cakes, cereals, pretzels, matzah, Passover flour, farfel, cream sauces, thickening agents, and breading. Gluten derivatives are also found in malt, modified food starches, hydrolyzed vegetable protein (HVP), hydrolyzed plant protein (HPP), textured vegetable proteins (TVPs), and dextrin, and they are used in the following unless labeled gluten-free: soy sauce, flavorings, instant coffee, some ketchups, mustards, commercial mixes, cake decorations, marshmallow crème, canned soups, deli meats, sausage, and hot dogs. Products labeled as corn bread or rice pasta may contain glutens. Breaded items contain glutens unless otherwise labeled. Gluten is also found in some of the binders and fillers found in vitamins and medications and even pastes and glues on envelope flaps.

Gluten problems are not new in medicine. A portion of gluten called gliadin is known to exacerbate a genetic condition known as celiac disease by damaging the small intestine villi and to cause dermatitis herpetiformis, a celiac-associated serious skin condition. Celiac and non-celiac gluten intolerances have increased. These conditions are not the same as the ADHD- or autism-related gluten intolerances that result in absorption of peptides from incomplete digestion of these foods. However, the information about gluten avoidance found in the celiac literature is still very helpful.

Note that a wheat-free food is not gluten-free unless all of the gluten sources are avoided. If the label does not state "gluten-free," then it is likely not gluten-free. It is not necessary to label foods that would not be expected to have gluten in them, such as meats, seafood, eggs, vegetables, fruits, beans, nuts, and seeds. Animal products are naturally gluten-free. Gluten is found only in gluten grains. For example, an unaltered chicken breast does not contain gluten; however, a marinated chicken breast may contain gluten in the marinade. Also, commercial soy sauce has gluten added and therefore would not be gluten-free.

How They Cause Problems: Don't Be a Gluten for Punishment

Glutens, casein, and soy can digest poorly in the intestinal tract to groups of undigested amino acid chains called peptides, some of which can have opiate-like activity. When these peptides are absorbed into the bloodstream, they can cross the blood-brain barrier and negatively affect mood, mental and neurologic function, and behavior. When these peptides are opiate-like, they can cause addiction to the food source. Hence, the child craves the foods causing the problem and begins to limit the diet to primarily opiate-forming foods. It is common for children to experience significant withdrawal symptoms when these foods are eliminated.

Symptoms Indicating Gluten-Free May Help

Because of the opioid effect from gluten opiate-like peptides, the most common symptoms are craving for the opioid source gluten foods and limiting food choices to the opioid-sources. Also common are silly behaviors, acting dopey, experiencing "brain fog," and seeming "zoned out." Obsessiveness and self-stimulation can increase and self-injury may occur. For some children, the brain effect is painful, causing the child to shake and bang his/her head as if a vise is applying pressure. Poor eye contact, inattention, and high pain tolerance are frequent symptoms. Digestive problems can include gas, diarrhea, indigestion, and constipation. When the symptoms are specific to gluten, then gluten-free is the right elimination diet.

What Is Left to Eat?

Grains that can be eaten on a gluten-free diet include rice of all varieties (white, brown, basmati, wild, sweet, and poha), millet, corn, quinoa, amaranth, tapioca, buckwheat (not related to wheat at all), sorghum (jowar), ragi, teff, corn (if tolerated), and Montina (Indian rice grass).

Nongrain substitutes for flours include potato starch and flours made from potato, taro, yam, arrowroot, almond, hazelnut, cassava, malanga, lotus, water chestnut, artichoke, chestnut, and beans, including chickpeas, peas, mung bean, and soy (if tolerated).

Since glutens provide the elastic quality needed in making baked goods, the substitutes must include safe ingredients that give the same result as gluten: xanthan gum, methylcellulose (indigestible polysaccharide of beta-glucose), or guar gum (soluble fiber from the Indian cluster bean). Substitutes for thickeners include the following: agar, arrowroot, bean flour, cornstarch, gelatin powder, guar gum, kudzu powder, sweet rice flour, tapioca flour, tapioca, and xanthan gum.

Remember to keep in your kitchen gluten-free baking powder and baking soda along with vanilla without alcohol (Frontier Vanilla). Successful gluten-free baked goods are possible; they just require a combination of flours, thickeners, and baking supplements to achieve an acceptable texture and flavor.

CATEGORY	SOURCES OF GLUTEN	GLUTEN-FREE (GF) SUBSTITUTES
Grains	**Wheat:** wheat berry, couscous, flour, graham, semolina, durum, bran, bulgur, cracked wheat, rusk **Oat:** oat bran, oat germ, oatmeal, oat flour, rolled oats **Barley:** flour, malt, starch, barley pearl **Rye:** rye starch **Triticale:** hybrid of wheat and rye **Spelt:** species of wheat **Kamut:** ancient wheat-like grain **Groats:** mixture of oat, wheat, buckwheat **Products of gluten grains:** bagels, biscuits, cakes, cereals, cookies, crackers, croutons, doughnuts, pasta, pretzels, stuffing, thickeners, tortillas, wafers, matzah, Passover flour, Communion wafers	**GF grains:** non-GMO corn, millet, Montina (Indian rice grass), rice (basmati, black, brown, sweet, white, wild), sorghum (jowar), teff, tapioca Exception: certified GF oats **Nongrain substitutes:** arrowroot, artichoke, cassava, lotus, malanga, sago, sweet potato, taro, water chestnut, yam **Pseudo Grains:** amaranth, buckwheat, quinoa **Nuts:** almonds, chestnuts, hazelnuts **Legumes:** beans, chickpeas, fava, mung bean, peas, soy **Thickeners:** agar, arrowroot, bean flour, gelatin, guar gum, kudzu powder, starch, sweet rice flour **Gluten-like elastic items:** guar gum, maltodextrin from corn or rice, methylcellulose, xanthan gum **Pasta/Noodles:** GF flours, rice noodles, spaghetti squash
Beverages	Malted drinks or malt in drinks Ovaltine, Postum, flavored tea or coffee Beer and ale (fermented) Some grain alcohols, especially if flavored Flavored water, seltzer Juice punch or drinks (additives, flavorings)	Water, including plain seltzer Herbal teas, tea, coffee (unflavored) Wines Distilled liquors Fresh or frozen juices
Sweets Sweeteners Flavoring Spices Baking aids	Artificial flavors Artificial colors Candy Caramel coloring—foreign brands Confectioners' sugar (flour, cornstarch) Commercial cake decorations Syrup (unless GF) Seasonings may have wheat Spice mixes (may have wheat) Nutritional yeast (may contain gluten), Brewer's yeast	Pure flavors, distilled or labeled GF Pure colors or labeled GF GF candy Caramel (US brands made from corn) GF confectioners' sugar GF cake decorations GF rice syrup Pure seasoning or labeled GF Single spices usually are pure Yeast (Baker's, Autolyzed)

CATEGORY	SOURCES OF GLUTEN	GLUTEN-FREE (GF) SUBSTITUTES
Condiments Sauces	Soy sauce	Wheat-free tamari soy sauce, liquid Bragg amino acids
	Worcestershire sauce	Lea & Perrins Worcestershire sauce
	Ketchup, mustard, mayonnaise	GFCF ketchup, mustard, mayo
	Flavored vinegar, malt vinegar	Distilled vinegar
	Yogurts and yogurt drinks with thickeners	Organic/natural yogurts/drinks w/o thickeners
Additives	Dextrin (foreign brands)	Dextrin (US brands made from corn)
	Monosodium glutamate (MSG)	No MSG of any kind
	Citric acid	Citric acid if GF (corn)
	Hydrolyzed plant protein (HPP) (if wheat sourced)	Hydrolyzed vegetable protein (HVP) (if not from wheat)
	Modified food starch can be wheat	Starch on food labels (means corn)
	Malt (barley)—assume "malt" means barley	Corn malt (must be labeled as such)
Foods	Canned soups, bouillon cubes, or powdered broth	Homemade GF soups, broths
	Deli meats, sausages, hot dogs	Fresh meat, poultry, fish, eggs, GF organic deli meats
	Flavored yogurts, malted milk	Pure milk products (if not intolerant)
	Imitation seafood and bacon	Fresh or frozen seafood and GF, casein-free (CF) bacon
	Processed cheese spreads	Natural cheeses (if not reactive)
	Pudding, marshmallow cream	100% natural oils, fats
	Stuffing mixes, breading	GF breading, stuffing
Other	Chewing gum	
	Glues—stamps, envelopes, stickers	
	Nutritional supplements (binders, fillers)	
	Play-Doh	Homemade GF Play Dough
	School glue	
	Nutritional supplements with alcohol if from a grain alcohol. (Note: Even if alcohol is "burned" off, grain residues will remain.)	

Milk Products and Casein: Where Are They Found?

Mammal milk (human, cow, and goat) has many components, including water, fats, protein, lactose, minerals, acids, enzymes, gases, and vitamins. Milk products include milk (from nonfat to whole), buttermilk, evaporated milk, yogurt, kefir, cream cheese, sour cream, cream sauces, cream dressings, ice cream, sherbet, cheese, curds, cottage cheese, whey, butter, and any food that contains any one of these products.

Milk products are hidden in many unexpected places, including canned tuna, nondairy creamers, whipped toppings, salad dressing, bakery glazes, breath mints, fortified cereals, high-protein beverage powders, infant formulas, nutrition bars, processed meats, and nutritional supplements. Remember the mantra "Read the label." Avoid products with the following ingredients: milk solids, lactose, galactose, lactalbumin, lactoglobulin, casein, and caseinate.

MILK PRODUCTS

Animal milk	Cream cheese	Powdered milk
Butter	Curds	Rennet
Buttermilk	Evaporated milk	Sherbet
Cheese—all	Half-and-half	Sour cream
Condensed milk	Ice cream, ice milk	Whey
Cottage cheese	Kefir	Yogurt
Cream	Nougat	

Read Labels & Avoid

Casein	Hydrolyzed vegetable protein	Lactose
Calcium caseinate	Lactalbumins	Magnesium caseinate
Caseinate	Lactic acid starter culture	Potassium caseinate
Galactose	Lactobacillus if not dairy-free (DF)	
Hydrolyzed milk protein	Lactoglobulin	

Non-Food Sources

Cosmetics

Pharmaceuticals (lactose)

Nutritional supplements

FOOD SOURCES OF MILK PRODUCTS

Not all listed items will contain milk products—read labels!

Baked Goods

Biscuits, breads	Mixes for baked goods
Cakes, cookies	Pancakes, waffles
Caramel coloring	Pie crust
Doughnuts, pastries	Soda crackers, Zwieback

Beverages

Chocolate milk	Ovaltine, chocolate
Cocoa	Sodas
Malt, malted milk	

Sweets

Creams in anything	Milk chocolate
Custards, puddings	Sorbet (not all)
Ice cream, sherbet	Spumoni
Gelato	

Sauces, Fats, Oils

Butter-fried foods	Mayonnaise (some brands)
Cream sauce	
Gravies	Salad dressing (some)
Margarine	

Meat/Fish/Other Proteins

Bisques, chowders	Egg dishes—omelets, scrambled eggs, soufflés, casseroles
Cheese—dairy-free (some have casein)	
Creamed foods	Processed meats, sausage, hot dogs
Cream soup bases	Tuna fish (canned)
Deli turkey	

Ingredients that sound like they contain milk products but do not contain them:

- Calcium lactate
- Calcium stearoyl lactylate
- Cocoa butter
- Cream of tartar
- Lactate
- Oleoresin
- Sodium lactate
- Sodium stearoyl lactylate

THE CASE AGAINST CASEIN

Casein, which accounts for 75% of the proteins in milk, is a major culprit in ADHD- or autism-related food sensitivities. It is found in all milk products, with the exception of properly clarified butter, also known as ghee, in which the milk solids have been removed. Dairy-free or milk-free does not mean casein-free. Even nondairy cheese substitutes from soy, almonds, or rice may have casein to improve the texture. Casein is commonly used in meat products such as deli meats, salami, sausage, hot dogs, and pepperoni, and caseinate is a common component in nutritional supplements.

What about Casein in Breast Milk?

Human casein proteins are different from the casein proteins in cow's or goat's milk. The alignment of the amino acids is different. Therefore, the negative effects from casein do not occur with breast-feeding. Breast-feeding is considered a protective factor in autism.

What about A2 Milk?

About one-third of the casein in cow's milk is beta-casein, of which there are several varieties, determined by the genes of the cow. The most common of these variants are A1 and A2. The percentage of A1 and A2 beta-casein protein varies between herds of cattle and between countries and provinces. While African and Asian cattle continue to produce only A2 beta-casein, the A1 version is common among cattle in the Western world. The A1 beta-casein type is the most common type found in cow's milk in Europe (excluding France), the United States, Australia, and New Zealand. On average, more than 70% of Guernsey cows produce milk with predominantly A2 protein while 46–70% of Holsteins and Ayrshires produce milk with A1 protein.

The difference between the two proteins is subtle, a change in only one amino acid in the sequence of the protein. However, as a result of this difference, when A1 milk is digested, it can produce an opiate-like molecule called beta-casomorphin 7 (BCM-7). For individuals with autism, opiate-like peptides can be problematic. (See page 21, "The Dope on Opiates.") The more critical point is that both A1 and A2 milks contain casein, so for individuals on a casein-free diet, both types of milk should be avoided.

What about Goat or Camel Milk?

Goat milk contains only the A2 beta-casein. However, goat milk is not allowed on a casein-free diet. Compared to cow's milk, camel milk contains lower fat, cholesterol, and lactose and higher vitamins and minerals. Regarding casein, camel milk has a different form of casein, and some believe that individuals who are otherwise sensitive to casein can tolerate camel milk. However, we recommend that during an initial casein elimination trial, all forms of animal milk be avoided, including camel milk. Once improvement is documented on a casein-free diet, camel milk could be introduced to see if it results in worsening of physical or behavioral symptoms.

Replacing Calcium, Vitamin D, and Protein When Milk Is Eliminated

When removing milk products from the diet, there is always the concern that calcium, vitamin D, and protein will be inadequate. In addition to other dietary sources of calcium, appropriate supplements can be used if needed: calcium and the necessary co-nutrients, which are vitamin D and magnesium. Vitamin D is of particular importance in that deficiencies are increasingly common, especially among those with autism.

Protein recommendations can be easily met by including sources other than animal milk products. Choices include seafood, poultry, meat, eggs, beans, nuts, and seeds. For those who cannot meet the dietary goals, protein supplements can be used. Sources include rice, coconut, hemp, nut, and bean protein powders.

Also, consider the following as worthy substitutes for 1 cup (235 ml) milk (300 mg of calcium): 1 cup (235 ml) rice milk, fortified; $1/3$ cup (80 g) tofu; 5 ounces (140 g) salmon, canned with bones; 2 $1/2$ ounces (70 g) sardines, canned with bones; 2 $1/2$ to 3 cups (175 to 215 g) green leafies, like broccoli; or supplements: calcium with magnesium and vitamin D.

The daily recommendation for calcium intake ranges from 210 mg for infants to 800 mg or more in older children. Calcium also needs to be balanced by adequate magnesium. We suggest consulting a practitioner with expertise in dietary advice and nutritional supplementation for dosing recommendations for your child. Vitamin D needs are best determined by blood testing.

WEIGHING IN ON WHEY

Whey is the serum, or watery, part of milk that is separated when milk protein/casein coagulates to become curd in the making of cheese. Whey is primarily lactose and soluble proteins. (There are pure forms of lactose-free whey.) Little Miss Muffet's curds and whey are known as cottage cheese. The lumps are the curds (cheese, casein) and the whey is the lactose-containing liquid. Unless the whey is pure and clearly stated as casein-free on the label, it is still to be avoided on the casein-free diet.

BUYER BEWARE—READ THE LABEL— CONTACT THE MANUFACTURER

For products manufactured in or after January 2006, manufacturers are required to declare in the ingredient list the name of any major food allergen that is contained in the product or product spices, flavorings, additives, and colorings:

- Milk
- Wheat
- Eggs
- Fish (must list specific kind)
- Crustacean shellfish (specific kind of crab, lobster, shrimp)
- Tree nuts (specific kind of almond, pecan, walnut)
- Peanuts
- Soy

If in doubt—find out. Contact the manufacturer.

What Is Left to Eat?

Substitutes for milk products include rice milk; soy milk; soy yogurt; potato milk; quinoa milk; and nut milks made from almonds, Brazil nuts, cashews, coconut, hazelnuts, macadamias, pecans, pine nuts, pumpkin seeds, sesame seeds, sunflower seeds, and walnuts.

Fermented Beverages

Julie Matthews (www.nourishinghope.com), in her *Cooking to Heal* workbook and recipes, emphasizes the importance of fermented foods in achieving excellent digestive and systemic health. Homemade fermented foods, such as yogurt (dairy and nondairy), kefir, raw sauerkraut, and kombucha (sweetened tea) are abundant with probiotics, a.k.a., the "good" bacteria. Whereas typical probiotic supplements may have 3 to 75 billion as a count, 1 cup (230 g) of homemade yogurt has 700 billion per cup. It is important to note that for those who are casein-free/milk-free, animal milk fermented products are to be avoided. For these purposes, only consume fermented products that are not from animal milk origins.

MILK-PRODUCT SUBSTITUTES

Beware: "dairy-free" does not necessarily mean "casein-free."

Milks/Yogurts

Coconut milk	Potato milk
Coconut Kefir and Yogurt	Rice milk
Hemp milk	Soy milk
Nut milks (almond, cashew)	Soy yogurt
	Tofu products

Chocolate

GFCF chocolate chips

GFCF semisweet chocolate chips

Ice Cream

Vance's DariFree milk	Italian ice
Fruit Popsicles	Non-GMO soy ice cream
Sorbets by Haagen-Dazs and Ben & Jerry's	Tofutti

Buttermilk Substitute

In recipes

1 cup (235 ml) buttermilk equivalent:

2 tablespoons (30 ml) lemon juice in

1 cup (235 ml) milk substitute

Butter

Coconut oil/butter	Kosher items— only pareve
Earth Balance Whipped Spread (GFCF, no trans-fats)	Applesauce can substitute for both milk and butter in mashed potatoes
Ghee (clarified butter— has no casein)	
Lard—excellent in baked goods	

For a complete listing of all combined GFCF foods, see The GFCF Diet: www.gfcfdiet.com

Coconut: The Wonder Food

- Coconut is actually a seed and fruit, and not a nut.
- Coconut water, the liquid inside the coconut, is a healthy electrolyte drink that is rich in nutrients. It was used in World War II as an electrolyte IV solution when saline solutions were not available.
- Coconut milk is made from the coconut "flesh." When chilled, the "cream" and "milk" separate and are useful substitutes for animal source milk products.
- Coconut gel is made via fermentation of coconut water.
- Coconut milk can be fermented into coconut kefir and yogurt, which are abundant in the good probiotics for the digestive tract.
- Coconuts, and the cream, milk, kefir, and yogurt made from the coconut, are health foods. They are helpful in promoting good immunity and alleviating digestive disorders such as gas, indigestion, diarrhea, vomiting, colitis, and ulcers.
- Coconut oil fatty acids do not raise cholesterol or contribute to heart disease. Fifty percent of the coconut oil fatty acids are lauric acid, which has antibacterial, antiviral, and antiprotozoal qualities.

The Kosher Connection

The kosher diet prohibits serving meat and dairy together; therefore, products are clearly labeled.

Kosher Abbreviation		For Dairy-free/Casein-free
UD	contains dairy	Avoid
KD	contains milk protein	Avoid
DE	produced with equipment shared with dairy	Avoid
P	Indicates for Passover use, but not necessarily pareve	Avoid
Pareve (or Parve)*	no animal ingredients	Include

*Most are dairy-free. Jewish law allows less than $1/5$ % dairy by volume.

Soy Sorry!

Soy has not been a common food in the American diet until recently. Soy foods include edamame (the immature soy bean harvested while still green and sweet) and fermented products such as miso, natto, tamari/soy sauce, tempeh, tofu, and yuba.

Soy is found in hydrolyzed vegetable protein (HVP), lecithin, mono- and diglycerides, monosodium glutamate (MSG), and vitamin E products (most all of which are soy-based). It may also be used in baked goods, canned tuna, cereals, infant formulas, margarine, mayonnaise, sauces, soups, vegetable broth, vegetable protein substitutes, and vegetable oils.

There is much controversy over soy and its suitability in the human diet. While other beans can be eaten if cooked properly, soybeans require fermentation due to the presence of natural toxins that can deplete or interfere with specific nutrients.

The processing of soy to render it acceptable as a food requires exposure to high heat and chemicals. Today, some soy is also genetically modified. Non-genetically modified sources are preferred and available. Soy remains a common allergen and is also not easily tolerated by many individuals. Like gluten and casein, it can also partially digest to form opiate-like peptides. The testing for this isn't reliable; therefore, the best testing is trial and response.

For those who are not allergic to soy and are able to tolerate it easily, the best soy sources are organic and include edamame and the naturally fermented soy products such as tempeh, natto, miso, soy sauce, tofu, and yuba.

SOY PRODUCTS
Read labels for soy and soy byproducts

Soybean oil, flour, milk	Tamari
Edamame	Tempeh
Miso	Tempura
Natto	Tofu
Sprouts (soy)	Yuba

Other

Lecithin	MSG
HVP	Vitamin E
Mono- and diglycerides	

FOOD SOURCES OF SOY

Baked Goods

Baking mixes, flours	Crackers
Bread, cakes, cereals	Pasta, pastries, rolls

Meats/Others

Baby foods	Luncheon/deli meats
Cheese substitutes	Sausage (not all)

Oils/Fats

Butter substitutes	Shortening
Oil, margarine	

Beverages

Coffee substitutes	Infant formulas
Soy milk	

Condiments

Butter substitutes	Nut mixes
Salad dressing, sauces, soy sauce	Vegetable broth
	Worcestershire sauce

Sweets

Candy and candy bars	Ice cream—Tofutti
Caramel, custard	

Soy substitutes are the same as those listed earlier as gluten and milk substitutes (with the exception of those containing soy).

Excessive soy consumption can be antagonistic to thyroid function (goitrogenic), and it is also known as an endocrine disruptor.

NOTE: *When first embarking on a casein-free diet, we recommend also removing major sources of soy, since many individuals who are sensitive to casein are also sensitive to soy. If soy products are used as the substitute for dairy, you may be replacing one problematic food with another, and may then mask any benefits that occur from removal of casein. If improvement occurs with removal of both casein and soy, then soy products can be gradually reintroduced to see if there is any worsening of symptoms.*

For a summary of Gluten-Free, Casein-Free, Soy-Free (GFCFSF) Diet, see page 32.

"For Joe, there were no overnight miracles. But when taken off glutens and milk products, and placed on nutritional and digestive supplements, he improved quickly and significantly within two months. Early in the diet, before going organic, I ran out of regular nitrate-containing hot dogs, and Joe went through withdrawal symptoms (hyperactivity, screaming, crying, whimpering). However, after the withdrawal, we noticed more improvement, so we switched to nitrate-free healthy hot dogs and cold cuts. Joe continued to improve steadily—better eye contact, interactive social skills, focus, attention, and language, and a steady decrease in perseverations. Each day he is better than the day before."

—Pauline,
mother of Joe, a five-year-old with autism

Eggs, Corn, and Nuts

Allergies or intolerances to these foods can occur. When casein, gluten, and soy are eliminated, consumption of foods containing eggs, corn, or nuts often increases in order to replace those foods that were eliminated. In some children, reactions to the increase in these foods may then appear.

EGGS

It is not always obvious that a product contains egg. Be aware that the following words on a label mean the product contains egg or egg byproducts: albumen, globulin, vitellin, livetin, ovoglobulin, ovamucin, ovamucoid, ovovitellin, ovovitelia, and lysozyme. See the chart below for a thorough listing.

EGG PRODUCTS

Read labels for eggs and egg byproducts

Egg whites, yolks	Ovamucin
Egg powder	Ovamucoid
Albumen, globulin	Ovovitellin
Vitellin, livetin	Ovovitelia
Ovoglobulin	Lysozyme

Nonfood Sources

Vaccines—those cultured in chicken eggs

FOOD SOURCES OF EGG

Not all of these products contain eggs. The egg source may not be obvious.

Baked Goods

Baking powder	French toast
Breading	Pastries
Breads, rolls, biscuits	Pancake/waffle mixes
Cake flour	Pastas
Cookies, doughnuts	Pie crusts and fillings

Beverages

Eggnog	Ovaltine

Sweets/Sweeteners/Flavoring

Protein powders	Marshmallows
Gelatin desserts	Meringues, macaroons
Frosting, icing, glazes	Puddings, pie fillings, soufflés
Ice cream, ices, sherbets	

Condiments/Sauces/Oils

Mayonnaise	Salad dressing
Hollandaise	Tartar sauce

Other Foods

Bouillon	Sausage, pâté
Meatballs, loafs, patties	Soup

SUBSTITUTES FOR 1 EGG

2 tablespoons (16 g) cornstarch

2 tablespoons (16 g) arrowroot flour

2 tablespoons (20 g) potato starch

1 tablespoon (8 g) soy milk powder

1 banana (good in cakes)

1/4 cup (62 g) tofu

Unflavored Gelatin:
Mix 1 envelope (1 tablespoon, or 7 g) in
1 cup (235 ml) boiling water.
3 tablespoons (45 ml) = 1 egg

Baby food (puréed apples or pears):
3 tablespoons (45 g) = 1 egg

CORN

Corn is one of the most common food allergens for children and adults in the United States, and it is also one of the most difficult to avoid. It is inexpensive and versatile and therefore abundant in processed foods. Approximately 90% of the corn in the United States has been genetically modified.

CORN PRODUCTS

Read labels for corn and corn byproducts

Cornstarch, cornmeal, flour	Fructose
Corn chips, popcorn	High-fructose corn syrup
Maize	Lecithin
Corn syrup	Maltodextrin
Corn oil	MSG
Dextrin	Salt (commercial)
Dextrose	Succotash
Glucose	Thickeners
Fruit pectin	Vegetable starch

Nonfood Sources

Aspirin	Laundry starch	Paper plates
Capsules	Livestock feed	Suppositories
Chalk	Medicines	Tablets (most)
Cosmetics	Nutritional supplements	Talcum powder
Glues: stamps, envelopes, stickers	Paper cups	Toothpaste

FOOD SOURCES OF CORN

Not all these products contain corn. However, most processed and prepared foods contain corn unless labeled "corn-free."

Beverages

Alcohol: distilled, ale, beer, bourbon, cordials, liqueurs, wine coolers	Ice cream, sherbets, sorbets
Coffee: instant, "designer"	Milk in paper cartons
Infant/toddler formulas	Sodas, soft drinks
Fruit-juice "cocktails" (not 100% juice)	Sweetened condensed milk
Soy milk	Sweetened/flavored drinks

Sweets/Sweeteners/Flavoring

Artificial sweeteners	Ice creams, sherbets, sorbets
Candy (almost all)	Jams, jellies
Caramel	Marshmallows
Carob	Powdered sugar
Chewing gum	Sorbitol
Custards, puddings	Syrups/corn syrup
Flavoring extracts	Gelatin desserts
Frosting, icings	Vanilla extract
Gelatin desserts	Vinegar (distilled)
High-fructose corn syrup	Yogurts (sweetened)

Baked Goods

Baking powder (most)	Grits, hominy
Breads, rolls, biscuits	Pancake/ waffle mixes
Cakes	
Cereals (prepared)	Pastries, pies
	Tortillas
Doughnuts (prepared)	Vegetable starch
Graham crackers	Xanthan gum

Condiments/Sauces/Oils

Gravies, sauces	Mustards
Ketchup, chili sauce	Salad dressings
Margarine	Steak sauce, tartar sauce
Mayonnaise	

Other Foods

Bacon (most)	Eggs: frozen, dried
Bean sprouts	Fried foods (in corn oil)
Canned foods (almost all)	Meats—cured, processed
	Oriental foods
Cheese spreads, cheese foods	Peanut butter (sweetened)
Coffee "creamer"	Pickles (sweetened)
Dehydrated soups	

NOTE: Most vitamin C supplements are sourced from corn. If your child is on a corn-free diet and needs vitamin C, look for a corn-free supplement.

NUTS

Of the nuts, the peanut, which is technically a legume, is the most common allergen. Allergic reactions to peanuts are considered the most common cause of anaphylaxis-related deaths in the United States. Identifying obvious sources of nuts is not difficult. It is more difficult to identify nut additives. It is even more challenging to determine which products have trace amounts, especially when not on the label. Cross-contamination occurs when nut parts or dust contaminate other foods during the manufacturing process. Nut oils should not contain nut protein, in theory, but this depends on the manufacturing process. The degree of allergy or sensitivity is the determining factor. Careful label reading is a must. When in doubt, call the company that makes the product. See the following charts for help.

KINDS OF NUTS

Almonds	Macadamia nuts
Brazil nuts	Peanuts (legume)
Cashews	Pecans
Coconuts	Pine nuts
Filberts	Pistachios
Hazelnuts	Walnuts
Hickory nuts	Black walnuts

PRODUCTS CONTAINING NUTS

These are nut products and foods commonly made with nuts:

Amaretto	Mixed nuts
Artificially flavored nuts	Nu-Nuts
Beer nuts	Nut butters, meal, pastes
Bitter almond	Nut oils, flavorings, syrups
Gianduja	
Gingko	Nutella
Ground nuts	Pesto
Loramine wax	Pignolia
Mandelonas	Pralines
Marzipan	

NUT-CONTAMINATED PRODUCTS

These are foods that may contain nuts or be cross-contaminated with nuts:

Baked goods	Frozen desserts
Baking mixes	Graham-cracker crusts
Barbeque sauce	HPP, HVP
Batter-dipped foods	Ice cream
Bulk bin foods	Milk formula
Candy	Nougat
Cereals	Oriental sauce
Chili	Pastry
Cookies	Pie crusts
Dessert toppings	Sauces
Egg rolls	Vegetable fat
Emulsifier	Vegetable oil
Flavoring	

Life Beyond Gluten, Milk, and Soy

In addition to the numerous substitutes for gluten, milk/casein, and soy, there is an abundance of healthy foods to eat. Remember, early humans ate fish, meats, fruits, vegetables, and nuts and seeds. They did not consume milk, grains, beans, or potatoes because milk products were not available and the other items could not be eaten raw without causing severe symptoms or illness. It was only 5,000 to 10,000 years ago that domestication emerged and created major dietary shifts. A GFCFSF diet returns us to the basic foods, which are easier for the body to digest. Here is the list of choices available (as long as they do not cause allergy or intolerance reactions and/or violate your beliefs):

- Meats—all varieties
- Seafood—fish, shellfish, and mollusks
- Fowl—chicken, turkey, hen, and duck
- Eggs—as tolerated
- Nuts and seeds—as tolerated
- Vegetables—all varieties
- Fruits—all varieties
- Grains—all varieties except for glutens, and non-soy corn unless tolerated

---

"Don't be afraid to take a big step if one is indicated.

You can't cross a chasm in two small jumps."

—David Lloyd George

Avoid:

- Gluten: wheat; barley; rye; spelt; kamut; triticale; groats; and commercial oat
- Milk: animal milk products including casein
- Soy: edamame; miso; natto; sprouts; tamari; tempeh; tempura; tofu; yuba; lecithin; HVP; MSG; and vitamin E

Why Is the Diet Needed?

- Incomplete protein digestion leading to partially digested food peptides including opiate-like peptides from DPP-IV enzyme deficiency
- Leaky gut allows partly digested peptides and opioid-like peptides to cross into the bloodstream and enter the brain, causing cravings for the food sources, and behavioral symptoms

Symptoms the Diet May Help:

- Cravings for opioid food sources (gluten, milk. casein, and/or soy); silly, "dopey" behavior; repetitive behaviors; OCD; self-injury; high pain tolerance; poor eye contact; and digestive symptoms

Diet Includes:

- Gluten substitutes: GF oats, non-gluten grains, pseudo grains (amaranth, quinoa, buckwheat), nut flours, and sweet potato
- Milk substitutes: milks from coconut, nuts, hemp, potato, rice, and non-GMO soy. Other substitutes for animal milk products: fruit ice, sorbets, fermented beverages, and smoothies using animal milk substitutes including plant protein powders
- Soy substitutes: legumes, vegetables, and other beans

Resources:

- Autism Research Institute (Dana Laake) www.autism.com/gfcf
- Autism Research Institute (Vicki Kobliner) www.autism.com/treating_diets
- The GFCF Diet www.gfcfdiet.com
- *Cooking to Heal* and *Nourishing Hope for Autism* by Julie Matthews

Note that some individuals may also be sensitive or reactive to eggs (see page 72) corn (see pages 73-74) and/or nuts (see page 74-75).

CHAPTER 5

Feingold and FAILSAFE Diets; Low Salicylate and Low Phenol Diets

WHAT ARE SALICYLATES? WHAT ARE PHENOLS?

Salicylates are chemicals found in plants and in many fruits and vegetables. They are also in medications including aspirin and other pain-relieving medications as well as in many common health and beauty products. Salicylates are thought to protect plants from insect damage and disease. Phenols are naturally occurring chemicals that are high in a number of foods such as apples, bananas, berries, grapes, tomatoes, cocoa, soy, and dairy products. Salicylates are a type of phenol; however, not all phenols are salicylates. (A more complete description follows.)

There are numerous foods that contain salicylates or phenols. However, defining the salicylate or phenol content of foods is not as easy as determining their presence or absence as can be done with the "all or none" foods such as gluten, milk/casein, soy, eggs, corn, and nuts. There are numerous factors that can affect the salicylate or phenol content of a food. These include:

- The season of the year or the location in which the food is grown
- Growth method
- Use of pesticides, preservatives, or additives
- The part of the food/plant tested
- Freshness or degree of ripeness
- Peeled vs. unpeeled
- Preparation and cooking method (e.g., raw vs. cooked)
- Differences based on the brand/variety of the food

In addition, the level in a particular plant may change. For example, according to the Feingold website, an organic fruit that has been attacked by pests will make more salicylates than other fruits. According to one research article, there can even be differences in the concentration of phenolic compounds in fruit grown on the same tree or on different sides of the same piece of fruit, based on exposure to sunlight.

To add to the confusion, there are multiple different ways in which levels of salicylates and phenols are reported. This makes review of the literature challenging and leads to resources and websites that offer differing lists. One reporting measurement is the amount of salicylates per 100 grams of the food/product. For salicylates, greater than 1 mg/100 grams

is considered high. People do not generally eat food by the gram. Another reporting measurement is the amount per "typical serving size" of a food. While you might eat several hundred grams of fruit in a typical serving size, you may consume far less than 100 grams of other salicylate-containing foods such as spices. Herbs and spices are not consumed in 100-gram amounts; however, their salicylate content is highly concentrated and extremely high even in very small amounts. Clinically, this is the reason we observe salicylate reactions to many of the spices.

Yet another confounding factor is the "bioavailability" of the salicylate or phenol based on the type of food. Bioavailability means how available that chemical is to the body based on metabolism by intestinal bacteria, absorption from the intestine, chemical structure, etc. Because of this factor, some foods that are high in salicylates or phenols on a list may not cause as many symptoms as might be expected because the chemical is not well absorbed. For example, pears are listed as a higher phenol containing food than tomatoes. However, in our clinical experience, tomatoes commonly cause phenol symptoms whereas pears are generally very well tolerated.

As authors, we reviewed numerous articles and listings of salicylate/phenol content and created our own grids and lists based on our best synthesis of currently available materials. The reader may find other listings or resources that differ somewhat from ours, because of the factors cited above. We have tried to include our best guidance, based on our decades of clinical experience, regarding which foods are commonly most problematic and which foods are generally tolerated, to help guide the reader in initiating these diets.

What Is the Feingold Diet?

The Feingold Diet was established by Benjamin Feingold, MD, a pediatrician and allergist who felt that hyperactivity was triggered in some children by an immunological reaction (not allergic reaction) to certain synthetic additives (such as colors, flavors, and preservatives) and foods containing salicylates. The Feingold Diet removes foods containing certain harmful ingredients or additives. In the Feingold Program, nonfood items containing problematic ingredients are also removed. Removal of these foods and items is a diagnostic trial to determine which are causing problematic behaviors. Stage I of the Feingold Program involves eliminating synthetic dyes, artificial flavors and specific preservatives entirely. It also involves removing naturally occurring salicylates from the diet until a favorable response is seen. Once improvement is seen, Stage II involves reintroducing some of the fruits and vegetables, with assessment of tolerance. Other ingredients and products can then be added back individually to help determine which are causing problems. Fortunately, most individuals are not reactive to all of the listed ingredients or additives. The success of the diet depends on the degree of a person's sensitivity to salicylates and the amount of exposure.

WHAT ARE THE CULPRIT FOODS OR INGREDIENTS?

Foods and additives that are eliminated include:

- Foods and products containing salicylates (see list below)
- Artificial food coloring (petrochemical dyes)
- Artificial flavors and fragrances

- Three preservatives (petrochemical preservatives: BHA, BHT, TBHQ)
- Artificial sweeteners (aspartame, acesulfame-K, cyclamates, saccharine, and sucralose)

What Foods Contain Salicylates?

There are numerous foods that contain salicylates. Foods are categorized as being either high, medium, or low salicylate foods. The amount of salicylates in a food can vary for numerous reasons, as described above. The chart on pages 82–83 lists high, medium and low salicylate foods based on our best synthesis of available data.

What Are Problematic Food Colorings, Flavors, or Fragrances?

ARTIFICIAL FOOD COLORINGS: Nearly all of the dyes in foods, medicines, toothpaste, beverages, vitamins, cosmetics, etc. are synthetic. Red 40 and Yellow 5 are the most used food dyes in the United States.

ARTIFICIAL SWEETENERS: Aspartame, acesulfame-K, cyclamates, saccharine, and sucralose.

ARTIFICIAL FLAVORS OR FRAGRANCES: For a complete list, see the Feingold Association's website, www.feingold.org

HOW DO I DO THE DIET?

For specific details on how to do the diet as recommended by the Feingold Association, see its website at www.feingold.org. With a membership, you can obtain a handbook, listings of potentially problematic and more allowable foods, and more specific guidance on doing this diet. A more general approach would be to first remove high salicylate foods that are common in your child's diet for at least 4 weeks. Also remove food dyes and artificial flavorings. If there is no obvious improvement or insufficient improvement, then consider removing medium and/or lower salicylate foods for an additional 2–4 weeks. After observing the response, you can reintroduce foods one at a time every 3–5 days and watch for negative reactions. This will help isolate/identify those foods that are causing problems.

WHAT SYMPTOMS MAY BE HELPED BY THE FEINGOLD DIET?

In our clinical experience, the most commonly reported symptoms that seem to be triggered by these foods are hyperactivity and behavioral outbursts. However, any negative behavior could be potentially triggered by these foods or chemicals including irritability, oppositional or defiant behaviors, temper tantrums, inattention, anxiety, mood swings, or learning problems. Some people with salicylate sensitivity also have physical symptoms such as nasal congestion, asthma-like symptoms, itching, skin rashes, hives, stomachaches, or headaches.

WHEN SHOULD I CONSIDER A TRIAL OF THE FEINGOLD DIET FOR MY CHILD?

We would suggest considering a trial of this diet if:

- You have observed reactions to foods containing certain dyes, additives, or flavorings (e.g., food dyes, MSG).

- Your child has symptoms often seen with sensitivity to phenols (see the Phenol section of this chapter), but the response to removal of phenols alone was ineffective or only partially effective.

- You have tried medications and the response was insufficient.

- You have tried the gluten-free casein-free diet and the response was insufficient.

What Is the FAILSAFE Diet?

The FAILSAFE diet was created by allergists at the Royal Prince Alfred Hospital in Australia. They felt that glutamates and biogenic amines found in foods had similar effects on the body as salicylates. This diet is similar to the Feingold diet, but with removal of additional potentially aggravating chemicals. FAILSAFE stands for Free of Additives, Low in Salicylates, Amines and Flavor Enhancers. The diet excludes:

- Approximately 50 artificial food additives: colors (such as food dyes), flavors, preservatives, and antioxidants (sulfites, nitrates, benzoates, sorbates, parabens)

- Salicylates and polyphenols found in a wide range of fruits and vegetables

- Phenolic free-glutamates (MSG) and other food source glutamates

- Neurotransmitters in food: amines (histamine, serotonin, dopamine, phenylethylamine, tyramine, and others) found in aged proteins and fermented foods (cheese, chocolate, game, hung meat)

- Aromatic (strong smelling and tasting) chemicals: Such as those found in perfumes, cleaning products, commercial cosmetics, and scented and colored toiletries, especially mint and menthol products

- Some pharmaceutical drugs including aspirin, NSAIDs and other COX II inhibitors (e.g., Ibuprofen and the methyl-salicylates found in decongestants and anti-inflammatory creams)

According to the website, www.failsafediet.com, this diet eliminates virtually all processed foods, many fruits and vegetables (with a small number of exceptions), aged or preserved proteins like ham, well-hung beef, game, and cheese. It also prohibits use of commercially manufactured cosmetics and perfumes (particularly mint and menthol products) that contain large amounts of salicylates and other chemicals that cross-react in salicylate-sensitive individuals such as benzoates. It also eliminates aspirin and COX II inhibitors; acetaminophen is allowed. The diet is composed mainly of very fresh (non-vacuum packed or hung) meat, chicken and white fish, eggs, fresh dairy products (if tolerated), many but not all grains (if tolerated), peeled potatoes, beans, peeled pears, and a number of green vegetables including cabbage and Brussels sprouts. Strong flavors, additives, many exotic fruits and vegetables, and spices are not allowed.

This diet is clearly very restrictive and would be very challenging to maintain for even the most motivated of families. In our opinion, this diet should be reserved for children who have significant behavioral issues not improved by other traditional or dietary/biomedical interventions. It should be done as a time-limited trial with the goal of identifying specific problematic foods.

WHAT IS A LOW PHENOL DIET?

Phenols are widely available, naturally occurring compounds found in high concentrations in a number of foods. Phenols have antioxidant qualities and protective functions, so some are beneficial and good to consume for most individuals. Foods that are particularly high in phenols include apples, bananas, berries, red grapes, tomatoes, oranges, cocoa, soy and dairy products. Fruits that are lower in phenols and better tolerated include pears, mangoes, and melons. Some individuals, particularly those on the autism spectrum, have difficulty handling phenols.

Phenols are cleared from the body by an enzyme in the liver, phenol sulfotransferase (PST). Enzymes in the body serve a number of functions, including converting one form of a chemical into another so it can be used in subsequent reactions or eliminated from the body. Enzymes require certain "cofactors" or nutrients to help them work most efficiently. Even if an enzyme is present in sufficient amounts, if the cofactor is deficient, the enzyme will be more sluggish. A helpful analogy is to consider that enzyme pathways are like roads or highways. If an enzyme does not have sufficient cofactors, there will be a traffic jam, much like a highway going from four lanes to two lanes. You can still get where you are going, just not very efficiently. If the nutrient the enzyme needs is given, the road construction blockade is lifted and the traffic jam resolves. The PST enzyme requires sulfate. Some individuals, particularly those with autism, do not have enough sulfate. The enzyme then does not work efficiently and phenols can become a problem. If sulfate is given, phenols will be cleared more efficiently. A good source of sulfate is Epsom salts, whose chemical name is magnesium *sulfate*. Epsom salts can be added to bath water. There are also several commercially available magnesium sulfate creams that allow sulfate to be absorbed through the skin; these have the advantage that they can be

SALICYLATE CONTENT OF FOODS

CATEGORY	HIGH-SALICYLATE FOODS	MEDIUM-SALICYLATE FOODS	LOW-SALICYLATE FOODS
Fruit	Apples (Granny Smith), apricots, avocado, berries, cantaloupe, cherries (sweet), coconut, cranberries, currants, dates, fig (dried), grapes (fresh or red), grapefruit, guava, mandarins, nectarines, oranges, peaches, pineapples (fresh), plums (canned), prunes, raisins, rockmelon, sultana, tangerines, tangelo	Apples (Jonathan), grapefruit juice, kiwi, loquat, lychee, nectarine (fresh), pear (with peel), plum (fresh), watermelon	Apples (golden & red delicious), bananas, cherries (sour, canned), fig, grapes (green), lemon (fresh), mango, passion fruit, pawpaw, pear (peeled), persimmon, pineapple juice, pomegranate, rhubarb, tamarillo
Vegetables	Alfalfa, artichoke, broad beans, broccoli, capsicum (green), champignon (canned), chicory, chili, corn (creamed), courgette, cucumber, eggplant, endive, fava beans, gherkin, mushroom (canned), okra, olives (green), pepper (sweet), radish, spinach (fresh), squash, sweet potato (white), tomato (paste, sauce & canned), water chestnut, watercress	Asparagus (canned), beetroot (canned), bok choy, choy sum, corn (canned), lettuce (other than iceberg), maize, olives (black), parsley, parsnip, potato (red), pumpkin, snow peas (& sprouts), sweet potato (yellow) rhubarb	Asparagus (fresh), bamboo shoots, beans, bean sprouts, beetroot (fresh), Brussels sprouts, cabbage, carrot (fresh), cauliflower, celery, chives, choko, corn (fresh), eschallots, French beans, horseradish. leeks, lentils, lettuce (iceberg), mung bean (& sprouts), mushroom (fresh), onion, peas (fresh or dried), pimento (canned), potato (peeled or unpeeled white), pumpkin, spinach (frozen), soybeans, swedes, tomato (fresh), turnip
Nuts and Seeds	Almonds, macadamia, peanuts, pine nuts, pistachio	Brazil nuts, coconut (desiccated), pumpkin seeds, walnuts	Cashews, hazelnuts, pecans, peanut butter, poppy seeds, sesame seeds, sunflower seeds

SALICYLATE CONTENT OF FOODS

CATEGORY	HIGH-SALICYLATE FOODS	MEDIUM-SALICYLATE FOODS	LOW-SALICYLATE FOODS
Spices	Allspice, anise seed, basil, cayenne, celery, cinnamon, cloves, cumin, curry powder, dill, fenugreek, five spice, garam masala, ginger, mace, mint, mixed herbs, mustard, oregano, paprika (hot or sweet), pepper, rosemary, sage, tarragon, turmeric, thyme, Vegemite, vinegars (red and white wine, cider, and others)	Cinnamon, cumin, oregano, sage	Chives, coriander, salt
Other	Clover honey, molasses	Honey (except for clover honey)	All grains (except maize), cocoa, dairy products, meat, seafood, brown and white sugars, golden and maple syrups, molasses

applied several times per day to provide more consistent sulfate to the enzyme than a once-daily bath. (See the authors' supplement book for more details.)

The PST enzyme system is an important part of the body's detoxification pathways, which remove toxins from the body that come from internal sources (metabolism) and from external sources (environmental chemicals, certain additives in foods). When the enzyme is not functioning well, phenols and salicylates from foods, toxins and chemicals that are high in these substances are not cleared well and the metabolite traffic backs up; this can cause a variety of behavioral symptoms. Remember, the phenols are *beneficial* to the system; it is the PST deficiency or decreased function that is the problem. Artificial coloring and flavorings are the most significant load on the PST system, but high-salicylate foods are significant too. This can be confusing because while salicylates are a type of phenol, not all phenols are salicylates. Environmental chemicals and toxins, especially petroleum byproducts, also weigh heavily on the PST system. Again, supporting the enzyme allows it to clear all of these chemicals more efficiently.

Symptoms and physical signs that suggest your child may have a phenol sensitivity include:

- Intermittent flushed red cheeks or ears that occur without obvious explanation
- Hyperactivity
- Unexplained silliness or laughing
- Disrupted sleep, especially unusual laughter when waking during the night
- Anger and/or aggression
- Sweating at night
- Large variations in functioning ability
- Regression in behavior after eating high phenol foods

For initial implementation of a low phenol diet, we recommend removing the following items, which we have found to be the biggest culprits:

- Artificial colorings, flavorings, and preservatives
- Fruits: apples, bananas, berries, oranges, red grapes, raisins, and tomatoes
- Chocolate and cocoa
- Milk products (animal source)
- Soy
- Vanillin

The best-tolerated fruits to use as substitutes include pears, mangoes, and melons.

There are three main categories of phenols: salicylates, amines, and glutamates.

- Salicylates: Includes aspirin and other salicylate medications, and phenolic salicylate foods
- Amines: Dietary amines come from protein breakdown in foods. They increase in meat, fish, and cheese as they age and in fruits as they ripen (bananas, tomatoes). Vasoactive amines are neurotransmitters present in foods: dopamine, histamine, phenylethylamine, serotonin, tyramine. Foods high in these are well-known triggers of migraines.

HIGH-PHENOL FOODS TO AVOID FOR A LOW-PHENOL DIET

*Note that bolded items are the most significant

PHENOL SALICYLATE SOURCES	PHENOL AMINE SOURCES	PHENOL FREE-GLUTAMATE SOURCES
Artificial: food coloring, flavoring, and preservatives	Aged meats	**Monosodium glutamate (MSG) Sources**
Apples, apple juice	Almond flour	Autolyzed yeast, yeast extract
Berries: blackberry, black currant, blueberry, chokeberry, elderberry, raspberry, strawberry	Avocado (ripened)	Bouillon
	Banana (ripened)	Calcium caseinate
	Berries	Carrageenan
Bananas	Bouillon	Citric acid
Beans: black, white	Broad beans (Fava)	Corn starch
Celery seeds	Canned fish	Corn syrup
Cherries	Cheeses (mature)	Flavoring
Chocolate (dark), cocoa	Cherries	Gelatin
Cloves	Chocolate	Hydrolyzed items
Globe artichoke heads	Citrus fruits	Maltodextrin
Honey	Coconut flour and milk	Milk powder
Grapes (especially red)	Deli meats	Modified food starch
Milk products (animal source)	Eggplant	Monopotassium glutamate
Nuts: Almonds, hazelnuts, pecans, walnuts	Fake crab meat/surimi	Pectin
Olives	Fruit flavored yogurt	Soy protein
Oranges, orange juice	Grapes	Soy sauce
Plums	Hummus	Textured protein
	Kiwi fruit	Whey protein isolate
	Mushrooms	(Chart continues on following page.)
	Nuts: most nuts and seeds	

- Glutamate: Glutamate is an excitatory neurotransmitter, affecting normal and abnormal brain function. Free (unbound) glutamate is problematic for many. Excesses of glutamate can cause migraines and contribute to hyperactivity.

If removing the most common phenol culprits from the diet has not resulted in improvement, consider avoiding more phenolic foods: more phenolic salicylates, phenolic amines, and/or phenolic glutamates.

NOTE: Different apples and grapes have different levels of salicylates. However, all apples are high in phenols so all types should be removed when doing a low phenol diet trial. While red grapes are higher in phenols than green grapes, both types showed be removed during a low phenol diet trial. Cocoa powder contains negligible amounts of salicylates but should be avoided on a low phenol diet.

HIGH-PHENOL FOODS TO AVOID FOR A LOW-PHENOL DIET (CONT.)

Note that bolded items are the most significant

PHENOL SALICYLATE SOURCES	PHENOL AMINE SOURCES	PHENOL FREE-GLUTAMATE SOURCES
Raisins	Oils: almond, avocado, coconut, extra virgin olive oil, sesame, walnut	**Natural Sources of Free-Glutamate**
Seasonings: cloves, dried peppermint, spice mixes, star anise	Olives	Aged, matured preserved foods
Soy	Passion fruit	Bone broths
Spinach	Pickled vegetables	Bouillon
Teas: black, green	Pineapples	Broad bean/fava
Tomatoes	Plums	Broccoli
Vanillin	Sauerkraut	Casein
	Soy	Deli meats
	Spinach	Dried fruits
	Tomatoes	Fish sauce
	Vegetable juice, stocks, soups	Gluten
		Grape juice
		Malted barley
		Mushrooms
		Peas
		Soy protein
		Soy sauce
		Spinach
		Tomatoes (ripe)

How Do I Know Which of These Diets to Do and in What Order?

We suggest first trying a low phenol diet, as it is the least restrictive of the above diets. If phenols are an issue for your child, the response to removal (or providing adequate sulfate) is often rapid and dramatic. If the improvements are negligible with removal of phenols or not sufficient, then removal of other high salicylate foods could be considered as a next, time-limited step. If you want to go further, removal of foods on the medium- or low-salicylate list or on the FAILSAFE list could also be considered. Once items have been removed, individual foods or products can be introduced individually, with at least 3–5 days in-between introduction of each, to try to identify which agents or foods are problematic. In regard to phenol sensitivity, if a child reacts to one high phenol food, he is likely to react to others; in this situation, most high phenol foods need to be removed, until or unless the enzyme that helps clear phenols can be adequately supported (e.g., by sulfate and other supportive nutrients). Fortunately, children who react to salicylates do not seem to react to all of them, so it is more common to be able to identify specific significant problematic foods or chemicals (such as MSG, for example).

What Else Can Be Done?

The PST enzyme is supported by a number of nutrients, most importantly sulfate, B6, and magnesium. Because B6 is interdependent with other B vitamins, a phenol-free multivitamin mineral supplement that provides B vitamins as well as other supportive nutrients can also be helpful. As previously noted, Epsom salt baths and/or magnesium sulfate creams are also good sources of sulfate to support the enzyme. Other sulfur-bearing nutrients can also be helpful. For those with more significant phenol problems, there may be benefit from phenol-targeting enzymes, available in supplement specialty stores and sites. Supporting enzyme functions can be complex; therefore, in order to design the most appropriate regimen for your child, we recommend a consultation with a health care practitioner who has expertise in these treatments.

Traditional medical doctors have been slow to accept the possibility that foods or food chemicals can adversely affect behavior. In 2008, the American Academy of Pediatrics published a Grand Rounds titled "ADHD and Food Additives Revisited." This was in response to an article published in the journal, *Lancet*, which was a randomized, double-blind, placebo-controlled trial regarding the effect of food additives on children's behavior. The authors of the study concluded that their results suggested that food additives and/or sodium benzoate increase hyperactive behavior in children. The Grand Rounds Editor's Note regarding this article stated, "The overall findings of the study are clear and require that even we skeptics, who have long doubted parental claims of the effects of various foods on the behavior of children, admit we might have been wrong."

What Are Salicylates and Where Are They Found?

- Salicylates are a type of phenol. They are found in plants, fruits, vegetables, aspirin, and other pain-relieving medications, and in artificial flavoring, preservatives, sweeteners, and fragrances.

Avoid:

- Environmental toxins and manufactured chemicals
- Artificial additives, preservatives, coloring, flavoring, MSG, and sweeteners
- Specific fruits and vegetables (especially brightly colored) and most spices

Why Is the Diet Needed?

- Insufficient sulfation and detoxification; inadequate gut flora

Symptoms the Diet May Help:

- Hyperactivity; behavior outbursts; irritability; oppositional/defiance; anxiety; and learning problems

Diet Includes:

- Organic foods! See Chapter 3 for detailed information on an organic, healthy diet.
- These foods have very little to no salicylates: cereal, meats, fish, eggs, and dairy products.

Resources:

- The Feingold Diet: www.Feingold.org
- *Cure Your Child with Food* by Kelly Dorfman
- My Child Will Thrive: www.mychildwillthrive.com/wp-content/uploads/Low-Phenol-Resource-V2-Final.pdf
- *Cooking to Heal* and *Nourishing Hope for Autism* by Julie Matthews

---

What is FAILSAFE?

- **F**ree of **A**dditives, **L**ow in **S**alicylates, **A**mines and **F**lavor **E**nhancers. It expands the Feingold Diet by also excluding glutamates and biogenic amines. It is the most rigid diet.

Avoid:

- Environmental toxins; manufactured chemicals; artificial additives, preservatives, colors, and flavors
- Sulfites, nitrates, benzoates, sorbates, and parabens
- Aromatic chemicals: perfumes, cleaning products, personal care products, mint, and menthols
- Aspirin, NSAIDs, and COX II inhibitors; salicylate-containing medications and foods
- Glutamates (MSG), MSG additives, and glutamate foods
- Neurotransmitter amines found in aged proteins and fermented foods
- All processed foods, many fruits and vegetables (with a few exceptions)

Why Is the Diet Needed?

- Insufficient sulfation and detoxification; inadequate gut flora (microbiota); chemical sensitivity

Symptoms the Diet May Help:

- Reactions to the items on the "Avoid" list
- Red cheeks/ears; hyperactivity; silliness; aggression; regressions; irritability; and poor sleep
- Night sweats; headaches; lethargy; and dark circles under eyes
- Behavioral problems (oppositional/defiance, tantrums, and mood swings); learning problems

Diet Includes:

- Organic is important.
- Fresh meat, chicken, white fish, eggs, fresh dairy products (if tolerated), grains (if tolerated), peeled potatoes, rice, beans, carrots, peeled pears, and many green vegetables including cabbage and Brussels sprouts

Resources:

- The FAILSAFE Diet: www.failsafediet.com/the-rpah-elimination-diet-failsafe
- My Child Will Thrive: www.mychildwillthrive.com/wp-content/uploads/Therapeutic_Diet-Cheat_Sheet_Final.pdf
- *Fed Up* and *The FAILSAFE Cookbook* by Sue Dengate

LOW PHENOL DIET   Chapter 5

What Are Phenols?

- Phenols have antioxidant qualities and are beneficial for most, but not for those who are intolerant. Phenols include phenolic salicylates, amines, and glutamates.

Avoid: Strictness is based on results. Some individuals must be rigid in adherence

- Environmental toxins, manufactured chemicals, and food coloring, flavoring
- Aspirin and salicylate-containing medications and foods
- Main food avoids: Apples, bananas, berries, cherries, chocolate, milk products, oranges, orange juice, raisins, red grapes, soy, tomato, and vanillin
- Other avoids: Beans (black, white), cloves, globe artichoke heads, honey, nuts (almonds, hazelnuts, pecans, walnuts), olives, plums, spinach
- If improvement is insufficient, try avoiding more phenolic salicylates, amines and glutamates
- See the chart in this chapter, on pages 84–85.

Why Is the Diet Needed?

- Defective phenol sulfotransferase (PST) enzyme necessary for sulfation and detoxification; inadequate gut flora, and high-sulfur food sources

Symptoms the Diet May Help:

- Reactions to the items on the "Avoid" list
- Red cheeks/ears; hyperactivity; silliness; aggression; regressions; irritability; and poor sleep
- Night sweats; headaches; lethargy; and dark circles under eyes
- Behavior and learning problems; oppositional; and mood swings

Diet Includes:

- Organic is important. Foods, low in phenol and high in sulfur: meat, poultry, seafood, eggs; garlic, onion shallots, leeks, broccoli, and cabbage
- Other foods: Grains (not rye and wheat); Beans/legumes (not black, white, soy); Fruit: pears, mango, melons; Vegetables: alfalfa, bean sprouts, Brussels sprouts, celery, chard, rhubarb, snow peas
- Nuts: all except almonds, hazelnuts, pecans, walnuts
- Spices: chives, cinnamon, curry, dill, fennel, ginger, mustard, oregano, pepper, rosemary, sage, tarragon, thyme, turmeric

Resources:

- Enzyme Stuff: http://www.enzymestuff.com/epsomsalts.htm
- Dana's View from the Inside: www.danasview.net/phenol.htm
- My Child Will Thrive: www.mychildwillthrive.com/wp-content/uploads/Low-Phenol-Resource-V2-Final.pdf
- *Cooking to Heal* and *Nourishing Hope for Autism* by Julie Matthews
- *Cure Your Child with Food* by Kelly Dorfman

"Ethan continues to improve. In the past week he has started to ask questions, which is the next step to being able to hold a conversation. I never thought I would be happy to hear 'why?' and 'why not?'"

—Bea Wolman, mother of four-year-old Ethan

The Specific Carbohydrate Diet (SCD) and Gut and Psychology Syndrome Diet (GAPS)

"Maintaining his special diet is very difficult, but not nearly as hard as living with a severely autistic child."

—Mother of a recovering autistic son

"MY SON HAD BEEN ON THE SPECIFIC CARBOHYDRATE DIET (SCD) for about a year, which means he couldn't (and still can't) have any starch, sucrose or lactose. After exploring the Air and Space Museum, we went into the food court and I unpacked the turkey burgers and almond cookies I'd made and brought along. Unfortunately, eating with hundreds of other people who didn't bring their own picnic means my son had to watch while all the other kids ate one of his favorite forbidden foods: French fries. Instead of going through the whole explanation of why he couldn't have them, when he asked, I let him have some. In my defense, after a year on the SCD, you're allowed to start slowly adding previously restricted foods back in to see how they're tolerated. But impulsively giving him both potatoes and probably gluten (I doubt they fry battered food in separate oil from the oil in which they fry French fries in the food court) at the same time didn't make sense. After thinking it through, I realized the reason for my lapse: I was mad that my son was deprived of something that most kids can eat. And as a parent, I felt deprived of having a kid who could not have something that most kids get to have. Apparently, this is normal."

—KATHRYN SCOTT, *in "Flirting with Disaster,"*
published in Living Without, *Spring 2006*

The Specific Carbohydrate Diet (SCD)

As previously discussed, many children with ADHD and autism have damage in their intestinal tracts. When the cells that produce digestive enzymes are damaged, fewer enzymes will be available for digestion. This occurs in the small intestine, where over 90% of digestion and absorption occurs. We have discussed the digestive problems resulting from gluten and milk products, but they are not the only potential culprits.

The SCD diet was developed by Sydney Haas and is described in the book by nutritional biochemist Elaine Gotschall, *Breaking the Vicious Cycle—Intestinal Health Through Diet*. It distinguishes between the two basic kinds of carbohydrates:

- Simple, monosaccharide sugars, including fructose, glucose, and galactose
- Double-sugar disaccharides, including lactose, sucrose, maltose, and isomaltose

Most people are familiar with lactose intolerance due to poor or no production of the enzyme lactase, which digests lactose sugar found in milk. When other disaccharide-digesting enzymes are missing, the symptoms and damage become more severe.

SCD is based on the principle that simple carbohydrates (monosaccharides) require minimal digestion, are well absorbed, and leave no undigested residues. The complex double-sugar carbohydrates (disaccharides) are hard to digest, especially for those who have damaged intestines and inadequate digestive enzymes. The residues of the undigested double sugars become food for intestinal "bad bugs" and yeast,

> "My children, Daniel and Ruth, are on the Specific Carbohydrate Diet and a casein-free diet. Daniel, who is eleven years old, has this to say about it: 'I think the diet has helped me with gut problems. My gut used to feel tight and now it doesn't.' Ruth, who is eight years old, says, 'I don't usually get stomachaches anymore, and I now like cauliflower and broccoli. I didn't used to eat them. I also like eating peas more than ever. The diet helped me read better, too.'"
>
> —Mother of Daniel and Ruth,
> *both of whom are on SCD and casein-free diets*

resulting in a "cesspool" within the gut. This leads to digestive distress, including gas, bloating, cramps, abnormal stools, constipation, and diarrhea. The result is poor absorption of nutrients. Disaccharide intolerance is common in many bowel conditions, including Crohn's disease, colitis, inflammatory bowel conditions, and irritable bowel syndrome.

Avoiding the disaccharide carbohydrates causes the bad bugs and their harmful byproducts to starve and decrease while the good bugs thrive and increase. The intestinal lining heals, digestion and nutrient absorption improve, and overall health benefits.

WHAT FOODS ARE ALLOWED AND PROHIBITED ON SCD?

The only carbohydrates allowed on the SCD are the simple sugars. Acceptable foods include honey, most vegetables, most fruits, and noncarbohydrates such as fats, oils, meats, eggs, fish, poultry, some hard cheeses, some legumes, and well-fermented yogurt. The foods to avoid include sugars; canned vegetables and fruits; all grains; breads; pastas and other starchy foods; processed, canned meats; and milk and most milk products, especially those with lactose. See the chart on the pages that follow for a more thorough listing.

There are a number of foods that are allowed on a gluten-free casein-free diet but are prohibited on SCD. These include:

- Grains: corn, rice, tapioca, and pseudo grains (amaranth, buckwheat, and quinoa)
- Starchy vegetables and some beans
- Double sugars (disaccharides): lactose, sucrose, maltose, and isomaltose

Lactose-free cheeses and well-fermented yogurt are not allowed on a casein-free diet but are allowed on SCD.

In addition to the diet, specific carbohydrate-digesting enzymes are prescribed in order to reduce the symptoms from minor infractions. The enzymes, however, cannot make up for not following the diet.

WHEN TO SPECIFICALLY CONSIDER THE SPECIFIC CARBOHYDRATE DIET

SCD, at least initially, is a very restrictive diet, especially if done along with gluten- and casein- elimination. This can be particularly challenging in children, who are often naturally picky about what they will eat. We suggest that SCD be considered as an additional treatment option for the following conditions or situations:

- Chronic GI symptoms such as gas, bloating, or diarrhea that have not improved with gluten, casein, or lactose elimination and provision of probiotics
- Intestinal yeast overgrowth that has not improved with

more foundational treatments such as probiotics and anti-fungal medications, herbs, or supplements

- Documented inflammatory bowel disease such as Crohn's disease or ulcerative colitis, or small intestinal bacterial overgrowth (SIBO)
- Children with autism whose behavioral and developmental symptoms have not improved in spite of pursuing other treatments such as special education and therapy supports, gluten- and casein-elimination, and biomedical treatments such as nutritional supplements

Gut and Psychology Syndrome Diet (GAPS)

The GAPS diet is a modification and expansion of the Specific Carbohydrate Diet and was developed by Dr. Natasha Campbell-McBride. According to Dr. Campbell-McBride's website, the GAPS program is divided into three protocols: the Nutritional Protocol, the Supplementation Protocol, and the Detoxification Protocol.

THE NUTRITIONAL PROTOCOL involves removal of the same foods as detailed for SCD. It also removes milk products/casein. In addition, it emphasizes the importance of the use of homemade broths and fermented vegetables. The protocols are complicated, and it is recommended that the reader refer to Dr. McBride's book, *Gut and Psychology Syndrome*, and her website, www.gapsdiet.com. For those individuals with severe GI issues (such as severe diarrhea or constipation, or inflammatory bowel disease), she recommends an "Introduction Diet" that is implemented in six stages, starting with homemade meat or fish broths and soups. She also recommends probiotic foods such as kefir (if dairy is tolerated) or home-made sauerkraut. The second stage adds raw organic egg yolks as well as stews and casseroles made with meat and vegetables. Fermented fish and homemade ghee can also be added. The third stage adds avocado, scrambled eggs, and "pancakes" (made from nut but-ter, eggs, and squash). Stage four incorporates addi-tional meats, but only roasted or grilled; introduces cold-pressed olive oil and freshly pressed juices; and adds homemade bread made with nut flours. In stage five, cooked apple as a purée and raw vegetables are added. Stage six introduces peeled raw apple and other raw fruits as well as cakes and other sweets that are permitted on the diet.

There is also a "Full GAPS diet" option, which is recommended after the Introduction Diet has been completed and the individual is having normal stools. The majority of the diet consists of fresh meats, animal fats, fish, shellfish, organic farm-fresh eggs, fermented foods, and vegetables. Baked goods made from nut flours and foods are eaten in moderation during the healing process. Dr. McBride's book and website give more information about the composi-tion, balance, and timing of foods and meals.

THE SUPPLEMENTATION PROTOCOL includes pro-biotics, essential fatty acids, cod-liver oil/vitamin A, digestive enzymes, vitamins, and minerals. General guidelines are provided, but please consult a qualified health professional for optimal treatment and indi-vidualized recommendations.

THE DETOXIFICATION PROTOCOL focuses on sup-porting the body's natural detoxification processes. It also discusses reducing the total toxic load on the body by restricting exposure to chemicals and toxins.

For those children who have severe GI issues and who need the Introduction Diet, we recommend consulting a nutritionist or functional medicine practitioner with familiarity with this diet to ensure that adequate nutrition can be maintained and that this can be done safely. For children who do not have severe GI issues, the introduction diet does not need to be done and the full GAPS diet may be imple-mented instead.

"My son, Robb, is on a gluten-free casein-free diet as well as the Specific Carbohydrate Diet. Although I saw nice improvements after several months on the GFCF diet, there was a remark-able change for him THE NEXT DAY after he started the SCD diet. He practically bounced out of bed and ran into our room—MUCH more energy."

—Mother of Robb
a six-year-old with autism and Down syndrome

THE SPECIFIC CARBOHYDRATE DIET

DOUBLE SUGAR	SOURCES	BREAKS DOWN TO	MISSING ENZYMES = DISACCHARIDASES
Lactose	Milk products	Glucose and galactose	Lactase
Sucrose	Sugars	Glucose and fructose	Sucrase
Maltose	Starch	Glucose and glucose	Maltase
Isomaltose	Starch	Glucose and glucose	Isomaltase

CATEGORY	AVOID	INCLUDE
Protein Animal	Preserved meats	Poultry, meat, seafood
	Processed meats (deli meats, hot dogs)	Gelatin: unflavored
	Canned meats & seafood	Eggs
	Flavored gelatin	Yogurt: well-fermented, homemade
	Milk products (most)	Dry curd cottage cheese
		Hard cheeses
Protein Plant	Bean sprouts, pinto, cannellini	Lima beans
	Chickpeas, fava, soy, mung	Almonds, Brazil, chestnuts, coconut, filberts/hazelnuts, pecans, pistachios, walnuts
	Processed nuts	Nut butters (w/o sugar added)
	Flours from beans, seeds	Nut flours
Vegetables Fresh or frozen May need to cook or steam	Canned vegetables (unless organic w/o added sugar)	Artichokes (French), asparagus, beets, broccoli, Brussels sprouts, cabbage, carrots, cauliflower
	Artichoke (Jerusalem)	Celery, cucumbers, eggplant, garlic
	Butter beans	Kale, lettuce, mushrooms, olives, onions, parsley, peas, peppers
	Garlic and onion powder	Pumpkin, rhubarb, snowpeas, spinach, squash, string beans
	Potato, sweet potato, yams	Tomato, watercress, zucchini
	Parsnips and turnips	
	Water chestnuts	

(Chart continues on following page.)

THE SPECIFIC CARBOHYDRATE DIET (CONTINUED)

CATEGORY	AVOID	INCLUDE
Fruits	Canned in syrup	May use fruit sauces (apple or pear) or steamed, baked fruits.
	Dried fruits!	Apples, apple cider, applesauce w/o sugar
	Plantains	Avocado, apricot, banana, berries, cherries, dates, coconut flesh, grapes, kiwi, lemons, limes, mangoes, melons, nectarines, oranges, papayas, peaches, pears, prunes, raisins, tangerines
Grains	All grains to be avoided	Nut flours
		Spaghetti squash
Sugar	All artificial sweeteners	Some honey
	Candy, carob, chocolate	
	Corn syrup, HFCS, dates	
	Maple syrup, molasses, Sucanat	
	Sugar alcohols, sucralose	
Other	Gums: guar, xanthan	Cellulose
	Fried foods	Homemade mayo
	Mayonnaise, margarine	Oils: avocado, canola, coconut, olive, safflower
	Oils: corn, soy	Ketchup (homemade)
	Commercial ketchup	Balsamic (homemade) vinegar
	Soy sauce, Tamari	Olives
	Corn starch, tapioca starch	
	Balsamic vinegar (commercial)	
Beverages	Sodas, fruit punch	Water, coffee, herb teas
	V8 juice, V8 fusion	Tea, coffee
	Frozen fruit juice, apple juice	Dilute pure juice (1/3 juice)
	Soy milk	Nut milks
	Alcohol (most)	Splash of 100% juice to flavor items, apple cider

What Else May Be Helpful?

Supplements must all be "SCD legal." SCD legal multiple vitamin mineral supplements are available. Probiotics and biotin are critical for improving the gut microbiota. Many benefit from the use of disaccharidase enzymes to improve digestion. Also commonly included are omega-3 fatty acids, methyl B12, and anti-fungal herbs.

SCD (SPECIFIC CARBOHYDRATE DIET) AND GAPS (GUT AND PSYCHOLOGY SYNDROME)
Chapter 6

Avoid:
- **SCD:** All disaccharides (lactose, sucrose, maltose, and isomaltose) found in sugars; grains, pseudo grains (buckwheat, millet, and quinoa); some beans, dried fruit, starchy vegetables, and some milk products
- **GAPS:** Expansion of SCD: additional removal of milk products and casein.

Why Are the Diets Needed?
- **SCD:** Deficiencies of disaccharidase enzymes that digest double sugars (lactase, sucrase, maltase, isomaltose); leaky gut; digestive and intestinal conditions; and bacterial overgrowth.
- **GAPS:** Persistence of inflammatory bowel disease (IBD); irritable bowel syndrome (IBS); and digestive problems

Symptoms the Diets May Help:
- **SCD:** Persistent belching; gas; cramping; constipation; diarrhea; yeast issues; celiac disease; diverticulitis; inflammatory bowel disease (IBD); SIBO; and other digestive problems
- **GAPS:** When the SCD has not been fully effective. GAPS is more strict.

Diet Includes:
- **SCD:**
- Protein: healthy seafood; pastured source poultry, meat, and eggs; some hard cheeses; dry curd cottage cheese; lentils; lima beans; nuts; and seeds
- Vegetables: artichoke (globe); asparagus; beets; carrots; celery; greens; pumpkin; string beans; snow peas; tomato; and watercress
- Fruits: apple; apricot; avocados; banana; berries; cherries; citrus; dates; grapes; papaya; peaches; pears; prunes; and tropical fruits
- Individual spices of all kinds. Avoid spice mixtures.
- **GAPS:** Add homemade broths and fermented vegetables.

Resources:
- *Breaking the Vicious Cycle* by Elaine Gottschall: www.breakingtheviciouscycle.info
- The SCD Diet: www.scdiet.net
- The GAPS Diet: www.gapsdiet.com
- The Best Method for Healing with SCD: www.PecanBread.com
- SIBO (small intestinal bacterial overgrowth): www.siboinfo.com/diet.html
- *Gut and Psychology Syndrome* by Natasha Campbell-McBride
- *Cooking to Heal* and *Nourishing Hope for Autism* by Julie Matthews

CHAPTER 7

The Anti-Yeast (Anti-Candida) Diet

THE UNDERLYING PROBLEM: IMBALANCED BACTERIA AND YEAST OVERGROWTH IN THE INTESTINE

As previously discussed, the intestine is home to trillions of bacteria. It is normal to have some yeast in the intestine, but their amounts are kept in check by the presence of the multitudes of beneficial bacteria. When this balance is disrupted, yeast can multiply. *Candida albicans* is the most common yeast. You may sometimes see this diet referred to as an "Anti-Candida" diet. However, there are other yeasts that live in the intestinal tract that are less commonly problematic.

Yeast can produce chemicals that are irritating to the intestinal lining. This, as well as other factors, can contribute to altering the permeability of the intestine (often referred to as "leaky gut"). If yeast toxins "leak" into the bloodstream, they may be delivered to the brain and interfere with brain function. Some of these yeast metabolites (such as tartaric acid) look similar to chemicals in an important chemical cycle (the Krebs cycle) in the energy-generating machinery of the cells called mitochondria. These "molecular mimics" have the potential to interfere with the functioning of this cycle. Lastly, yeast chemicals may also trigger inflammation in the intestinal lining. It is thought that GI inflammation is one of the triggers for inflammation elsewhere in the body, including the brain.

WHAT CAN CAUSE OVERGROWTH OF YEAST IN THE INTESTINE?

The most common cause of intestinal yeast overgrowth is the use of antibiotics. Antibiotics are necessary treatments for a number of infectious conditions and we support their use. However, an unintended consequence of antibiotics is that they do not only attack the organisms for the infection for which they were prescribed. As they pass through the intestine, they also kill off intestinal bacteria. It is important to take a probiotic ("beneficial" bacteria) when on antibiotics, in order to maintain good intestinal balance.

Another common cause of imbalanced bacteria is insufficient fiber in the diet. The intestinal bacteria feed on fiber. Without enough fiber, they will gradually die off, resulting in imbalance of the organisms. Another dietary factor is excessive sugar in the diet. Sugar is believed to "feed" yeast.

WHAT SIGNS AND SYMPTOMS CAN INDICATE THAT MY CHILD HAS PROBLEMS WITH YEAST?

Physical signs and symptoms of yeast include:

- Diaper rash
- Thrush (yeast on the tongue or mucus membranes of the mouth)
- Circular red ring around anus
- Abdominal bloating
- Loose or smelly stools

- Sugar cravings
- Skin rashes
- Nausea
- Headache
- Fatigue
- Dizziness

It is important to note that it is not uncommon to have intestinal yeast overgrowth without any obvious outward physical symptoms. Sometimes, the only clues to yeast overgrowth are behavioral symptoms that may include:

- Silly or inappropriate laughing. Some have described the conditions in an imbalanced intestine as an "auto-brewery."

- Inattention

- "Brain fog"

- Irritability and mood changes

WHEN SHOULD I CONSIDER AN ANTI-YEAST DIET?

It is our opinion that anti-yeast diets should not be done routinely for individuals with autism or ADHD, as they become very restrictive when done in combination with other diets. It is common sense, and good for overall health, to use sugar in more limited amounts than is typical in most children's diets. However, strict elimination of sugars, fruits containing sugar, etc., should be considered in more limited situations. Our general approach is to first try to make the intestine "inhospitable" to yeast (e.g., by improving the balance of beneficial bacteria, with either probiotics or fermented foods such as kefir, and eliminating excessive yeast with anti-fungals) before eliminating foods that feed yeast or contain yeast.

We would suggest considering an anti-yeast diet when:

- You have tried the Specific Carbohydrate Diet (SCD) and yeast remains problematic. One of the specific indications for SCD is persistent yeast.

- Intestinal yeast overgrowth and the associated symp-toms persist *in spite of* adequate probiotics and anti-fungal medications, herbs, or supplements.

- Physical symptoms (e.g., chronic diarrhea) persist that are not better explained by other factors.

- Behavioral symptoms known to be associated with yeast overgrowth (e.g., unexplained laughing, inattention) persist in spite of other behavioral and biomedical treatments and that are impairing to the child's life.

Note that "die-off" symptoms can occur due to the toxins being released as yeast die or are killed off. Symptoms can include nausea, headache, swollen glands, bloating, gas, digestive problems, chills, fever, sweating, and flare-up of infections in the rectal and vaginal areas. Worsened behavior can also occur, often in the form of irritability.

WHAT FOODS NEED TO BE AVOIDED ON AN ANTI-YEAST DIET AND WHY?

The main intent of the anti-yeast diet is to avoid foods high in sugar. The following list includes obvious and more hidden sources of sugar as well as yeast promoting foods.

- All sugars and sweeteners (except stevia): These include sugar, agave, corn syrup, honey, malt, maple syrup, molasses, aspartame, and sorbitol.

- High sugar fruits: These include bananas, dates, grapes, mangos, and raisins. The high sugar content in fruit is a good food source for yeast, even though the sugars are natural sugars. Most, if not all, fruits should be avoided in the early stages of the diet.

- Dried fruit: The act of drying fruits dramatically increases their sweetness. The dehydration process removes most of the water content and concentrates the natural sugars found in the fruit.

- Fruit juices and sweet vegetable juices

- Starchy vegetables: These include potatoes, sweet potatoes, yams, corn, winter squash, beets, peas, parsnips, and beans.

- Breakfast cereals that are high in sugar: Even those with "healthy sounding" names often have sugar as a significantly high percentage ingredient. Also read labels on food bars (e.g., granola bars) as many are high in sugar.

- Energy drinks and soft drinks

- Processed meats like lunch meat and SPAM: They often contain dextrose, nitrates, sulfates, and sugars.

- Dairy products: Most dairy products should be avoided except ghee, butter, kefir, and probiotic yogurt. Dairy foods tend to contain a lot of natural sugars (e.g., lactose).

- Condiments with added sugars: These may include barbeque sauce, horseradish, ketchup, mayonnaise, soy sauce, and white vinegar. Many salad dressings are also high in sugar.

- Grains: Some experts recommend avoidance of classical "true" grains from the "grass family," which includes barley, corn, kamut, millet, oats, rice, rye, sorghum, spelt, sugarcane, cane sugar, raw sugar, molasses, teff, triticale, wheat, and bulgur. Individual patients may respond differently to grains. There are many grain substitutes called pseudo grains (amaranth, buckwheat, and quinoa). See the next section, "What Foods Are Allowed on This Diet?"

- Moldy foods such as cheeses (blue cheese, Camembert) and nuts that are high in mold: peanuts, cashews, pecans, walnuts, and pistachios. Also avoid nut butters made from these nuts. Molds release toxins that can be damaging to the gut lining and encourage yeast overgrowth.

- Fermented food advice also varies among the experts. Some recommend avoiding all fermented foods; however, our advice is to include the healthy fermented foods (see list on page 56). Some recommend avoiding the wild strains of fermentation like those in kombucha, whereas others recommend including them. Individuals may have different reactions. Brewer's yeast and baker's yeast are best avoided, especially when an individual has a serious candida/yeast infection that is unresponsive to initial dietary changes and supplementation.

NOTE: *The Specific Carbohydrate Diet eliminates foods containing complex carbohydrates and allows more simple carbohydrates. It is often helpful for those individuals who have persistent yeast overgrowth. It is a very structured diet, with some similarities to the anti-yeast diet but also some differences. See Chapter 6 for details on this diet.*

WHAT FOODS ARE ALLOWED ON THIS DIET?

Foods that are allowed on this diet include:

- Non-starchy vegetables: These include artichoke, asparagus, avocado, bok choy, broccoli, Brussels sprouts, cabbage, cauliflower, celery, cucumber, eggplant, fennel, garlic (raw), greens, hearts of palm, jicama, kale, kohlrabi, okra, olives (not in white vinegar), onions, parsley, radish, rutabaga, spinach, tomatoes, turnips, water chestnuts, watercress, and zucchini.

- Low sugar fruits: Lemons, limes, grapefruit, and if tolerated, apples, berries, peach, and pears. *Note that the following allowed fruits are typically considered vegetables: avocado, eggplant, cucumber, olives, peppers, and okra.*

- Organic and pastured chicken, eggs, beef, turkey, lamb, venison, and organic unprocessed deli meats

- Healthy seafood includes herring, salmon (wild), and sardines. Consider more variety in noncontaminated seafood by purchasing seafood produced from RAS fisheries. See page 54 for more information.

- Some dairy products: Butter, ghee, and cultured foods such as kefir and yogurt (probiotic)

- Low-mold nuts and seeds: These include almonds, coconut, flaxseed, hazelnuts, pumpkin seeds, sunflower seeds, and chia seeds.

- Herbs, spices, and condiments: These include apple cider vinegar, basil, black pepper, cinnamon, cloves, coconut aminos, dill, garlic, ginger, oregano, paprika, rosemary, salt, thyme, and turmeric.

- Healthy fats and oils: Coconut oil (virgin), flax oil, olive oil, avocado oil, and sesame oil

- Grain substitutes, known as pseudo grains, include quinoa (legume family), amaranth (beet family), and buckwheat (buckwheat family). Other grain substitutes include flours from almonds, hazelnuts, coconut, macadamia, arrowroot, hemp, and chickpea/garbanzo. Some may tolerate sourdough bread. Most of these have high protein and are low in starch; however, there may be individuals who may not tolerate any or most of the substitutes.

- Mushrooms (shiitake, maitake, reishi, and others) may be included. They are fungi that are beneficial to immunity and considered anti-yeast. Some experts recommend avoiding all mushrooms. Again, this is a food that some individuals may need to avoid.

- Fermented foods that are beneficial include apple cider vinegar, sauerkraut (homemade), kimchi, fermented vegetables, and young coconut kefir. They improve the microbiota with friendly bacteria and friendly yeast that protect against yeast overgrowth. According to Julie Matthews, CNC nutrition consultant and author of *Nourishing Hope for Autism*, individuals who have lab evidence of IgG reactions to yeast may not tolerate any fermented foods and should proceed cautiously.

- Nutritional yeast may be included because unlike brewer's yeast and baker's yeast, it does not contribute to yeast infections/overgrowth because it is derived from a different species that has been deactivated. Again, individual reactions may vary.

- Consumption of sufficient water is essential. We recommend half the body weight in pounds as the number of ounces of fluids to consume (water, herbal teas, and coconut water).

WHAT SUGAR SUBSTITUTES ARE RECOMMENDED?

Stevia is recommended as a substitute for sugar. Stevia (organic) comes from the *Stevia rebaudiana* plant. Many stevia brands contain maltodextrin or dextrose. Read labels and try to find a brand made of 100% pure stevia leaf. Xylitol is often recommended because it has a low glycemic index. Xylitol is a natural sugar alcohol, found in raspberries, oats, mushrooms, and other foods. Commercially available xylitol is typically derived from corn; however, non-GMO corn sources are widely available. While there are health benefits from xylitol (reduced tooth decay, improved dry mouth problems), it is not digested in the gut and can ferment and create an unfavorable environment in some individuals including those with yeast overgrowth. Xylitol can also destroy some good gut bacteria and contribute to dysbiosis. Symptoms from excess xylitol include gas, bloating, and diarrhea.

INGREDIENTS ON LABELS THAT MEAN SUGAR

According to The Candida Diet website, www.thecandidadiet.com, the following can indicate that a product contains sugar:

- barley malt
- Barbados sugar
- beet sugar
- brown sugar
- buttered syrup
- cane juice
- cane sugar
- caramel
- carob syrup
- castor sugar
- confectioners' sugar
- corn syrup
- corn syrup solids
- date sugar
- dehydrated cane juice
- demerara sugar
- dextran
- dextrose
- diastatic malt
- diatase
- ethyl maltol
- free flowing brown sugars
- fructose
- fruit juice
- fruit juice concentrate
- galactose
- glucose
- glucose solids
- golden sugar
- golden syrup
- grape sugar
- high fructose corn syrup
- honey
- icing sugar
- invert sugar
- lactose
- malt
- maltodextrin
- maltose
- malt syrup
- mannitol
- maple syrup
- molasses
- muscovado
- panocha
- powdered sugar
- raw sugar
- refiner's syrup
- rice syrup
- sorbitol
- sorghum syrup
- sucrose
- sugar (granulated)
- treacle
- turbinado sugar
- yellow sugar

WHAT FOODS ARE HELPFUL FOR FIGHTING YEAST?

Coconut oil contains lauric acid and caprylic acid, which have anti-fungal effects. Also helpful is young coconut kefir. Olive oil contains oleuropein, which also has anti-fungal properties. Other foods reported to have anti-yeast benefits include garlic, onions, and rutabaga.

WHAT OTHER INTERVENTIONS ARE HELPFUL REGARDING YEAST?

It is ideal to have the guidance of a health care practitioner with experience in treating intestinal yeast overgrowth when pursuing these supportive treatments.

Providing beneficial bacteria through the use of probiotic supplements helps to rebalance the intestinal flora. Specific Carbohydrate Diet (SCD) legal probiotics should be used and appropriate digestive enzymes as needed. Biotin is also an important nutrient. Although it is produced in the gut by specific gut microbiota,

that production is reduced significantly by antibiotic destruction of biotin-producing microbes. Biotin maintains stability in the gut and reduces the overgrowth of pathogenic yeast. It is also important to systemic immunity and epithelial health.

The following have been documented as effective anti-yeast agents: oregano, myrrh, and lavender oils in addition to Pau D'arco tea, astragalus, olive leaf, black walnut, neem, and garlic concentrates.

Your health care practitioner may recommend antifungal medications.

It is also important to have daily, healthy stools in order to eliminate bacterial and yeast toxins from the body. If there are not daily stools, speak with your health care practitioner about using magnesium and vitamin C.

It is important to introduce new supplements or special foods one at a time in order to determine if they are helpful or not. Each person is unique. Regardless of what you may read about suggestions for resolving yeast overgrowth, if your health steadily declines, please rethink what you are consuming. The body does not lie!

If the anti-yeast diet and other recommendations described here are not sufficiently successful in resolving yeast/candida overgrowth, consider the Body Ecology Diet by Donna Gates, which is more restricted in allowable foods. The strategy also includes combining foods in a compatible manner in order to improve digestion, maintain a healthy acid/alkaline pH for body balance, support detoxification, and individualize the diet. It is important to have guidance from a nutritional professional with expertise in this diet. More information is available through Body Ecology: www.bodyecology.com

ANTI-YEAST (ANTI-CANDIDA) DIETS   Chapter 7

What Is Yeast/Candida? Yeast is a normal fungus in the intestine and *Candida albicans* is the most common yeast. The problem is the overgrowth of yeast, which produces toxins that cause damage.

Avoid: Consider the SCD diet first; if not sufficient, add this anti-yeast diet:

- All sugars and sweeteners (except stevia); high sugar fruits (bananas, dates, grapes, mangoes, raisins, and ripe fruit)
- Fruit juices and sweet veggie juice; starchy veggies (potatoes, yams, corn, beets, peas, parsnips, and beans)
- Processed foods; deli meats
- Grains (wheat, oat, barley, rye, spelt, kamut, corn, millet, rice, sorghum, and bulgur)
- Most dairy (especially moldy cheeses); moldy nuts (peanuts, cashews, pecans, walnuts, and pistachios)

Why Is the Diet Needed? Yeast overgrowth from intestinal microbiota imbalance, known as dysbiosis. Antibiotic use and/or poor fiber intake increase yeast overgrowth. Yeast can produce inflammatory chemicals damaging to the intestinal lining.

Symptoms the Diet May Help:

- Abdominal bloating; loose or smelly stools; sugar cravings; fatigue; and dizziness
- Rashes; thrush; diaper rash; red ring around the anus; and rectal and vaginal itching
- Silly or inappropriate laughing; inattention; "brain fog"; and mood and behavior changes

Diet Includes:

- Proteins: healthy seafood; organic pastured source meats, poultry, and eggs
- Butter; ghee; organic, homemade yogurt; and kefir
- Low mold nuts and seeds (almonds, coconut, flaxseed, hazelnuts, pumpkin seeds, sunflower, and chia seeds)
- Non-starch veggies, low sugar fruits, fermented foods, grain substitutes, and healthy oils
- Spices and herbs: wide variety, many of which are also anti-inflammatory
- Recirculating Aquaculture System technologies, or low-toxin seafood (salmon, mackerel, lake trout, herring, and sardines)

Resources:

- The Yeast Connection: www.yeastconnection.com
- The Candida Diet: www.Thecandidadiet.com
- Body Ecology (Donna Gates): www.bodyecology.com
- *Digestive Wellness:* 4th edition, by Elizabeth Lipski
- *Feast Without Yeast* by Bruce Semon
- *Cooking to Heal* and *Nourishing Hope with Autism* by Julie Matthews

CHAPTER 8

The Low Oxalate Diet (LOD)

WHAT ARE OXALATES?

Oxalates are organic acids that come from three main sources: diet, fungi/yeast, and the body's own metabolism. Oxalates are particularly high in soy products, spinach, beets, chocolate, peanuts, wheat bran, tea, cashews, pecans, almonds, and berries. Plants make oxalates to protect themselves against infection or from being consumed.

WHY ARE OXALATES A PROBLEM?

Normally, oxalates are metabolized by bacteria in the intestine or bound by fecal calcium and eliminated via the stool. In the presence of insufficient calcium, imbalanced intestinal flora, or altered intestinal permeability (known as "leaky gut"), oxalates can be absorbed from the gut into the bloodstream.

When oxalates are high in the blood, they can combine with calcium and form crystals that deposit in tissues and cause severe pain. Crystals may deposit in bones, joints, blood vessels, lungs, and brain. They may also form kidney stones. The crystals may cause tissue damage and are also thought to lead to inflammation in the tissues.

Excessive oxalates have a number of negative effects on the body. These include:

- Formation of kidney stones

- Pain

- Inflammation

- Oxidative stress

- Depletion of glutathione, a potent, sulfur rich, antioxidant that is already deficient in a number of children with autism

- Negative effects on the function of mitochondria, the energy machinery in cells

- Interference with biotin, an important B vitamin

- Interference with sulfation, a process that is important for detoxification

Oxalates may be a particular problem for individuals with autism. According to data reported by Dr. William Shaw at Great Plains Laboratory, oxalates in the urine are much higher in children with autism than in neurotypical children.

Research has shown that a subset of individuals with autism have differences in the pathways that make glutathione, which is critical in sulfation and detoxification. Excessive oxalates affect glutathione production and interfere with sulfation. Therefore, it is possible that oxalates may have even more of a negative effect in individuals with autism. Individuals with hypomethylation problems may also experience sulfation deficits.

WHAT INCREASES OXALATES OR OXALATE ABSORPTION?

Factors that can increase oxalates include:

- Diets high in high oxalate foods

- Insufficient sulfate and impaired sulfation, which are needed to rid oxalates

- Excessive intestinal yeast (especially *Aspergillus*)

- Genetic disorders called hyperoxalurias

Factors that can increase oxalate *absorption* include:

- Insufficient calcium in diet

- Insufficient sulfur in diet

- Excessive fat intake in diet if fatty acids are poorly absorbed due to deficiency of bile salts. These free fatty acids can bind calcium, leaving less calcium available to bind to oxalates.

- Altered intestinal permeability (also known as "leaky gut")

- Vitamin A deficiency

- Deficiencies of magnesium and zinc

WHAT KIND OF SYMPTOMS CAN OXALATES CAUSE?

Oxalates can cause a variety of types of pain including:

- Urinary pain, including pain with urination or pain from passage of kidney stones
- Genital pain (especially vulvar pain)
- Headaches
- Joint or muscle pain
- Gastrointestinal pain
- Eye pain

WHEN SHOULD THIS DIET BE CONSIDERED?

We recommend that a trial elimination of oxalates be considered in a child with the following symptoms that have not responded to traditional medical diagnosis and treatment:

- Extreme pain with urination
- Eye-poking behaviors not explained by visual loss or other clear ophthalmologic reason
- Self-injurious behavior (SIB), especially in a nonverbal child, in whom the cause of SIB is not clear
- Kidney stones (Calcium oxalate stones are the most common type of kidney stone.)
- Worsening of symptoms or behavior when on the Specific Carbohydrate Diet (since nut flours are high in oxalates)

WHAT IS A LOW OXALATE DIET AND HOW IS IT DONE?

The initial step is to remove foods that are high in oxalates. Then, if necessary, medium oxalate foods can also be removed. Oxalates should be removed gradually from the diet, as some children will have worsened pain or discomfort if they are removed too rapidly.

WHICH FOODS ARE AVOIDED?

Oxalates are high in almost all seeds and nuts. Foods especially high in oxalates include soy, spinach, beets, chocolate, peanuts, wheat bran, tea, cashews, pecans, almonds, and berries. See the table on page 108 for detailed information. The table includes very high and high oxalate foods; foods highest in oxalates are indicated by an asterisk.

Most flour substitutes for gluten are high oxalate, but rice flour, coconut flour, and pumpkin seed flours are not. Most milk substitutes are high in oxalates, such as brown rice milk, almond milk, and potato milk. Coconut and goat milk are acceptable substitutes.

It is interesting to note that the oxalate content of some foods varies based on the form it is in. For example, some are higher in oxalates when eaten steamed, but lower when eaten raw or boiled. Tomato paste, sauce, and purée (canned) are high in oxalates but fresh tomatoes are medium. Lemon peel is high in oxalates but lemons and lemon juice are low. Lime peel is high in oxalates but lime juice is low. In some lists, zucchini is listed as high in oxalates while on others, it is very low. We would recommend avoiding zucchini initially until it is clear whether your child reacts to it. Other factors that can affect the oxalate content of food include growth season (whether plants are picked early or late in a season), nutrients in the soil, and the length of time the plant is grown.

FOODS HIGH IN OXALATES

LEGUMES, NUTS, AND SEEDS	GRAINS	VEGETABLES	FRUITS	OTHERS
Almonds *	Amaranth	Beets *	Blackberries *	Chocolate *, cocoa powder *, chocolate milk
Black beans *	Buckwheat *	Broccoli (steamed)	Currants	
Cashews *	Durum flour *	Brussels sprouts (steamed)	Dates	V8 Juice
Filberts (Hazelnuts) *	Kamut	Carrots *	Dewberries	Sesame oil *
Macadamia nuts*	Millet *	Celery *	Gooseberries	Spices/Herbs: Cinnamon, oregano, black pepper, turmeric*
Navy beans *	Rye *	Chard *	Kiwi *	
Peanuts *, peanut butter *	Wheat *	Chili peppers	Lemon peel	Sweeteners: Date sugar, stevia *
Pecans *		Collard greens (steamed)	Lime peel	
Pine nuts *		Dandelion greens	Oranges and orange peel	
Pinto beans *		Okra *	Persimmons	
Pistachio nuts		Olives (black and green) *	Raspberries:	
Sesame seeds *		Potatoes *	black *, red	
Soy, soybeans, * and soy milk *		Rhubarb *	Star fruit *	
Tahini *		Sorrel		
Walnuts *		Spinach *		
		Sweet potatoes *		
		Tomato paste, purée, or sauce (canned)		
		Yellow dock		
		Zucchini (see previous page for more information)		

Indicates foods that are very high in oxalates.
Source: The Autism Oxalate Project

WHICH FOODS ARE ALLOWED ON A LOW OXALATE DIET?

Foods that are very low in oxalates and allowed on the diet include:

- Meats (except cured meats), fish, and dairy products
- Fruits: apples, avocados, cherries, citrus, cranberries, melons (cantaloupe, honeydew, watermelon), seedless grapes, peaches, and plums
- Vegetables: asparagus, cauliflower, cucumbers, lettuce (iceberg and romaine), mushrooms, onions (yellow and white), radishes, red sweet peppers, squash (acorn and yellow), turnips, and water chestnuts
- Beverages: spring and filtered water, chamomile tea, ginger ale, apple juice, and apple cider
- Chocolate: white chocolate
- Grains: white and wild rice; barley
- Herbs and spices: basil, cilantro, mustard, nutmeg, white pepper, saffron, tarragon, vanilla, and salt
- Condiments: mustard, mayonnaise, and vinegar
- Nuts, peas, and seeds: coconut, black-eyed peas, green peas, yellow split peas, and flaxseeds
- Fats and oils: butter and vegetable oils including olive, and safflower
- Sweets and sweeteners: sugar (white), maple syrup, corn syrup, and honey

WHAT ELSE MAY HELP?

Good hydration and daily stools are both important to help promote elimination of oxalates. Citrus juices can also be helpful in oxalate elimination. Taking a calcium citrate supplement 20 minutes before meals containing high oxalate foods may be helpful. Calcium binds oxalate in the intestine, which prevents it from being absorbed so that it can be eliminated in the stool. It is important to provide additional minerals such as magnesium and zinc, which can also bind with oxalates to be eliminated in the stool. Probiotics, prebiotics, and biotin support can be helpful by providing sufficient beneficial bacteria that can metabolize oxalates in the intestine. Vitamin B6 may also be helpful by supporting the enzyme that degrades oxalates. The guidance of a health practitioner with experience with the low oxalate diet is recommended for determining appropriate amounts of these supportive nutrients and supplements.

For a summary of the Low Oxalate Diet, see page 110.

What Are Oxalates? Oxalates are in foods, in fungi and yeast, and made by the body. Plants make oxalates to protect against infection and consumption.

Avoid:

- Nuts, seeds, and legumes/beans: almonds; black beans; cashews; hazelnuts; macadamia; navy beans; peanuts; pecans; pine nuts, pinto beans; pistachios; poppy seeds; sesame/tahini; soy; safflower and sunflower seeds; walnuts
- Grains: amaranth; buckwheat; durum flour; kamut; millet; rye; wheat
- Fruits: berries; citrus (orange, lemon, and lime peels), currants; dates; kiwi; persimmons; star fruit
- Vegetables: beets; broccoli; Brussels sprouts; carrots; celery; chard; chili peppers; greens; okra; olives; potatoes; rhubarb; sorrel; spinach; sweet potatoes; tomatoes; V8 juice; yellow dock; zucchini
- Spices/herbs: black pepper; cinnamon; oregano; turmeric
- Other: chocolate; sesame oil; sweeteners (date sugar, stevia); some teas

Why Is the Diet Needed? Problems occur when there are insufficient good bacteria (microbiota) to metabolize oxalates and prevent the overgrowth of yeast. Inadequate fecal calcium impairs elimination of oxalates. Oxalate crystals can damage the GI tract, cross into the bloodstream, and damage tissues, causing inflammation and pain.

Symptoms the Diet May Help:

- Kidney stone formation; pain; inflammation; urinary and genital pain; headaches; joint and muscle pain; digestive tract inflammation; eye pain; and self-injurious behavior (common in autism)
- Oxalates cause oxidative stress; depletion of the antioxidant glutathione; poor energy metabolism; depletion of biotin; and interference with sulfation/detoxification

Diet Includes:

- Pastured meats; poultry; eggs; fish; cheese and milk products (if tolerated and milk permitted)
- Seeds and legumes; flaxseeds; coconut; peas; black-eyed peas; green peas; and yellow split peas
- Vegetables: asparagus; broccoli; cauliflower; cucumbers; lettuce; mushrooms; onions; radishes; squash; red sweet peppers; turnips; and water chestnuts
- Fruit: apples; avocados; cherries; citrus; cranberries; grapes (seedless); melons; peaches; and plums
- White/wild rice
- Herbs/spices: basil, cilantro; mustard; nutmeg; white pepper; saffron; tarragon; Vanilla; and salt
- Fats/oils: olive; butter; and safflower

Resources:

- Autism Oxalate Project (Susan Owens): www.lowoxalate.info
- *Low Oxalate Fresh and Fast Cookbook* by Melinda Keen

Other Helpful Diets:

- Anti-Inflammatory Diet
- FODMAP Diet
- Rotation Diet

The Anti-Inflammatory Diet

INFLAMMATION, IMMUNITY, AND AUTOIMMUNITY

Inflammation in the brain and the gut is a hallmark of autism and an important focus in research. There are indications that inflammation of the brain can be an issue in ADHD as well. Inflammation is part of the body's immune response. It is an important biological response defense mechanism in the body's attempt to deal with damage, irritants, and pathogens. Inflammation is a beneficial and protective response when there is an injury because it is critical to wound healing. For external problems, it is recognized by pain, redness, swelling, heat, and sometimes immobility in the area involved. When inflammation is internal, only some of the signs may be noticed: generalized aching, fatigue, digestive problems, and skin conditions. Diagnoses of inflammatory bowel conditions or autoimmunity are signs that chronic inflammation has worsened. Acute inflammation, which is obvious, starts rapidly and becomes more severe quickly, lasting for days to weeks. Chronic inflammation is problematic and may start quickly or slowly and last for months to years. It is the immune system gone rogue and can be caused by or aggravated by viruses; bacteria; fungi; toxins; foreign bodies remaining in the system; medications; foods and food components; and autoimmune antibodies. The autoimmune-damaging antibody attacks against the body organs and systems, including the neurological system, can profoundly affect function. In autism, the maternal antibodies to the developing fetal brain can be measured. They may be initiated by the culprits listed and also from brain inflammation. The effects of the autoimmune attack can include changes in the individual's function, cognition, mood, behavior and self-injury.

The concepts of cumulative effects and "total load" can apply to the neuroinflammatory responses in autism, and to a much lesser extent, ADHD. "Leaky membranes" are also known to play a role: the "leaky gut" allows foreign molecules from poor digestion and exogenous sources to cross into the bloodstream, and then the "leaky blood brain barrier" allows them to enter the brain.

Why do some respond so poorly while others are unaffected? The answer lies in "environmental modification of gene expression." This involves the underlying genetics of the individual and how the environment affects them, both positively and negatively. Environment includes everything from the womb on—diet, lifestyle, toxin exposures, medications, stressors, etc. There are gene variants that can increase susceptibility to environmental challenges, which can then trigger the cascade of negative influences. In other words, we are all unique in our genetic makeup and our environmental experiences.

WHAT FOODS, FOOD COMPONENTS, AND ADDITIVES CAN CAUSE OR INCREASE INFLAMMATION?

The problem additives are described in chapter 3. They include artificial additives, preservatives, sweeteners, flavoring agents, and coloring. There are foods listed in this section that are well known to be inflammatory. In addition, there are food components that can be inflammatory, such as oxalates, phenols, salicylates, fructans, polyols, lectins, purines, glutamates, amines, and others. Those with autoimmunity and/or "leaky gut" problems are more likely to be sensitive to many of the culprits in inflammation. Observe the responses and adjust the diet changes accordingly.

NIGHTSHADES

The nightshade plant family known as Solanaceae includes edible nightshade vegetables, harmless flowers, trees, and toxic herbs. The nightshades contain a natural group of substances called alkaloids; the most notable in the nightshade vegetables are solanine, capsaicin, and nicotine. High intakes of foods with solanine and the other alkaloids can disrupt cell membranes and negatively affect mitochondrial potassium channels. This varies according to the individual and the amount consumed.

REACTIONS: All of the nightshade vegetables have benefits such as nutrient density and antioxidant effects; however, they also have alkaloids (which are pro-inflammatory) and some are high in pro-inflammatory phenols and/or salicylates. In addition to causing inflammation, the alkaloids can irritate the gastrointestinal system, increase headaches, inflame

muscles and joints, and in severe cases of excess consumption, cause nausea, vomiting, and diarrhea. It is not always easy to identify reactions because they may not show up for several days.

SOLANINE is found primarily in potatoes (white inside) and solanine-like tomatine in tomatoes. The green leaves of these plants, the green sprouts on potatoes, and green tomatoes are highly concentrated in solanine (potato) and tomatine (tomato). Sunlight increases the solanine in potatoes.

CAPSAICIN is the active ingredient in hot peppers, often noted for its anti-inflammatory effects; however, as an alkaloid, it can increase inflammation.

NICOTINE, found primarily in tobacco, is also present in all parts of the nightshade vegetables.

What Affects the Concentration of Solanine in Nightshades?

- Cooking in water lowers the alkaloid content of nightshade foods by about 40 to 50%.

- As the plants ripen, the solanine/tomatine content declines.

- Green and sprouted spots on potatoes should be discarded or removed before cooking.

- Sunlight exposure increases solanine content of potatoes. Keep them in a dark drawer. Avoid consuming mushy potatoes.

Tips on Reducing Inflammation via Nightshade Avoidance

- Absolute avoidance is the best test.

- Check all labels. Prepared foods often contain potato starch or tomato paste. Relish may contain peppers or paprika. Any time you see "spices" listed under ingredients, the food may contain paprika or pepper.

FOODS TO AVOID IF INFLAMMATION IS PRESENT

- **NIGHTSHADES**

  - Potatoes (white inside)—especially green potato skins, sprouts

  - Tomatoes—especially green

  - Eggplant

  - Okra

  - Peppers, cayenne, capsicum, paprika

  - Tomatillos

  - Sorrel

  - Gooseberries

  - Ground cherries

  - Pepino melons

  - Tobacco exposure

- Also avoid the following foods that contain alkaloids similar to solanine: blueberries, Goji berries, and huckleberries

- **COMMERCIALLY PROCESSED FOODS** including grains and meats and contaminated seafood

- **ARTIFICIAL ADDITIVES**, preservatives, sweeteners, taste enhancers, artificial flavoring and coloring agents, and excitotoxins

- **PARTIALLY HYDROGENATED TRANS-FATTY ACIDS:** These are mutant plastic fatty acids that promote inflammation; harden cell membranes; interfere with essential fatty acid metabolism, cell function, reproduction, fetal development, brain structure and development, breast milk quality, and metabolic enzymes; and increase the risk for inflammation, immune disorders, cancers, and autism. The commercial fatty acids certainly increase the total load in ADHD and autism via the detrimental changes in brain structure and function.

- **GENETICALLY MODIFIED ORGANISMS**—GMO foods

- **SUGARS AND A GLYCEMIC (SUGAR-RAISING) DIET** affect immunity and contribute to the "total load." This includes sodas and caffeine, which can raise glucose easily.

- **GLUTEN** grains (wheat, oat, barley, rye, spelt, kamut, farro, durhum and bulgur) are major culprits in inflammation and autoimmunity. For some individuals, all of the grains and even the pseudo-grains (amaranth, quinoa, and buckwheat) can be inflammatory. Information on identifying sources and substitutes can be found in chapter 4.

- **ANIMAL MILK PRODUCTS,** especially from cows from industrial dairies that produce the problematic A1 milk, are also culprits in inflammation and autoimmunity for many individuals. See chapter 4 for detailed information on identifying sources and substitutes.

- **SOY** is not easily handled by many individuals. Reactions can include inflammation. For information on sources and substitutes, see chapter 4.

- **CORN, ESPECIALLY GMO CORN**, is pro-inflammatory for many people.

- **NUTS** are common reaction culprits. Seeds are far less of a problem.

- **LEGUMES** can cause problems due to their lectin content. Lectins can increase inflammation and damage the gut barrier. Lectins are reduced in legumes (and grains) by soaking, cooking, and fermenting.

- **ANY REACTION-PROVOKING FOODS** should be avoided. Reactions to foods can increase inflammation. Note that most of the culprits described in this book (e.g., gluten, casein, soy, nuts, corn, phenols, oxalates, salicylates, lectins, and purines) are pro-inflammatory. Even if the food is listed as healthy, if there is a significant reaction, it must be avoided. Make sure you are reacting to the food and not the additives and/or contaminants in the food before eliminating it.

FOODS TO REDUCE INFLAMMATION

Also see chapter 3.

- Choose organic foods that have the USDA Organic seal.
- Oils: olive, avocado, and omega-3 fish or krill oils
- Pastured poultry, lamb, pork, venison, eggs, and beef if tolerated
- Bone broths from pastured animals
- For omega-3 fatty acid sources, use high-quality non-polluted seafood or safest choices of low toxin seafood: salmon, mackerel, lake trout, herring, and sardines.
- White rice (not brown rice)
- A2 milk if tolerated (not A1 milk)
- Based upon the elimination diet(s) being used, include the following as tolerated:
  - Non-nightshade vegetables
  - Fruits
  - Garlic, onions, leeks, and scallions
  - Substitute sweet potato and squash for grains, pseudo grains, and legumes (beans and peanuts).

METHODS TO REDUCE INFLAMMATORY EFFECTS OF CULPRIT FOODS

- Cooking in water or pressure cooking
- Fermenting foods
- Sprouting foods
- Peeling and de-seeding fruits and vegetables

WHAT ELSE CAN BE DONE?

Omega-3 seafood sources are important in counteracting inflammation. Consider probiotics and biotin to support a healthy microbiota, nutrients to support a healthy gut barrier, and nutrients specific to the individual's nutritional needs.

What Is Inflammation? Chronic inflammation is not as obvious as short-term acute injury. It may develop slowly and can last for months to years. Contributors include pathogens; toxins; foreign bodies; foods; food components; GMO foods; trans-fatty acids; and autoimmune antibodies. Plants have more inflammatory components than animal products. Plants that are nightshades, alkaloids, and lectins are among the most inflammatory foods. Oxalates, phenols, salicylates, phytases, FODMAPs, and purines also contribute to inflammation. Individuals will vary on reactions to these food components.

Avoid:

- Nightshades/solanine/tomatine and alkaloid foods: white potatoes; tomatoes; tomatillos; eggplant; okra; gooseberries; ground cherries; pepino melons; capsicum plants (bell peppers; cayenne peppers; and paprika); and tobacco (nicotine) exposure; blueberries; Goji berries; huckleberries

- High lectin foods: legumes (beans, soy, peas, lentils, peanuts), corn; nuts; seeds; squash; grains; and some fruits; and some seafood sources

- High lectin/inflammatory spices: allspice, caraway, cardamom, juniper berry, marjoram, nutmeg, peppermint, white pepper, pink peppercorns, and vanilla bean

- Commercially processed foods; artificial additives; GMO foods; trans-fatty acids; sugars; gluten; other grains;
  A1 cow milk products

- Other pro-inflammatory groups to limit/avoid if helpful: oxalates; phenols; glutamates, phytates; purines; and/or salicylates

Why Is the Diet Needed? Chronic inflammation of the gut and brain is a hallmark in autism and known to be an issue in ADHD. This involves "leaky gut" and "leaky blood brain barrier." In autism, maternal antibodies against the fetus can contribute to inflammation. Removing pro-inflammatory foods can reduce the inflammation and allow for healing and improvement.

Symptoms the Diet May Help: Digestive problems including "leaky gut"; brain inflammation, which increases the risk for behavior changes; poor cognition and function; self-injury; mood disorders; and joint and muscle pain.

Diet Includes:

- Organic, nutrient-dense foods and healthy oils (olive, avocado, coconut, and omega-3 fish and krill oils)

- Pastured animal source foods (meats, poultry, eggs)

- If seafood is tolerated, use high-quality, nonpolluted seafood from Recirculating Aquaculture System technologies, or low-toxin seafood, salmon, and sardines being the lowest in seafood lectins.

- Based upon the other elimination diets being followed, include these as tolerated:
  -Grains—well cooked
  -Non-nightshade, low-lectin vegetables and fruits: asparagus; avocado; bok choy; broccoli; Brussels sprouts; carrots; cauliflower; celery; garlic; leeks; leafy greens; onions; mushrooms; olives; pumpkin; scallions; sweet potatoes; apples; some berries; and citrus (not the skins)

- Spices: include a wide variety of non-nightshade low-lectin spices; basil, bay leaves, chives, cilantro, cinnamon, cloves, rosemary, saffron, thyme, turmeric, and more.

Resources:
- The Green Farmacy Garden: www.thegreenfarmacygarden.com (James Duke, Ph.D.)
- Dr. Duke's Phytochemical Database: https://phytochem.nal.usda.gov/phytochem
- Arthritis Nightshades Research Foundation: http://www.noarthritis.com/news.html
- Lectin information: *The Plant Paradox* by Steven Gundry

The FODMAP Diet

WHAT ARE FODMAPs?

FODMAPs are short-chain carbohydrates (a type of sugar), that if poorly digested, can ferment in the gut to cause digestive distress. These FODMAPs are found in many natural foods as well as in food additives. The Low FODMAP diet is a highly restrictive diet, designed to temporarily avoid the amount of FODMAPs consumed. Nutritional supplements are included in the treatment protocol in order to maintain overall health and restore the digestive tract to optimal health.

F—FERMENTABLE. The gut bacteria ferment undigested carbohydrates (oligosaccharides, disaccharides, monosaccharides, and polyols) and produce gas, which can cause gastrointestinal discomfort and symptoms.

O—OLIGOSACCHARIDES. Fructans, fructo-oligosaccharides (FOS), and galacto-oligosaccharides (GOS)

D—DISACCHARIDES. Lactose and other low fructose double sugars (glucose, dextrose, and palm sugar)

M—MONOSACCHARIDES. Fructose

P—POLYOLS. Sorbitol and mannitol, xylitol, and isomalt

OLIGOSACCHARIDES include foods that are high in *fructans* (FOS, inulin, barley, rye, wheat, shallots, spring onion [white part], onion [Spanish, brown, white, and onion powder], leeks, garlic, Jerusalem/Globe artichokes and GOS legumes [chickpeas, bortolotti beans, kidney beans, and baked beans]).

DISACCHARIDES include foods that are high in *lactose* (soft unripened cheeses such as ricotta, cottage cheese, cream cheese, and mascarpone), yogurt, milk powder, evaporated milk, condensed milk, dairy desserts, custard, ice cream, and milk.

MONOSACCHARIDES include foods that are high in excess *fructose* (high fructose corn syrup, watermelon, pear, mango, apples, and honey).

POLYOLS are found in foods (mushrooms, prunes, plums, pears, nectarines, apricots, and apples) and additives including sugar alcohols (isomalt, maltitol, xylitol, mannitol, and sorbitol), which are found in artificial sweeteners and chewing gum.

HOW FODMAPS AFFECT DIGESTIVE HEALTH

These saccharides and polyols, if digested poorly, can ferment in the lower part of the large intestine, drawing water into the bowel and producing carbon dioxide, methane, and/or hydrogen gas. This causes the bowel to stretch and expand, contributing to bloating and abdominal distension. Unhealthy digestive bacteria take advantage of the situation and interact with FODMAPs in the gut, causing many symptoms such as bloating, gas, and pain.

SYMPTOMS THAT INDICATE THE FODMAP DIET MAY HELP

Prevalent signs include gastrointestinal symptoms occurring with most meals and snacks. Symptoms typically include recurrent bloating, burping, gas, cramps, diarrhea, constipation, abdominal distension, undigested food material in the stool, and abnormally loud bowel sounds. Motility problems can include delayed gastric emptying (gastroparesis), which leaves a sense of fullness initially and far beyond the meal, and also increased gastric emptying, which contributes to a feeling of fullness, abdominal cramping or pain, nausea or vomiting, severe diarrhea, sweating, flushing, light-headedness, and rapid heartbeat. The more symptoms present, the more likely there are problems with the foods listed in the avoids. Among the most problematic are garlic, onions, leeks, and scallions.

The diet can be particularly helpful in those diagnosed with irritable bowel syndrome (IBS). However, there are many other conditions for which the diet may be useful. Other forms of functional gastrointestinal disorders (FGID) affecting the esophagus to the rectum may benefit. Inflammatory bowel diseases (IBD) are chronic inflammatory conditions in the digestive tract. Ulcerative colitis and Crohn's disease are the most common. Small intestinal bacterial overgrowth (SIBO) has been noted as a condition in which the bacteria in the small intestine are excessive. It is the lower bowel (large intestine) that contains most of the good bacteria that make up the microbiome. Risk factors for SIBO include intestinal infections, chronic antacid use, immunodeficiency syndromes, celiac disease, gastroparesis, and aging. Other conditions that may benefit from the diet include autoimmune conditions, chronic migraines, and even eczema.

FOODS TO AVOID AND INCLUDE
Vegetables and Legumes

- **AVOID HIGH FODMAP**—Asparagus, artichoke, beans (black, broad, kidney, lima, and soya), beets, bok choy, broccoli, Brussels sprouts, cauliflower, fennel, garlic, Jerusalem artichoke, leeks, mushrooms, onions, savoy, scallions/spring onions (white part), shallot, snow peas, and sugar snap peas

- **INCLUDE LOW FODMAP**—Alfalfa, artichoke hearts, arugula, bamboo shoots, beans (green), bean sprouts, beets, bell pepper (capsicum, red, and green), cabbage (common, red), carrot, celery (2 inch [5 cm] stalk), chickpeas (1/4 cup [60 g] max), chives, corn (1/2 cup [80 g] max), cucumber, eggplant/aubergine, endive, ginger, green beans, kale, lettuce (butter, iceberg, and rocket), legumes (most), olives, parsnip, potato, pumpkin, scallions/spring onions (green part), squash (small servings), sweet potato, turnip, yam, and zucchini

Fruits

- **AVOID HIGH FODMAP**—Apples, apricots, avocados, bananas (ripe), blackberries, dried fruit, cherries, figs, mangoes, nectarines, papaya (dried), peaches, pears, plums, pomegranate, prunes, raisins, sultanas, tamarillo, watermelon, and canned fruit in fruit juice

- **INCLUDE LOW FODMAP**—Bananas (unripe), berries (blueberry, boysenberry, cranberry, raspberry, strawberry), cantaloupe, citrus (clementine, lemon, lime, orange, tangelo, and tangerine), currant, grapes, guava, kiwi, melons (honeydew and cantaloupe), papaya (paw paw), passion fruit, pineapple, and rhubarb

Dairy and Alternatives

- **HIGH FODMAP**—Buttermilk, cow's milk and cow milk products, soy milk (made from whole soybean), cheeses (soft, unripened: cottage cheese, cream cheese, mascarpone, and ricotta cheese)

- **INCLUDE LOW FODMAP**—Almond milk, butter and ghee, cheese (hard cheeses, brie, and Camembert), coconut milk, gelato, sorbet, hemp milk, lactose-free milk, oat milk (30 ml max), rice milk (200 ml max), soy milk (made from soy protein), sour cream, and yogurt (homemade and lactose-free)

Protein Sources, Meat, and Substitutes

- **HIGH FODMAP**—Bone cartilage broths, chorizo, sausages, some processed meats, and some marinated meat, poultry, and seafood (check ingredients)
- **INCLUDE LOW FODMAP**—Bacon, beef, bone broths, cold cuts (ham and turkey breast), eggs, plain cooked meats (beef, chicken, lamb, pork, and poultry), plain cooked seafood, tempeh, and tofu (firm)

Plant Source Protein: Legumes, Nuts, and Seeds

- **HIGH FODMAP**—Baked beans, chickpeas, hummus dip, kidney (red) beans, lentils, navy, white, haricot, and split peas; Nuts: cashews, pistachios, and higher intakes of almonds (>20), hazelnuts (80), pine nuts (1/2 cup/ 70 g), pumpkin seeds (1/2 cup/80 g), sesame seeds (1/2 cup, 72 g), and sunflower seeds (1/2 cup/70 g)
- **INCLUDE LOW FODMAP**—Lentils (brown, green, and red); Nuts: almonds (15 max), chestnuts, coconuts, hazelnuts, macadamia, peanuts, pecans (15 max), pine nuts, poppy seeds, pumpkin seeds, sesame seeds, sunflower seeds, and walnuts

Breads, Cereal, Grains, and Pasta Products

- **AVOID HIGH FODMAP**—Barley (bread, cereal, and pasta), biscuits, bran, breakfast cereals, couscous, gnocchi, granola, muesli, muffins, rye (bread, cereal, and pasta), semolina, snack products, spelt, wheat foods (bread, cereal, and pasta)

- **INCLUDE LOW FODMAP**—Arrowroot, biscuits (savory), buckwheat, chips/crisps (plain), corn flour, gluten-free foods (breads/pasta), oats/oatmeal (1/2 cup [40 g] max), pasta (quinoa, rice, and corn), plain rice cakes, polenta, popcorn, pretzels, quinoa, quinoa flakes, rice (basmati, brown, and white), sorghum, sourdough spelt bread, tapioca, tortilla chips, wheat-, rye- and barley-free breads

Oils

- **INCLUDE LOW FODMAP**

  - All of the fats and oils are low FODMAP foods: bacon fat, butter, coconut oil, cod liver oil, duck fat, garlic-infused oil, ghee, lard, tallow, medium-chain triglycerides (MCT oil), olive oil, and red palm oil (not palm kernel oil)
  - Omega-3 oil sources: fish oils (cod liver oil, fish oils, and krill oils), algae, and precursors from nuts and seeds (flaxseeds)
  - Plant oil sources: avocado, almond, coconut, borage, flax, grape seed, hemp, pumpkin, sesame, sunflower, and walnut

Sugars, Sweeteners, and Confectionary—small amounts please!

- **AVOID HIGH FODMAP**—Agave, fructose, fruit sugar, high fructose corn syrup (HFCS), honey, inulin, isomalt, maltitol, mannitol, sorbitol, molasses, sugar-free confectionery, xylitol, and yacon syrup
- **INCLUDE LOW FODMAP**—Limited amounts of beet sugar, brown sugar, coconut sugar, corn syrup, dark chocolate, dextrose, glucose, golden syrup, pure maple syrup, palm sugar, rice malt syrup, stevia (pure organic only), sucrose/table sugar, and sugarcane

Condiments

- **AVOID HIGH FODMAP**—Jam (mixed berries), pasta sauce (cream based), relish, and tzatziki dip

- **INCLUDE LOW FODMAP**—All spices (except onion and garlic), barbeque sauce, chutney (1 tablespoon [16 g] max), garlic infused oil, golden syrup, strawberry jam/jelly, mayonnaise, mustard, soy sauce, tomato sauce, wasabi, and vinegar (apple cider, distilled, white, red, and white wine vinegar)

Drinks

- **AVOID HIGH FODMAP**—Coconut water (8 ounces, or 235 ml), apple juice, pear juice, mango juice, sodas with HFCS (high fructose corn syrup), fennel tea, and herbal tea (strong)

- **INCLUDE LOW FODMAP**—Coconut water (less than 4 ounces, or 118 ml) cranberry juice (pure), fruit juice from low FODMAP fruits, herbal tea (weak), peppermint tea, and water

Prebiotics (fuel for beneficial bacteria)

- **AVOID HIGH FODMAP**—Wheat and rye breads, couscous, wheat pasta, barley, gnocchi; Jerusalem artichokes, garlic, onion, leek, asparagus, beetroot, peas, snow peas, and sweet corn; nectarines, peaches, watermelon, persimmons, rambutan, grapefruit, pomegranate, dried fruit, custard apples; cashews and pistachios; and foods containing inulin

- **INCLUDE LOW FODMAP**—Chicory leaves, fennel bulb, green section of leeks and spring onion, red cabbage, banana, rhubarb, kiwifruit, dried cranberries, pomegranate, and non-gluten oats

THE LOW FODMAP DIET HAS THREE PHASES and should be overseen by a licensed nutritionist, registered dietitian nutritionist, or other nutrition professional.

PHASE 1 involves following a strict diet that removes all high FODMAP foods for a period of four to six weeks. You should keep a diary to track all the food that is consumed as well as any symptoms or improvements experienced. At the end of Phase 1, you should meet with the nutritionist/dietitian to review the diary and symptoms. This information should be used to design the next phase of the diet.

PHASE 2 involves gradually reintroducing the FODMAP foods that were eliminated during Phase 1. The type and amount of FODMAP foods that the person can tolerate will be tailored to them. The nutritionist will provide guidance through the reintroduction process to help maximize the dietary variety of foods consumed while minimizing the gastrointestinal symptoms.

PHASE 3 involves establishing your longer term, personalized FODMAP diet. Reintroduce foods and FODMAPs that were tolerated well and avoid only the foods that triggered symptoms.

The goal is to have a final diet/lifestyle that includes some FODMAP foods as tolerated, but not as restrictive as Phase 1 recommendations.)

This diet is so complex that it requires the supervision and guidance of nutrition practitioners with expertise in the diet. The Monash University FODMAPs website provides more detailed information and recipes (www.monashfodmap.com.) It also provides a FODMAP app.

Supplement Recommendations

Beyond the dietary changes, there are digestive and nutritional supplements that are helpful. It is important to include an appropriate probiotic along with biotin for improving the good digestive microbiota. To improve digestive ability, SCD legal digestive enzymes are helpful. Also important is a multiple vitamin/mineral supplement specific for FODMAP problems, omega-3 fatty acids, and curcumin to reduce inflammation.

What are FODMAPs? **F**ermentable **O**ligosaccharides, **D**isaccharides, **M**onosaccharides, and **P**olyols
This is an intense elimination diet of these short-chain carbohydrates that, if poorly digested, can ferment in the gut to cause digestive distress. They are also in natural foods and food additives.

Avoid:

- Processed meats and deli meats, bone cartilage broths, marinated meat and poultry.
- Oligosaccharides: Fructo-oligosaccharides (FOS), inulin; barley; couscous; rye; wheat; garlic; leeks; onions; shallots; Jerusalem and globe artichokes; and legumes; chickpeas (fresh); split peas; beans; nuts and seeds.
- Disaccharides: high lactose soft unripened cheeses (cottage cheese, ricotta, cream cheese, and mascarpone); yogurt; milk (liquid, condensed, evaporated, powder); dairy desserts; custard; ice cream; and milk
- Monosaccharides: high fructose corn syrup; apples; honey; mangoes; pears; and watermelon
- Polyols: Sugar alcohols in artificial sweeteners and chewing gum (sorbitol, xylitol, isomalt, mannitol). Food source polyols: apples; apricots; nectarines; mushrooms; pears; plums; prunes
- Commercially processed foods, artificial additives, GMO foods, trans-fatty acids, sugars, gluten, and possibly other grains and grain substitutes, cow milk products, soy, corn, nuts, and legumes

Why Is the Diet Needed? The diet is for those who have symptoms consistent with sensitivity/reactions to many foods noted to be culprits in many of the elimination diets. The more types of reactions and symptoms present, the more likely the FODMAP diet will help.

Symptoms the Diet May Help: Multiple digestive conditions and symptoms: irritable bowel syndrome (IBS); inflammatory bowel disease (IBD); colitis; gas and bloating; and small intestinal bacterial overgrowth (SIBO)

Diet Includes:

- Organic is important.
- Animal protein: pastured source meats; poultry; eggs; bone broths; healthy sliced meats; hard cheeses; lactose-free milk (if tolerated); homemade lactose-free yogurt and sour cream; if tolerated, tofu; tempeh. Seafood: nonpolluted seafood (Recirculating Aquatic System technologies) and low-toxin seafood.
- Milk/dairy alternatives: nut milks from almond, coconut, hemp, oat, and rice gelato and sorbet Fats: all fats and oils are low FODMAP foods: all animal and plant source fats, lard, tallow; and oils; butter; ghee; coconut; fish oils; and oils of avocado, almond, borage, flax, grapeseed, hemp, pumpkin; sesame; sunflower; and walnut
- Grains: amaranth; arrowroot; buckwheat, non-GMO corn; millet; polenta; popcorn; quinoa; rice; sorghum; tapioca; and basmati, brown and white rice
- Legumes: chickpeas (canned); lentils and small amounts of a wide variety of nuts (almonds, hazelnuts, macadamia, peanuts, pecans, pine nuts, walnuts); and small amounts of seeds (poppy, pumpkin, sesame, sunflower)
- Vegetables: alfalfa; artichoke hearts; arugula; bamboo shoots; bell pepper (capsicum); bok choy; cabbage; carrots; celery; chives; choko; corn; cucumber; eggplant; endive; green beans; kale; lettuce; olives; parsnips; potatoes; pumpkin; silver beets; scallions/spring onions; squash; and tomatoes

- Fruits: bananas; berries; citrus (clementine, lemon, lime, orange, tangelo, tangerine); cranberry juice; currants; grapes; guava; kiwi; melons (cantaloupe, honeydew); passion fruit; papaya (paw paw); pineapple; and rhubarb
- Spices and Other: All spices except onion and garlic. Sweets: golden syrup; maple syrup; gelato, sorbets and any sweetener other than polyols and artificial sweeteners. Sauces: barbeque, mayonnaise, mustard, soy sauce, tomato sauce, wasabi, and vinegars.

Resources:
- FODMAP Everyday: www.Fodmapeveryday.com
- Monash University Site and Low FODMAP App: https://www.monashfodmap.com
- "Low FODMAP Food Chart": www.IBSDiets.org.
- *The Complete Low-FODMAP Diet* by Sue Shepherd and Peter Gibson
- *Healthy Gut, Flat Stomach: The Fast and Easy Low-FODMAP Diet Plan* by Danielle Capalino

ROTATION DIETS

WHAT IS A ROTATION DIET?

Technically, the rotation diet is not a diet, but is instead a method used to change a person's dietary consumption by consciously rotating certain foods. Rotation diets can be used to expand variety, nutrient availability, and balance in the diet, or they may be used as treatment for those with numerous food reactions. This book focuses on the therapeutic elimination diets. The following foods are eliminated from the rotation plan choices: the avoid foods from chapter 3; high reaction-provoking foods; and problem foods based on testing and elimination diet avoids. Permitted foods include mild reaction-provoking foods and all other remaining healthy, organic, and nutrient-dense foods (from chapter 3). Once consumed, a specific food is not repeated for a set interval, which may be four, five, or seven days. The most common is the four-day rotation, which is a good place to start.

WHY USE A ROTATION DIET?

In chapter 1, we discussed many of the ways people can react to foods including allergies, sensitivities, and intolerances. As we noted, there is no testing that can identify all of the potential reactions individuals may experience. Beyond test-positive findings, individuals may be aware that a food causes a reaction, even though tests are negative. People who are living with many food reactions tend to limit their food choices and may get into a habit of eating the same foods repetitively. The poor diversity increases the risk for nutrient deficiencies and reactions to the most frequently consumed foods. For those who have multiple reactions to any one or many foods, complete avoidance can be too difficult. When a mild reaction-provoking food is consumed daily, the negative effects are more significant than when the food is rotated based upon a timetable in which the food is eaten every four, five, or seven days.

Eating based on a rotation diet can be beneficial to a person's health. In addition to fewer and less severe food reactions, the diet improves nutrient intake. The rotation diet also helps to heal the gastrointestinal tract and may be helpful in identifying food intolerances that may not show up on the usual food allergy and food reaction tests. Food reactions include many kinds of intolerances and sensitivities, for which there are no reliable tests available. Undiagnosed food sensitivities and/or intolerances can cause inflammation in the body. When food is not digested properly and the gut barrier is "leaky," some of the byproducts of maldigestion can cross into the bloodstream and trigger inflammation, immune suppression, and/or autoimmunity. In this book, we have discussed the many effects from many kinds of food reactions including digestive problems, dysbiosis (imbalanced gut bacteria), fatigue, sleep disorders, weight changes, skin conditions, inflammation, depression, anxiety, behavioral problems, inattention, learning problems, neurological symptoms, and more. Rotation dieting is one of the strategies to address these issues.

WHAT ARE FOOD FAMILIES?

Food families are groupings of foods based on their biological similarity. Foods that are closely related are from the same species and will possess similar proteins. The chart that follows shows how the foods are grouped into families within categories: primary proteins, vegetables, fruits, grains, nuts/seeds, oils, and seasoning/spices. Rotation allows a person to eat certain foods during a 24-hour period. Those foods may not be consumed again for four, five, or seven days.

ROTATING BY FAMILIES allows all of the choices within a family as options to consume. For example, "Bird" day allows all poultry and their eggs—and "Gourd" day allows melons, cantaloupe, honeydew, and watermelon.

ROTATION BY FOODS is more restrictive, allowing only one food from each family in a 24-hour period. There are different families each day of the four-, five- or seven-day rotation. The food can be repeated during the day. The other foods in the family are not included on that same day.

In the following chart, we provide a list of the food groups, food families, and the most common edible foods within a family. In the seafood group, there are more than 48 separate fish families, some of which include only one species in the family. This permits multiple seafood choices for a month without repeating a family.

FOOD GROUP	FOOD FAMILY	FOODS IN THE FAMILY
Primary Proteins	Bird	chicken, duck, and turkey (and their eggs)
	Bovine	beef/bison, beef/bison products, milk, and dairy products (butter, cheese, and ice cream)
	Legume	tofu
	Fish	freshwater, saltwater
	Mollusk	clam, oyster, mussel, periwinkle, scallop, snail, and squid
	Crustacean	crab, crayfish, lobster, and shrimp
	Ovis	lamb, mutton, and sheep
	Mammal	deer
	Swine	pig, hog, bacon, ham, and pork
Vegetables	Algae	dulse, kelp
	Aster	artichoke, chicory, escarole, endive, Jerusalem artichoke, lettuce, and stevia
	Fungus	mushrooms, truffle, beet, beetroot, chard, spinach, and sugar beet
	Goosefoot	beet, beetroot, chard, spinach, and sugar beet
	Gourd	casaba, cucumber, marrow, pumpkin, squashes, and zucchini
	Legume	green beans, navy beans, and peas
	Lily	asparagus, chives, garlic, leek, and onion
	Mallow	okra
	Morning Glory	sweet potato, yam
	Mustard	broccoli, Brussels sprouts, cabbage, cauliflower, greens, kale, mustard greens, radish, turnip, and watercress
	Nightshades	bell peppers, eggplant, hot peppers, potato, tomato, and tomatillo
	Parsley	carrots, celery, fennel, parsley, and parsnips
	Sedge	water chestnuts

FOOD GROUP	FOOD FAMILY	FOODS IN THE FAMILY
Fruit	Actinidiaceae	kiwi
	Banana	banana, plantain
	Cashew	mango
	Citrus	grapefruit, kumquat, lemon, lime, and orange
	Custard Apple	custard apple, paw-paw
	Ebony	persimmons
	Gourd	cantaloupe, honeydew, melons, and watermelon
	Grape	grapes, raisins, wine, and wine vinegar
	Heath	cranberry, blueberry
	Honeysuckle	elderberry
	Laurel	avocado
	Mulberry	breadfruit, figs
	Palm	coconut, date, and sago
	Papaya	papaya
	Pineapple	pineapple
	Plum	apricot, cherry, chokecherry, nectarine, peach, plum, and prune
	Pomegranate	pomegranate
	Rose Berries	blackberry, raspberry, and strawberry
	Rose Pomes	apple, apple cider vinegar, loquat, pear, and quince
	Saxifrage	currant, gooseberry
Grains	Amaranth	amaranth seeds, amaranth flour
	Arum	arrow root
	Buckwheat	buckwheat flour
	Composite	artichoke flour
	Ginger	East India arrowroot starch
	Grain	barley, bulgur, kamut, rye, spelt, and wheat (durham, graham, and selemon).
	Grass	cornmeal, cornstarch, millet, oats, popcorn, rice, sorghum, and wild rice
	Legume	carob, chickpeas, lentil flour, soy (soymilk/tofu), and sprouts
	Nightshade	potato flour
	Spurge	cassava flour, tapioca starch

FOOD GROUP	FOOD FAMILY	FOODS IN THE FAMILY
Nuts/Seeds	Aster	sunflower seed
	Beech	chestnut
	Birch	hazelnut
	Cashew	cashew, pistachio
	Conifer	pine nuts
	Gourd	pumpkin seeds
	Pedalium	sesame seeds, tahini
	Protea	macadamia
	Rose Stone	almond
	Sapucaya	Brazil nut
	Walnut	butternut, pecan, walnut
Oils	Aster	sunflower oil
	Bovine	butter, ghee, lard
	Bird	bird fat
	Flax	flaxseed oil
	Grass	corn oil
	Laurel	avocado oil
	Legume	peanut oil, soy oil
	Mallow	cottonseed oil
	Mustard	canola oil
	Olive	olive oil
	Palm	coconut oil
	Pedalium	sesame oil
	Rose Stone	almond oil, apricot oil
	Walnut	walnut oil

FOOD GROUP	FOOD FAMILY	FOODS IN THE FAMILY
Seasonings and Condiments	Aster	chamomile, chicory, goldenrod, and tarragon
	Citrus	orange blossom honey
	Fungi	baker's yeast, brewer's yeast
	Ginger	cardamom, ginger, and turmeric
	Grass	corn sugar, corn syrup, and rice sweetener
	Laurel	bay leaf and cinnamon
	Legume	carob, clover, fenugreek, honey, and licorice
	Madder	coffee
	Mint	basil, mint, oregano, rosemary, sage, savory, summer, and thyme
	Mustard	allspice, clove, paprika, pimiento, and mustard seed
	Nightshade	cayenne, chili peppers, paprika, and pimiento
	Nutmeg	mace, nutmeg
	Orchard	vanilla
	Parsley	caraway, celery seed, coriander, cumin, dill, and parsley
	Pepper	pepper, peppercorns
	Poppy	poppy seeds
	Rose Stone	almond extract

TIPS ON HOW TO ACCOMPLISH A ROTATION DIET

1. *WHICH ROTATION DIET STYLE:*

Determine the type of rotation diet you want to start with: four-day, five-day, or seven-day, the most common being the four-day rotation. Also determine how you want to select the foods. We suggest rotating food families, which permits more choices than rotating singular foods.

- Days 1, 2, 3, 4—different food choices by families
- Day 5 is a repeat of Day 1

2. *WHAT TO REMOVE FROM THE ROTATION PLAN:*

- The avoid foods from chapter 3: artificial additives, refined and processed foods, partially hydrogenated oils, sugars, and contaminated food and water
- High reaction foods by lab test findings and/or observed reactions
- Foods based on your elimination diet avoids list
- If there are more than 2 high reactions within the family, avoid all foods in that family.

3. *WHAT TO INCLUDE IN THE ROTATION PLAN:*

- Organic, nutrient-dense foods as described in chapter 3

- Foods that are mildly reaction-provoking (by lab test results)

- All other remaining non-reaction-provoking foods

- In choosing foods for each day, select those which belong together based on your recipes, so that the rotation effort will be far more efficient and successful.

4. *FOODS TO INCLUDE:*

- Three different foods groups at each meal

- Per day:
  - 3 to 4 protein foods: seafood, meat, poultry, eggs, A2 milk products, beans/legumes, nuts, and seeds
  - 2 to 3 fruits
  - 3 to 5 vegetables
  - whole grains as tolerated

5. *ORGANIZATION TIPS*

- Color code the menu days. Then, use containers for the foods that match the color codes. Post the color-coded meal plan in a convenient place.

- Try storing all nonperishable foods for each day in a large container made easily accessible.

- Record the food eaten, the time it was eaten, the amount of the food eaten, and liquids consumed.

- Also document any changes in aches, alertness, attitude, fatigue, hearing, mood, pains, pulse, skin, or vision. Record the time these changes/symptoms occurred. It is common to experience food withdrawal symptoms the first few days.

6. *READ LABELS*

Read all food labels. Make sure you know the alternative names that a food may be called (see chart in this chapter). The intolerant food may be hidden on the label under a different name. Commercially prepared supplements and foods may contain fillers or additives.

Buying fresh produce is the best option. However, this can be expensive and the produce may spoil before it is used. If using fresh produce, only buy enough to get through that rotation cycle. Typically, frozen produce is less expensive than fresh. Use frozen foods that are plain (no sauces or seasoning).

7. *FREEZE LEFTOVERS*

When meals are cooked, if there are any leftovers, make sure to freeze them. Once the food has cooled to room temperature, place it into a freezer bag or container, labeled and color coded.

8. *KEEP HYDRATED*

It is important to maintain adequate hydration to keep the body systems functioning properly. Fluids include water, water flavored with natural juices, and herb teas—not sodas! A good daily goal is to consume a minimum of half of the person's body weight in ounces per day. For example: A 150-pound [68 kg] person would drink a minimum of 75 ounces [2.2 L] of water throughout the day. A 50-pound [23 kg] child would drink at least 25 ounces [0.7 L] throughout the day.

9. *CONSIDER NUTRITIONAL SUPPORT*

To support digestion and a healthy digestive microbiome, consider fermented foods (if tolerated), probiotics, prebiotics, and biotin. Digestive enzymes and additional nutritional support based upon deficiencies in intake and lab testing may be helpful. Consult with a physician, dietitian/nutritionist, or other health practitioners with expertise in supplementation specific to the individual.

What Is a Rotation Diet? The diet avoids repetition of foods based upon a four- to seven-day rotation by food families.

Families are how biologically related foods are grouped. Rotating by food families provides more options. The diet can reduce reactions to mildly reactive foods and help identify problem foods.

Avoid:

- Artificial additives, processed foods, GMO foods, trans-fatty acids, oils, sugars, contaminated food and water
- Food identified as highly reactive by lab testing, observation, or elimination diet responses
- Food families that include many foods that are reaction-provoking

Why Is the Diet Needed? When there are multiple food reactions and very limited choices, rotation is helpful. It expands nutrient diversity. Rotation permits the inclusion of mildly reaction-provoking foods and any other non-reaction-provoking foods.

Symptoms the Diet May Help:

- Persistent digestive problems (gas, diarrhea, constipation, reflux, and motility problems); dysbiosis; irritable bowel syndrome (IBS); inflammatory bowel disease (IBD); autoimmunity; inflammation; skin problems; depression/anxiety; behavioral problems; and inattention

Diet Includes:

- Organic, nutrient-dense foods which are mildly to not reaction-provoking
- Safe foods based on testing, observation, and any elimination diet or diets being used

Resources:

- www.drsallyrockwell.com complete information on rotation diets, tools, self-help products
- www.thesuperallergycookbook.com/PDF/FoodFamilyChartbyFamily.pdf
- *The Super Allergy Girl Cookbook* by Lisa Lundy

CHAPTER 10

Getting Started and Bumps Along the Way

"The person who moves a mountain begins by carrying away small stones."
—Chinese proverb

Getting Started—Easy Does It!

Modifying your child's diet can feel like an overwhelming and almost impossible task. Most parents are already exhausted from the full-time job of seeking appropriate services and therapies. Adding a specialized diet can put some people over the edge. Know that you are not alone in this feeling. Know that, as with most difficult tasks in life, the hardest part is getting started. Often, the worry about the challenge of the diet is worse than actually doing it. There is a lot of support available for you in doing an elimination diet. In addition to this cookbook, there are websites and parent

"We cannot do everything at once, but we can do something at once."
—Calvin Coolidge

Listservs that can provide lots of good information. Talk with other parents in your community; there are others who have done this ahead of you, and most are more than glad to make your road easier than theirs was. Most of all, do the best that you can and focus on what you *are* doing for your child rather than what you aren't doing. Some children are easy to get on these diets, but most require time and effort. Even cleaning up the diet by eliminating artificial additives and toxic contaminants is a good start. Then, simply decreasing the amount of offending foods can often be helpful. Remember that your child is different from all other children with ADHD or autism. Your family structure is unique, and you need to do what works best for your child and family. This section will provide you with guidelines and helpful hints for starting the diet.

If You're Feeling Overwhelmed, Start Here

There are many ways to start the elimination diet. Some practitioners advocate taking the child off the offending foods cold turkey. This approach feels right for some parents, who "want to get it over with." In general, however, this approach results in more significant withdrawal symptoms. For many children, the only foods in their diet are the foods that cause the problems, and they will not eat when all of those foods are removed.

For these children, we advocate a gradual removal of offending foods by substituting foods similar to the problem foods. The rate of removal is dictated by both the ease with which your child accepts the new foods and the degree of withdrawal symptoms. Again, the most common offending foods are casein, gluten, and soy, in that order. Casein is the easiest protein to remove, as there are many acceptable substitutes. Often, changing the type of milk is the easiest place to start. Casein-free rice, almond, coconut, and potato-based milk substitutes are available in both vanilla and chocolate flavors. (See chapter 4 for more details about substitute foods.) Except for coconut milk, these milks provide the same amount of calcium as cow's milk and, in some cases, even more. However, they do not contain significant protein. This can be an issue for children whose main protein source is dairy protein in milk. This topic will be addressed in the sections that follow.

An important note about removing casein: We recommend that you do not use soy as a replacement for casein foods because soy is also such a common offending food. If you replace cow's milk–based products (milk, cheese, yogurt, and ice cream) with soy versions, you will be significantly increasing your child's soy intake. For some children, this means you are taking out one problem food and substituting it with another, possibly equally problematic food. This may mask any potential benefit from removing casein, and you will not be able to tell whether casein was a problem. Initially, it may be too difficult to completely remove soy from your child's diet, as soy lecithin is found in many food products. There are options for replacing some cow's milk products with non-soy alternatives.

As you remove casein, you will often also be decreasing gluten. All of the recipes in this book are casein-free and gluten-free. Many commercially available products are also free of both proteins. Once you have removed casein, you can focus on more completely removing gluten. This is a more challenging task, since gluten is found in so many foods. It is found in a variety of grains, not just wheat. (See chapter 2 for details.) However, again, you will find that there are a variety of recipes and commercially available products that are not just palatable but actually enjoyable.

Variety Is Not Always the Spice of Life

People tend to be fairly routine about what they eat. When we shop, we tend to buy the same foods week after week. And although what we eat on a given day varies, in the bigger picture, we tend to eat the same foods week in and week out. This actually works in your favor when trying to change your child's diet. Your child's main motivation is not that food is good for him or her, but that it tastes good. So, if your child loves chocolate chip cookies and you always make or buy one particular type, your challenge is to find a GFCF version of that cookie. Once you find it and your child accepts it, that cookie is the type of cookie you buy or make week in and week out. The same applies to main courses, side dishes, snacks, and desserts. The challenge is starting the diet and finding the substitute foods. Maintaining the diet is much less difficult.

How Strict Does an Elimination Diet Have to Be, and How Long Should It Last?

There is no single answer to these questions. It really depends on the individual child. Most books written or lectures given on this subject emphasize the importance of completely and strictly eliminating the problem foods. There is no doubt that this is the purest approach. However, authors and lecturers are generally talking about the "generic" child with ADHD or autism; they are not talking about your child with ADHD or autism. They are also not talking about the family of the child with these disorders. It is important to look at each child as an individual and as a member of a family to determine the best approach for that child. We have never seen a "generic" child. There is a bumper sticker that jokingly says, "I'm unique—just like everyone else." In treatment of children with special needs, this is actually a very serious statement. While children with ADHD or autism can have similar underlying biochemistry, no children are exactly alike in the way symptoms present themselves through behavior and development.

Some children with ADHD or autism truly require a strict elimination diet to show benefit. Even small exposures can result in significant negative behaviors. Other children seem to benefit from even a decrease in the problem foods. Still others require strict elimination initially but are eventually able to loosen up on the diet once the leakiness of their intestine has healed and it has become a good barrier again. The use of digestive enzymes specifically designed to digest casein and gluten has also allowed some children to eventually eat foods they previously needed to avoid completely. While there is no enzyme that can equal the complete elimination of foods, for some children, "mimicking" the elimination diet by use of enzymes can allow some "cheating" on the diet and can even allow some to eat a normal diet. Again, this mostly relates to how well the leaky gut has healed, since this is what allows the problem foods to get into the blood.

In most cultures, much social experience revolves around food. When a child's autism symptoms are severe, he has no awareness that his diet is different from other kids' diets. However, as autism symptoms lessen and awareness improves, a child may start to care that he is different from other children or that he can't eat the same cake as other kids at a birthday party. He may want to eat pizza on "pizza Fridays" at school. These are all good signs, as they show improved social awareness and a desire to be like peers. It would certainly help social development if a child who has been on a strict elimination diet were able to eat "normal" foods in these social situations. For some children, once the intestine has healed sufficiently, and especially with the use of digestive enzymes before meals, broadening the diet to include other foods is possible. For other groups of children, unfortunately, this is not possible, as any intake of problem foods, however small, results in unacceptable side effects on brain functioning. The only way to tell is to try. The ideal timing for reintroduction of foods is best discussed with the health care practitioner (doctor or nutritionist) who is guiding your child's dietary treatment.

What Kind of Improvements Can We Expect?

It is our experience that about two-thirds of children with autism improve when gluten and casein are removed from their diets. With soy removal, there may be even further improvement. Some children have immediate and dramatic improvement, whereas others have slower but steady improvement. Less than one-third of children with autism do not respond to the diet, and the GFCF diet does not appear to be a contributing factor to their symptoms.

In general, improvements from removal of casein and soy occur more quickly than gluten, though in some children, gluten removal results in rapid improvement as well. It is our experience that a one-month trial of casein or soy removal is usually sufficient to determine benefit, though the trial may need to be longer in children with autism, due to the frequent presence of other contributing biomedical imbalances. However, benefits from gluten elimination may take longer to become evident, especially for children with autism, and we recommend at least a 3-month trial of gluten elimination to best determine if the elimination is helpful. This prolonged time to benefit with gluten elimination may possibly occur in those children with autism who have brain inflammation which may be triggered by gluten. Improvement from a decrease in brain inflammation occurs more slowly than improvements seen from a decrease in casein or gluten opiates, for example. In general, we recommend a 3-month elimination trial of casein, gluten, and soy to determine if your child is having a significant enough improvement from the trial to warrant a continuation of the elimination diet.

How Long Before We See Results?

It could be days, weeks, or months depending on the:

- Child's age
- Presence of other conditions
- Co-existing additional food allergies or sensitivities
- Health of the gut
- Amount of gluten and dairy previously in the diet
- Degree of elevation of opiates from casein or gluten
- Diet compliance and strictness
- Nutritional supplements used (including digestive enzymes)

What to Do for Mistakes

Authors Karyn Seroussi and Lisa Lewis offer the following helpful advice about what to give your child, and what to do when you make a mistake with the diet:

- Extra enzymes, as soon as possible—if within 1 hour of eating the food
- Alkalize! Alka Seltzer (gold) or Vitaline Alka Aid or Prelief as soon as the reaction is evident. This may work on some reactions and not others.
- Increase fluids.
- Benadryl or other antihistamine (for a problematic histamine reaction)
- Investigate reason and create a safeguard.

CHAPTER 11

Dealing with the Diet and Common Concerns

"My stomach does not hurt anymore. Now, I can go places. I love to go places. I made honor roll twice this year. I love to read and I can now do math easier. School is much easier. I am no longer in speech therapy. My teachers are proud of me and say I am a role model. I feel GREAT!"

—Ashley Stilson

"Right now my life is just one learning experience after another. By the end of the week, I should be a genius."

—Jeannette Osias

Picky Appetites, Texture Issues, and Odd Food Choices

A common problem in children with autism is picky eating. This can show itself in a variety of ways. Children may limit themselves to only dairy and wheat foods. They may decide what to eat not based on taste, but by the smell or the look of foods. They may become brand-specific.

They may limit themselves to unusual categories of food, such as eating only food that is white or brown. Some like only crunchy foods, while others like only soft or mushy foods. Some like both types but cannot stand having them mixed together or even on the same plate together. They may be sensitive to any change in food or to hiding supplements in food. Children with autism can often detect even the subtlest difference in foods. All of these factors combine to make adequately nourishing these children a challenging task.

There are many reasons why children develop these picky appetites. Many children, not just children with autism, are deficient in zinc, which is a critically important nutrient in the body. One important consequence of zinc deficiency is a change in taste and smell. The taste of a food is what makes eating pleasurable. If you are unable to taste or smell a food, or if the food has an unpleasant odor and taste, the main sensation you would be aware of when eating the food is its texture. You can well imagine that this can be unpleasant or intolerable. Many of us have experienced a negative response to a food, such as developing food poisoning. These types of "sense memories" can be strong, resulting in a complete lack of desire for that food for a long time, even if you can convince yourself that the reaction was temporary. Even when zinc deficiencies are corrected and taste normalizes, there may be a strong behavioral component to avoidance of specific foods that may need to be addressed. Often, the best treatment is time and patience, though in severe situations, specific feeding therapy interventions may be needed. Monosodium glutamate (MSG), which is found in

processed foods, also affects the brain's perception of taste. Routine exposure can result in craving food sources that tend to be low in nutrient content and restricting unprocessed foods.

As previously described, opiate-like reactions from food can also lead to picky appetites. Children may not know why they are choosing particular foods; they may simply be responding to an awareness that certain foods make their brain feel good. They may then want to eat only those foods, due to a physically based craving for those foods or to an "addiction" to the pleasurable feelings they get from them. Once this addiction is broken—either by eliminating those foods from the diet or by digesting them more efficiently (through the use of digestive enzymes)—children's dietary choices may broaden.

Another possible side effect of zinc functional deficiency is sensory integration dysfunction or sensory processing disorder, which occurs in a large number of children with autism and a subset of children with ADHD. This refers to problems handling the variety of sensations that bombard our bodies every day. Zinc is critical in sensory development. We sense the environment through touch, sound, smell, taste, and movement. In some children with sensory disorders, these senses are heightened, so that sounds that don't typically bother people are too loud or smells are too strong. If severe enough, this can be painful for children. Related to eating, if a child does not process taste or smell or touch normally, certain foods may be unpleasant. Mild tastes may seem strong, mild smells may be overwhelming, or particular textures may be intolerable. In these cases, occupational therapy can be helpful to normalize a child's ability to process sensory feelings in a more normal and tolerable way. Zinc supplementation may be helpful, as described above, and can be discussed with a nutritional professional.

Picky Appetite: The Trojan Horse Technique

Remember Odysseus from seventh-grade mythology? Seeking to gain entrance into Troy, he cleverly ordered a hollow wooden horse so large that the Greek army could hide inside. What looked like a huge horse was really a disguise to conquer the city. We have used this concept for decades to hide nutritious food to nourish picky eaters.

In the recipe sections, we provide clever ways to introduce and hide new foods, especially vegetables. Mix, blend, or purée a very small amount (1 tablespoon [15 g]) of the new food with a well-liked food. As the child accepts the taste, more can be included. The key is to start small. Blended foods may also be better tolerated by those children who have oral sensory issues regarding food textures. Their sensory development may be younger than their age. It is better to adapt to the sensory level and return to purées until the sensory issues have improved. It is important to have the child eat rather than encourage progression to foods that are not tolerated because they are "lumpy" or unpleasant to chew.

Vegetables must be cooked and puréed well with a food where it will not change the overall color, texture, or taste. If there is nothing but white food in the diet, then start with very light-colored vegetables (squash, cauliflower, and corn). If the child likes ketchup or tomato sauce, then you can introduce deeper-colored vegetables (beets, greens, peas, and beans). First, the vegetable must be well cooked and puréed completely with the child's favorite food. You can also use baby food purées. Puréed vegetables can be included in batter for pancakes, muffins, brownies, and cookies or in sauces such as tomato sauce, pizza sauce, and ketchup. Blend puréed vegetables into fruit sauces, meatballs, and even peanut butter.

Many of our patients' families have developed what we call "muffin casseroles." One child would eat only breads and muffins. His resourceful mother developed a GFCF muffin he liked and then gradually started adding fruit purée to the batter. As that was tolerated, she added vegetable purée and finally added puréed meat. Until he was able to transition to eating foods more traditionally, he had these muffins at every meal and snack—and loved them.

You can also add a vegetable juice to a fruit juice. The color change will not matter if you serve it in a sippy cup. Try carrot juice with orange juice and then add a small amount of another vegetable juice. Again, start with only 1 teaspoon (5 ml) or less. Expand as tolerance improves.

There are dried vegetable powders that can be added easily to various foods and dishes. And if none of the above works, consider natural gummy bears made of vegetables and fruits. As your child expands to eating vegetables, try vegetables dipped in honey or GFCF mayo/ketchup mix or hummus. It's a start. But remember to carry out the Trojan Horse technique out of sight of your child!

If more protein is needed, there are many clever ways to increase it. If eggs are tolerated, add more eggs, especially the high-protein whites, to foods. This works for batters, breads, and meatballs. Heat-stable rice protein powders can be added to batters, breads, and smoothies made of rice milk and fruit. Do not add raw eggs to smoothies. Taste and texture determine acceptance.

Keep trying this sneaky manner of introducing new foods. Eventually, he or she will accept the food alone—we promise! All it takes is patience, and a lesson from Greek mythology. There is more advice on this technique in the next chapter.

Withdrawal Symptoms from Foods

Some children, especially those who are making opiate-like peptides from their foods, are physically addicted to those foods. When the foods are removed from the diet, they can experience symptoms similar to drug withdrawal. The most common symptoms are irritability, anger, or rage. Children may also temporarily regress in their behavior or in their developmental skills. Withdrawal symptoms can be viewed as a good sign, as this indicates the foods were having some effect on the child. Anytime there are negative symptoms from removing a food from the diet, the food is a problem. Not having withdrawal symptoms does not necessarily mean the food is not a problem. Some children have resilient personalities and bodies and can tolerate withdrawal symptoms well, without obvious side effects.

Some children can tolerate abrupt removal of the offending foods. However, most do best with gradual removal of the foods, as this allows their body to adjust with fewer side effects. From a practical standpoint, gradual withdrawal is usually a necessity if your child is a picky eater, as you need to find substitute foods your child is willing to eat.

What Can Be Done for Withdrawal Symptoms?

The best treatment for withdrawal symptoms is time. Food-withdrawal symptoms often subside within a few days and usually not longer than a week. In some cases, they may last longer, again depending on the particular child. As the body becomes clear of the offending foods, there will be a period of time when the child is more sensitive to those foods. If there are unknown dietary infractions during that time, the child's behavior may worsen. If withdrawal symptoms seem prolonged, they may not be withdrawal but rather reaction to intake of problem foods.

It is worth then carefully reviewing possible sources of exposure to the eliminated foods in case unknown infractions are occurring. One commonly overlooked source of gluten is play dough at school. Play dough is often made out of flour. One of our patients had prolonged behavioral regression without any obvious cause. The cause of his regression became clear only when he came home from school with flour all over his clothes from the play dough.

Time may seem to pass slowly as you try to survive your child's withdrawal symptoms, but try to remember that there is a light at the end of the withdrawal tunnel.

Is the Diet Helping?

The best test for determining response to the diet is the change in the child's physical and behavioral symptoms. For some children, this is easy: Within days or weeks, there is an obvious and dramatic improvement noticed by a variety of people in the child's life. In other children, the response to an elimination diet is slow and subtle, especially if there are other complicating factors (significant nutritional deficiencies, untreated food allergies/sensitivities, or toxic metals). When the total load is great, it takes longer and more effort to overcome it.

Parents often ask if they should keep data in order to tell whether the diet is working. As a general point, it is our opinion that if the only way to tell the diet is working is by minute inspection of data, then it is probably not worth doing the diet long-term. The goal of the diet is noticeable change that results in an improved quality of life for the child.

Elimination diets result in increased expense and effort, and the benefit needs to be worth that effort. Parents are usually the best people to determine whether the improvements seen are worth the challenge of the diet. Most children with ASD have multiple adults involved in their care who can provide helpful feedback. Feedback from those who are not aware there has been any change in diet is the most valuable. Their observations are less influenced, consciously or unconsciously, by awareness that something has been changed. This type of feedback may come from relatives or friends who have not seen the child since the elimination diet was started and who spontaneously comment on positive changes. Teachers and therapists often need to be informed about the dietary changes because food is often part of the school day or the therapy sessions. However, they can also provide good feedback on apparent changes.

Another way to tell if the diet is helping is through dietary infractions. These may be planned but are often unplanned. Children are exposed to foods that are not on their diets. This can occur at home, school, restaurants, and therapy offices. You can guarantee that if a classmate leaves a gluten-containing snack unattended, your child will be the first one to grab it. This will result in an unplanned "challenge" to your child's system. Often, in the initial months on an elimination diet, these challenges will result in obvious worsening of symptoms. This is evidence that the food is a problem. It often gives parents motivation to continue the diet, as these infractions often occur around the time parents are tiring of these diets, especially if there has not been convincing improvement by that point. When the child is further along in the healing process, these accidental dietary infractions also provide information. If digestion has improved and/or the intestine has healed enough and is no longer leaky, the same infractions that caused significant symptoms in the past may no longer cause the same degree of symptoms. This is evidence that less of the bothersome food peptides are reaching the brain and causing it problems.

In general, the timing of planned food challenges is best discussed with the practitioner who is guiding your child's care. Some individuals believe that it is best to challenge the body with a large amount of the offending food so that any reactions will be obvious.

We would not recommend that approach because some children are exquisitely sensitive and may be miserable for a significant period of time after a large challenge. Rather, we would suggest an initial challenge with a single serving of one type of offending food (such as casein). For example, we would suggest a challenge with a single slice of cheese rather than an unlimited amount. In addition, we would not recommend a combination food such as pizza, since this contains both casein and gluten. The single serving should be given and no further offending foods given over the next three days. The child's behavior should then be monitored over these three days, remembering that food sensitivity reactions can occur anytime within 72 hours of eating the food. Reactions most commonly appear the next day or two days after eating the offending food. If no reaction is obvious, a second challenge can be done with a larger serving of the food, again with monitoring of behavior for three days. If still no reaction, servings can be given every two days, then every day, until you are sure there is no negative reaction. The most common negative reactions are irritability or regression in behavior or development (such as reappearance of ADHD or autism symptoms, decrease in language, etc.). There are many fine points to food challenges and interpretation of reactions, and these challenges are best done under the guidance of a knowledgeable practitioner (functional medicine physician, nutritionist).

There is also debate about how long of an elimination period is necessary to determine whether particular foods are a problem. There seems to be general agreement that casein clears out of the system more rapidly than gluten. Recommendations regarding casein elimination have ranged from five days to three weeks; however, in children with autism, longer elimination trials are usually necessary because of the combinations of offending foods and the complexity of the other nutritional and medical factors affecting the brain. Some say that gluten can take six to twelve months to completely clear the system and that one cannot say a gluten elimination trial has failed until it has been done for that period of time. Again, a knowledgeable practitioner can discuss this with you as part of your child's overall treatment plan.

"After my son Dorian was evaluated and diagnosed with Asperger's syndrome, he went on the gluten-free, casein-free diet and supplements. Within a month, we began noticing changes. By three to six months later, he was a different child. He was able to focus and participate in class so well that his teachers were amazed. He was playing basketball with the other kids and was chosen team captain! He was even chosen for the starring role in his school play. I can proudly say that Dorian has become an honor-roll student who has a fun group of close friends he has hung out with through middle school and now into high school. He is well known at school and well liked everywhere. Granted, he does still have some quirkiness and his special interests but he has been able to transform all of these points into assets rather than liabilities!

Had anyone ever told me that having an autistic child would be the least of my concerns as a parent of special-needs children, I would have never believed them. But last year when we went to adopt in Ukraine, they were amazed that we were willing to take on a child that had gluten-free, casein-free dietary needs. We said, 'No problem, we know all about it.'"

—Natalie Sirota

In general, we recommend elimination of casein and gluten for at least three months.

Are Elimination Diets Healthy?

Concern: My child's doctor is concerned that the GFCF diet is not healthy.

Your physician's goal is to make sure your child is healthy. Your doctor is right to raise the question of whether your child is being adequately nourished. The concern is usually that two "essential food groups" are being removed from the diet. What is factual, but not well known, is that milk products and grains are not mandatory food groups for human survival.

What most physicians do not realize is that children on the GFCF diet often eat much healthier diets than those who eat "regular" diets. Children on the GFCF diet eat much less fast food and processed food, which often contain casein or gluten. Not much attention is paid to what typical children are getting in their diets, other than ensuring they get enough calcium for bone health. Given the pace of today's lifestyle, many children eat too much in the way of processed food or fast food and often eat in ways that do not support healthy digestion.

When removing milk products from the diet, there is always the concern that calcium, vitamin D, and protein will be inadequate. As described in chapter 4, there are other sources of protein, calcium, and vitamin D in addition to dietary supplements, which can be used as needed. There is also a concern that gluten-free breads and cereals may not be fortified with

nutrients. It is important to note that appropriate use of nutritional supplements is one of the support strategies in achieving successful elimination diets. See chapter 2 for details. In addition, refer to *The ADHD and Autism Nutritional Supplement Handbook.*

A testimony to the resilience of the human body is its miraculous ability to afford adequate brain function for most children and adults despite poor nourishment. For children on elimination diets, it is just as important to pay attention to what is being put back into the diet as it is to what is being taken out. When this is done, children's diets are healthy, and often more healthy, than those of their typically developing peers.

Elimination Diet—Worth It or Not?

Concern: My child's doctor feels the elimination diet is a waste of time.

Physicians are also concerned that parents of children with special needs do not get taken advantage of in their desire to help their children. They are concerned that parents may have false hope or undertake treatments that are harmful or expensive. These can be positive qualities in a physician. However, most physicians do not receive much education about nutrition during their formal training. They may only hear that you are removing foods from your child's diet and may not be aware of the potential health benefits. An elimination diet, done correctly, will not be harmful to your child and will hopefully be helpful. All physicians take the Hippocratic Oath, which states, "First do no harm." It may help to tell your physician that you are aware of this and that you will be pursuing the diet in a way that "does no harm." Even if your physician feels the diet may not help, at least you can make him or her aware that it will not harm your child if done thoughtfully.

Getting Support from Family and the School Team

Concern: What can we do to get more support from family and the school?

It is important that all caregivers involved in the child's life be aware of the diet and be committed to supporting it. Especially when starting the diet, it is important to be as strict as is reasonably possible so that you can feel you've given the diet an adequate trial. Again, some children improve simply with a decrease in the amount of offending foods. However, other children need to be taken completely and strictly off the offending foods before improvement is seen. If other adults involved with a child give nonpermitted foods, this may sabotage the elimination trial.

Some people, such as grandparents, teachers, or other family members, may think a small amount of a prohibited food couldn't hurt. In this case, it may help to compare the GFCF diet to a diet for a child

with diabetes or a life-threatening peanut allergy. In those situations, no adult would contemplate giving just a little bit of an impermissible food. Similarly, while food infractions on the GFCF diet are not life-threatening, they can have serious negative effects on brain functioning. The adults in your child's life who know and love your child and want the best for him or her may be better able to support the diet if they understand what problems the foods can cause in the brain.

One additional challenge in convincing other caregivers about the consequences of cheating on the diet is that the effects of the cheat often do not occur immediately. Effects of infractions often occur the next day or two days later, when the adult who gave your child the food is no longer present. Some parents have jokingly told their child's grandparents that they were welcome to give the child an offending food but then they would have to keep the child for the weekend. Many a grandparent has probably become aware of the reactions to food when babysitting a grandchild for the weekend.

"I think a hero is an ordinary individual who finds strength to persevere and endure in spite of overwhelming obstacles."

—Christopher Reeve

CHAPTER 12

From Yucky to Yummy: Finding the Right Kid-Friendly Foods

"You don't have to cook fancy or complicated masterpieces—just good food from fresh ingredients."

—Julia Child

BEYOND OUR OWN RECIPES AND ADAPTED RECIPES, many have been graciously contributed by the parents of our patients and by some of the children themselves. There are also recipes inspired by others who have expertise in cooking for those on special diets.

We are grateful for the collective wisdom of those who have been through the journey that so many are now beginning, including Julie Matthews, Vicki Kobliner, Lisa Barnes, Lizzie Vann, Lori Skalitzky, Joyce Mulcahy, Jeannie Fritz Godbout, Michael Thurmond, Elaine Gottschall, Linda and Bill Schmidt, Iris, Bette Hagman, Tracey Smith, Lori Brown Tremper, Travis Martin, Lisa Lewis, Pauline McFadden, Marie Donadio, Jody Cutler, Sue Chubb, Angela Lowry, Nicole Young, Diana Hann, Kathy Rivers, Bobby Warfield, Sue and Dick Redding, Leonardo Hosh,

Mollie Katzen, Jennifer Richardson, Sally Fallon, Jeanne Wilson, Barbara Rees, Glenda Ingham, Colleen Godbout, Bonnie Gutman, Anne Evans, Jane Ruane, Doug and Jeannette DeLawter, Lisa Compart, Marilyn Lammers, Vivian Cavalieri, Maria Ribaya Than, Wendy Higgins, Carla and Aidan Hancock, Sharon Dahn, Vivian Duckett, Erika Melton, Melissa Kemp, Elynn Demattia, Sueson Vess, Christina Godbout, Welby Griffin, and Sara Keough.

We, as authors, have tried to provide recipes that can meet differing needs from Quick N Easy to gourmet and take into account the variation in appetite and food tolerances within families. There are Quick N Easy recipes for those who want to provide their families with healthy food and still juggle the extremely stressful demands of everyday schedules. The more complex recipes may appeal to those with the culinary skills and desire to create interesting dishes. For many of the complex recipes, we have offered Quick N Easy alternatives as well.

We repeatedly hear parents describe their children's appetite changes as follows: "He ate all kinds of foods as a baby and when we moved to more solid foods, he developed an extremely picky appetite." The food needs to be adapted to the child's preferences until the child is ready to advance to the next stage. Limited appetites and food aversions are not behavioral choices; they result from the way a food's appearance, smell, color, taste, and texture are perceived.

One Person's Yummy Food Is Another Person's Yucky Food

In previous chapters, we have described the many factors that can contribute to picky appetites and other feeding challenges. These include zinc deficiency, craving foods due to the creation of opiate-like peptides from casein and gluten, and sensory sensitivities. The negative outcome of this combination of factors can be faulty messages from the sensory receptors to the brain and dysfunctional interpretation of those messages by the brain. Perception is the "truth" for that person. That is why begging, bribing, and punishing do not and will not work.

How to Go from Yucky to Yummy—Perfecting the Trojan Horse Technique

For those with texture issues, it is important to adapt the diet to the child's oral and food developmental stage. If textures are a sensory issue, no matter how tasty the food, it will not be consumed. By providing the food in a sensory-pleasing form, the child benefits nutritionally and begins to find mealtime more pleasant and rewarding. Purées are generally helpful. They are better tolerated and can open the door for getting more types of foods into the diet. Many family dishes, including soups, casseroles, or the meat and vegetable main dish, can also be served puréed for the child who has sensory texture issues. In this way, the whole family is enjoying the same meal.

Many of the recipes in this book have been selected to expand nutritional intake, especially using the Trojan Horse Technique—hiding a small amount of the new food (especially vegetables and proteins) within a very well tolerated and acceptable food. This technique is described in more detail in chapter 11. Each child is different and, therefore, it is important to identify what foods will work as "carriers" to get the new foods in.

Purées can be made from cooked fresh or frozen vegetables and/or purchased baby foods. If your child is offended by being served baby food, simply keep it well hidden. Create interesting new names for the foods and see that others in the family join in consuming them. The secret to success in introducing these new foods is to combine a small amount with the food the child already likes. For many children, this is the only way new foods can be introduced.

Start with 1 tablespoon (15 g) or less and then increase when tolerated. Hide the cooked vegetable purées anywhere you can, selecting colors that are not obvious when added to the carrier food. The carrier food needs to be one that the child enjoys. It may even be a food that is being slowly eliminated. Include puréed fruits to improve the taste. Here are some examples of places to hide foods (and even supplements):

- **SPAGHETTI SAUCE.** Blend the puréed vegetables thoroughly with at least three times as much spaghetti sauce; then hand-mix the new blend in with the rest of the sauce. Carrots, beets, sweet potatoes, turnips, squash, green beans, and peas are easy to hide in spaghetti sauce. Watch the amount of green if it is a food color that your child rejects.

- **MUFFINS, CAKES, AND BROWNIES.** Well-puréed foods are easy to hide in these batters, including puréed chicken and turkey. A chicken/vegetable/fruit muffin becomes a healthy meal!

- **PANCAKES.** Not only can puréed vegetables and fruits hide in the batter, but also pancakes are a good hiding place for supplements such as protein powders (if heat-stable), calcium, magnesium, and zinc.

- **PEANUT BUTTER.** If a child likes peanut butter, it is an excellent medium for adding small amounts of protein and nutritional supplements.

- **MEATBALLS.** If these are well liked, especially with spaghetti sauce, the job becomes a whole lot easier. Well-puréed vegetables and fruits are an excellent thickener/filler for meatballs. Make many and freeze them and then bring them out for snacks.

- **JUICES.** Juices with a strong flavor, such as pineapple juice, grape juice, nectars, apple cider, and orange juice, are particularly good for hiding supplements. Use 100% juice with no sugar added. Avoid frozen and concentrate.

- **SMOOTHIES, FRUIT PURÉES, AND APPLESAUCE.** These offer an unlimited opportunity for expanding nutrition and an excellent way to hide supplements. Protein powders can be included to expand protein intake, especially for those with texture issues who avoid meat, beans, and other sources of protein. Always start with the fruit your child favors and then expand.

- **CHOCOLATE.** Let chocolate be your friend. There are sources of GFCF chocolate chips, sauces, powders, and so forth. Check the product search section of the GFCF Diet website (www.gfcfdiet.com/directory.htm).

Feeding a Child Who Won't Eat
Rules to Make

- Turn off phones, cell phones, and unpleasant noise or upsetting programs.
- Put a note on the front door that you are not available.
- Keep the mealtime pleasant and happy.
- Allow no one at the table to speak negatively about the food or meal.
- Prohibit any gross talk at the table.
- Always have a favorite food as part of the child's meal.
- Provide a small portion of the favorite food to be followed by new or less-liked foods.
- Finish the meal with the favorite food.
- Provide a reward for any effort toward eating or participating. Be casual about this—parent anxiety undermines success.
- If one parent is more effective with feeding, have that parent do the feeding.
- If there is a well-liked sitter or relative, have that person participate.
- There are no "breakfast police"! Start serving lunch and dinner foods for breakfast.

A Rule to Break

Allow a child to watch TV or a favorite tape during mealtime. This results in a positive association with the meal and eating. The attention to the show reduces the sensory focus on the food. It can allow for more food consumption and slipping in the well-disguised new foods. It is temporary—it's not forever—and it works!

Gelatin

Gelatin itself is a health food. The presence of gelatin in foods improves digestion by attracting digestive juices to the surface of food particles. According to Sally Fallon and Mary Enig in *Nourishing Traditions*, gelatin has been used throughout history in the treatment of many digestive and intestinal disorders.

Include it in meat broths, soups, stews, vegetable purées, fruit salads, vegetable salads, and gelatin desserts. The vegetarian gelatin source, carrageenan, does not have the same healthy effect and can hinder the actions of digestive enzymes. The recipes in this book use only unflavored gelatin.

Substitutions: What to Use and How to Do It

Please note that you may need to modify the substitutes used depending on your child's particular elimination diet(s). Please see the individual chapters on specific diets for recommendations for foods to avoid and include.

SUBSTITUTES FOR SUGAR AND GUIDELINES ON SWEETENERS

The natural sweeteners are preferred over table sugars (sucralose). Some of the substitutes are too acidic and require the addition of baking soda to compensate. The information that follows comes from multiple sources, two of which are Sally Fallon and Mary Enig's *Nourishing Traditions*, which provides excellent information, and Carol Fenster's *Special Diet Celebrations*, which also provides detailed information for food substitutions.

SWEETENERS	EQUIVALENT TO 1 CUP SUGAR	INFORMATION
Brown Rice Syrup	**1¹/₃ cups (425 g)** Add ¼ teaspoon baking soda per cup. Reduce liquid by ¼ cup (60 ml) per cup (235 ml).	Less sweet than sugar, it is excellent for baking. Be certain it is GF.
Agave Nectar (organic only)	**³/₄ cup (255 g)** Reduce liquid by ¼ cup (60 ml) per cup (235 ml).	This sweet liquid is from the cactus plant. The texture is similar to honey. It has a lower glycemic index and less effect on blood glucose. It works well in baked goods, puddings, and beverages.
Raw Honey	**¹/₂ –³/₄ cup (170–255 g)** Add ¼ teaspoon baking soda per cup (340 g) of honey. Reduce liquid by ¼ cup (60 ml) per cup (235 ml).	Honey should not be heated above 117°F (47°C). It is loaded with beneficial enzymes that digest carbohydrates, including grains. Local honey is best. When used in heated recipes, it will not have the enzyme activity. Lower oven temperature 25°F (4°C) to prevent overbrowning. Avoid honey in any form in babies up to age 1 year.
Maple Syrup, Maple Sugar	**²/₃ –³/₄ cup (160–175 ml)** Add ¼ teaspoon baking powder. Reduce liquid by ¼ cup (60 ml) per cup (235 ml).	This syrup (distilled sap) from deciduous maple trees is rich in trace minerals. The sugar is dehydrated syrup. Both have a distinct flavor and are best used in creamy desserts and baked goods. Use organic only.
Fruit Juice Concentrate (Liquid)	**²/₃ cup (160 ml)** Add ¼ teaspoon baking soda. Reduce liquid ¹/₃ cup (80 ml) per cup (235 ml) juice.	This has a negative impact on glucose control in the same way sugar does. Avoid high-fructose corn syrup (HFCS) in foods. Reduce oven temperature 25°F (4°C) and adjust baking time for slightly longer period. Orange juice is more acidic.

SWEETENERS	EQUIVALENT TO 1 CUP SUGAR	INFORMATION
Fruit Juice Concentrate (Frozen)	½ cup (140 g) Add ⅛ teaspoon baking soda. Reduce liquid ½ cup (120 ml) per cup (235 ml) juice.	Frozen concentrate must be 100 percent pure juice whether one juice or a combination. Use less when using the liquid juice concentrate. See information above.
Fruit Purée	1 cup (250 g)	This is a good way to provide nutritional sweetener in baked goods. It works best if used to replace only ¼ to ½ of the sugar in the recipe.
Molasses	½ cup (170 g) Reduce liquid by ¼ cup (60 ml) per cup (235 ml).	This "waste" product from the production of refined sugar has a strong, moderately sweet taste and is rich in minerals.
Brown Sugar	1 cup (150 g)	This is refined cane or beet sugar with molasses still on the sugar crystals. It is no healthier than white sugar.
Date Sugar	⅔ –1 cup (150–220 g)	Made from dehydrated dates, this sweetener is nutritious but does not dissolve easily. It is best sprinkled on a food or used in combination with other sugars. Dissolve in hot water before using in batters. Lower baking temperature 25°F (4°C).
Fructose	½ cup (100 g)	This is refined simple sugar made from fruit juices, corn, or corn syrup. Know the source! It is less glycemic (sugar-raising) than sucrose and glucose. Avoid HFCS.
Sucanat	1 cup (200 g)	This is dehydrated cane sugar juice that is rich in nutrients. It is the most similar to sugar.
Stevia Powder or Liquid	1 teaspoon (5 ml) May need to increase dry ingredients. 1 teaspoon sugar = 2–4 drops liquid stevia or pinch stevia powder.	A little bit goes a long way. This sweet-tasting herb is 30 times sweeter tasting than sugar (and has an aftertaste). It does not affect blood glucose. Substitution is not easy. Baked items with stevia do not brown well. It is best used in recipes requiring very little sugar or as part of the sugar replacement.

SUBSTITUTES FOR WHEAT FLOUR

SUBSTITUTE	EQUIVALENT TO 1 CUP (125 G) WHEAT FLOUR
Buckwheat flour	⅞ cup (1 cup – 2 tablespoons [105 g])
Corn flour	1 cup (120 g)
Cornmeal, cornstarch	¾ cup (105 g cornmeal, 98 g cornstarch)
Chickpea flour	¾ cup (105 g)
Nut flours (ground fine)	½ cup (60 g)
Potato flour	1 cup (160 g)
Potato starch	¾ cup (105 g)
Rice flour, sorghum	⅞ cup (140 g rice flour, 125 g sorghum)
Tapioca flour or starch	1 cup (120 g)

SUBSTITUTE THICKENERS

SUBSTITUTE	EQUIVALENT TO 1 TABLESPOON (8 G) WHEAT FLOUR
Arrowroot	1 ½ teaspoons
Bean flours	1 tablespoon (9 g)
Cornstarch	1 ½ teaspoons
Gelatin powder (unflavored)	1 ½ teaspoons dissolved in water
Guar gum	1 ½ teaspoons mixed in liquid
Potato starch	½ tablespoon (5 g)
Tapioca flour	1 ½ tablespoons (12 g)

SUBSTITUTES FOR MILK PRODUCTS

MILK PRODUCT	SUBSTITUTE
1 cup (235 ml) milk	1 cup (235 ml) milk substitute: rice, coconut, non-GMO soy, nut, hemp
1 cup (230 g) yogurt	1 cup (230 g) yogurt substitute: coconut, non-GMO soy
1 cup (235 ml) light cream	¾ cup (175 ml) milk substitute + ¼ cup (55 g) butter substitute, melted
1 cup (235 ml) heavy cream	⅔ cup (160 ml) milk substitute + ⅓ cup (75 g) butter substitute, melted
1 cup (225 g) cottage cheese	1 cup (250 g) crumbled tofu (better flavored with dressing)
1 cup (235 ml) buttermilk	2 tablespoons (28 ml) lemon juice in 1 cup (235 ml) milk substitute

SUBSTITUTES FOR BUTTER

- Earth Balance Whipped Spread 100% vegan, non-hydrogenated (no trans-fat)
- GFCF, organic, non-GMO expeller-pressed oils, no artificial flavor or color
- Lard (excellent in baking, 4 parts lard for 5 parts butter)
- Coconut Butter/Coconut Oil (excellent for baking), healthy, non-hydrogenated unrefined good vegetable fat
- Spectrum Palm Shortening (excellent in baking and ice creams)
- For melted butter, substitute oil (safflower, almond, avocado, coconut) or melted ghee

SUBSTITUTES FOR EGG

SUBSTITUTE	EQUIVALENT TO 1 EGG
Unflavored gelatin 1 envelope (1 tablespoon or 7 g) unflavored gelatin in 1 cup (235 ml) boiling water	3 tablespoons (24 g)
Puréed fruits, mild flavors only—apple or pear	3 tablespoons (45 g)
Ener-G Egg Replacer (egg-free)	2 tablespoons (10 ml) + 2 tablespoons (30 ml) water
Cornstarch	2 tablespoons (16 g)
Arrowroot flour	2 tablespoons (16 g)
Potato starch	2 tablespoons (20 g)
Non-GMO soy milk powder	1 tablespoon (8 g)
Banana (good in cakes)	¼ cup (60 g)
Tofu naturally fermented	¼ cup (60 g)
Flaxseeds	Egg White Substitute: ½ cup flaxseeds + ¾ cup water Blend for 2–3 minutes. Refrigerate for ½ hour.

GENERAL SUBSTITUTES

ITEM	SUBSTITUTE
1 clove garlic	⅛ tablespoon garlic powder
1 cup (240 g) ketchup	1 cup (245 g) tomato sauce + ¾ cup (255 g) agave + 2 tablespoons (30 ml) vinegar
1 medium lemon	3 tablespoons (45 ml) lemon juice
1 tablespoon (15 g) mustard	1 tablespoon (9 g) dry mustard
1 small onion	2 tablespoons (20 g) fresh chopped or minced
1 medium onion	4 tablespoons (40 g) fresh chopped or minced
2 cups (300 g) chopped tomatoes	1 (16-ounce [455 g]) can chopped tomatoes, drained
1 cup (235 ml) wine	1 cup (235 ml) apple juice, apple cider, or chicken or beef broth
1 cup (330 g) corn syrup	1 cup (235 ml) maple syrup or 1 cup (340 g) honey

Quick Online Resources

- GFCF product finder: www.gfcfdiet.com/directory.htm

- Troubleshooting for Baking with Substitutes: Miss Roben's site: www.missroben.com/id1171.htm

Key to Recipe Icons

Throughout the recipe section, icons and short descriptors are used to indicate potentially problematic foods and food chemical components that are ingredients in the recipe or may be optional. Please refer to the guide below for assistance in determining whether a recipe is compatible with a particular elimination diet.

Icons for Gluten, Milk, Soy, Egg, Corn, and Nuts

This means that the recipe contains the food.

A solid circle with a slash indicates that the recipe **does not** contain the food.

Dashed lines with a slash indicates the recipe may contain the ingredient in some situations. For example, xanthan gum is sometimes derived from corn.

Low Phenol, Low Salicylate, Low Oxalate, and SCD (Specific Carbohydrate Diet)

- If a recipe is compatible with any of these diets, this will be indicated in writing below the icons. Look for the following labels:

  SCD Legal

  Low Phenol

  Low Salicylate

  Low Oxalate

  Modified for SCD

  Modified for Low Phenol

  Modified for Low Salicylate

  Modified for Low Oxalate

- If there is no mention of these diets, the reader should assume that the recipe is **not** compatible with those diets.

CHAPTER 13

A Complete Guide to Making Breakfast and Packing Lunches

THE MEAL TO FOCUS ON FIRST IS BREAKFAST. Studies have shown that the first food or drink of the day is the most important. It sets the pattern of eating for the day. Typical breakfast foods include too many refined carbohydrates, which raise blood sugar too quickly: breads, bagels, muffins, cold cereals, and instant hot cereals. This results in a pattern throughout the day of mood swings, frequent hunger, and cravings for more sweets and refined carbohydrates. Studies on the effect of breakfast quality on children's performance repeatedly reveal that the sweet and sugared breakfasts impair focus, attention, and performance.

Breakfast Like a King

The ideal breakfast should start with a protein or mix of proteins such as fish, poultry, meat, eggs, beans, nuts, seeds, and milk products if tolerated. Protein is critical for making brain neurotransmitters, strengthening immunity, and maintaining lean muscle mass and good muscle tone. Lunch and dinner leftovers are perfect choices for breakfast and certainly Quick N Easy. There are no "Breakfast Police"; you can improve the quality of breakfast by moving toward nontypical breakfast foods. Make a little extra at dinner and refrigerate enough for a serving at breakfast.

Eggs are the most nutrient-dense food available and have the highest-quality protein. Do not use egg substitutes. Humans have enjoyed and benefited from eggs for more than 400,000 years. Please read "The Good Egg" in chapter 3. As long as there are no allergies, include eggs!

The breakfast ideas below will need to be adjusted and adapted based on your child's individual elimination diet needs. Please see the specific chapters on the individual diets for recommendations regarding foods to avoid or include.

BREAKFAST IDEAS

Hardboiled eggs + fruit
Christina's Delicious Deviled Eggs
(p. 203)

Egg salad on tomato slice or egg salad + fruit
Simple Egg Salad (p. 287)

Scrambled eggs with or without vegetables + fruit
Scrambled Veggie Eggs (p. 200)

Vegetable omelet + fruit
Ground Vegetable Omelet (p. 200)
Mexican Breakfast Pizza (p. 201)

GFCF Quiche + fruit
Crustless Spinach Quiche (p. 199)

Hearty soup + fruit
Erika's Chicken Noodle Soup (p. 313)
Turkey Noodle Soup (p. 301)
Jane's Lentil Vegetable Soup (p. 301)
Best Beef Soup Ever (p. 304)

Breakfast sausage + fruit
Breakfast Sausage (p. 198)
Best's Kosher Sausage Links
(www.bestskosher.com)

Applegate Farms Turkey Apple or Turkey
Maple Sausage (links)
(www.applegate.com)

Other meat dishes + fruit
Shepherd's Pie (p. 227)
GFCF Chicken Nuggets (pp. 205, 214)
Fruity Rice Chicken or Turkey (p. 211)
Chicken Purée (p. 210)
Meatballs with Vegetables (p. 231)

Waffles, bars, granola, or oatmeal + additional protein (nuts, egg, GFCF sausage)
High-Protein Waffles (p. 190)
Crispy Breakfast Bars (p. 190)

Nuts and other options
Peanut butter on apple slices
Lentil Loaf (p. 243) + fruit
Dahl (Vegetarian or With Chicken) (p. 244)
Fruity Good Shake (p. 164)
Connor's Peanut Butter Blast Shake (p. 165)
Creamy Custard Drink (p. 166)

Packing School Lunches

THE CHALLENGE

With only twenty minutes to eat lunch, kids with autism spectrum disorder should be given "fast" foods that are not only easy to eat, but healthy, tasty, loaded with nutrients, and free of the culprits that are common problems: gluten, milk products, soy, and artificial additives and coloring. Compounding the time challenge are sensory issues involving food texture, color, and taste along with unusually picky appetites so common in ASD. Now, the task seems insurmountable. Beyond the challenges with foods themselves are the safety issues concerning the food containers, especially plastics containing phthalates and bisphenol A (BPA). And, of course, there is the "cool" factor, which affects preschoolers through high schoolers. Food that is different is totally uncool for kids who already face so many social and learning stigmas.

Knowing the challenges, we can now focus on the solutions.

THE SOLUTIONS

Basics

As is the case with any meal, there are some basics to follow. Protein, fiber, and good fats are needed to stabilize blood sugar. Blood sugar control is critical. All people are affected by rapidly rising blood sugar, which then cascades down too quickly and too low. The most noticeable effects are on brain function, especially mood and attention. When the blood sugar drops too quickly and/or too low, there can be irritability, hunger headaches, lack of focus, behavior problems, and cravings for a "quick sugar fix" that keeps the cycle going. This interferes with learning and can be disruptive to the class. See chapter 3 for more detailed information.

Additional Suggestions

- **SEEK THE ELIMINATION DIET(S) RECOMMENDED FOODS AND GIVE THEM A TEST RUN.** There are numerous resources for foods and recipes online and in many books. Use all of these to find the organic, commercially available foods your child will eat as well as recipes that are also nutritious and delicious.

  Test new items at home, however, not in the school lunch.

- Establish three to five basic lunches that work. If your child is willing and interested, engage him or her in the process. Use freezer packs for keeping foods cold and a thermos for hot foods. Include nontoxic hand sanitizers, which are commercially available (avoid the commercial sanitizers). You can also send two paper towel pieces—one moistened with soap and one moistened with water.

- **TOSS IN A FAVORITE FOOD.** Promote more interest in the meal by including at least one food that your child considers "a favorite."

- **PACKAGING: A GOOD OPPORTUNITY TO GO GREEN**

  Again, follow the marketer's lead—jazz it up! Select a lunch container your child loves. Young children love to decorate a lunch box with stickers and paints. Make the lunch box the child's own work of art, personalized with a name. Reusable containers and boxes are the green way to go. Older children will definitely want to select whatever is considered cool. The coolest may be a paper bag or small recycled bags carried in a backpack. Go with the trend and your child's own choice.

There are companies that make safe, BPA-free, lunch box sets with inserts for the different foods.

Avoid plastic wraps and sandwich bags for sandwiches; instead, use wax paper or parchment paper. Avoid containers with BPA by avoiding items with the recycle number 7. There are many BPA-free containers which can be washed and reused. Your child will need to be reminded to bring these back home rather than throw them away.

For napkins, use washable cloth napkins or dishcloths or choose processed chlorine-free (PCF), post-consumer-waste (PCW) paper napkins available in stores and online. If utensils are needed, use stainless steel appropriate to the child's skill level and age.

- **ADD TO THE FUN-FACTOR.** Take a tip from the fast-food marketers and include a surprise gift in the lunch. It might be a small collectible such as a car, baseball card, character, hair clip, sticker, ring, or bracelet. Homemade "giftlets" (tiny gifts) are perfect.

Nutritious Can Be Delicious

Recall what we discussed in chapter 11 and use the Trojan Horse concept as a way to sneak nutrition into your child's lunches. Disguise the new foods within the usual, well-liked foods. We can't emphasize enough the importance of matching the color and texture, mixing vegetable juice with fruit juice, and including muffin "casseroles" that mask puréed fruits, vegetables, and even meat. Your goal is to get a child to eat nutritious food, however you can. If an opaque sippy cup is used, the color of the beverage will not be noticed.

Assuming the new food is a vegetable, use organic baby food purées or make your own. Purée the vegetable into an established food in such a fashion that it does not change the overall color, texture, smell, or taste of the well-liked food. If a child eats nothing but white food, start with very light-colored vegetables such as squash, cauliflower, and corn. Vegetable choices may need to be adapted depending on your child's particular elimination diet(s). If the child likes ketchup or tomato sauce, then introduce deeper-colored vegetables such as beets, greens, peas, and beans. Puréed vegetables can be beaten into batter for pancakes, muffins, brownies, and cookies or into tomato and other pasta and pizza sauces, and even into ketchup.

Five Simple and Delicious Lunch Suggestions

Use the following five lunch suggestions (on pages 156–158) as they are written, or feel free to mix and match the pieces to find the perfect lunchtime combination for your child.

DRINKS: All of these lunches should be accompanied by either water or other drinks compatible with the elimination diet(s) being used: vegetable juice, juice box, or fortified organic rice-milk drink box.

CONTAINERS: Use BPA-free containers to store foods.

LUNCH INGREDIENTS WILL NEED TO BE ADAPTED BASED ON YOUR CHILD'S PARTICULAR ELIMINATION DIET(S). Please see the individual chapters on specific diets for suggestions for foods to avoid or include.

Lunch #1: BBQ Chicken for Champions

- **Chicken strips**
- **BBQ dipping sauce**
- **Steamed vegetables**
- **Veggie dipping sauce**

Snack, if needed: GFCF chips and 1 cup (260 g) Fruity Salsa (recipe below)

Toy surprise ideas: yarn bracelet, mini toy figure

Chicken Breast

- $^1/_2$ chicken breast

Add salt and pepper to taste and pan fry in olive oil on medium-high heat for six minutes on each side. Cut into strips. Serve with $^1/_4$ cup (65 g) serving of BBQ Dipping Sauce.

Steamed Vegetables

- 1 broccoli stalk (or frozen single-serving package)

Steam broccoli florets for 7 minutes. Run cold water over them.

BBQ Dipping Sauce

- 1 cup (240 g) organic ketchup
- 1 tablespoon (15 ml) lemon juice
- 1 teaspoon Worcestershire sauce (GFCF)
- 1 tablespoon (20 g) honey
- Dash of black pepper

Blend all of the above until smooth.

YIELD: *1$^1/_4$ cup (300 g)*

Fruity Salsa

- 1 cup (250 g) salsa
- ^{1} cup (80 g) grape, blueberry, or raspberry fruit spread

Mash the fruit spread into the salsa.

YIELD: *1$^1/_4$ cup (330 g)*

Lunch #2: DLT

- **DLT sandwich**
- **GFCF Potato Salad, $^1/_3$ cup (85 g)**
- **Fruit (e.g., apple or grapes)**

Snack, if needed: Hummus on rice crackers

Toy surprise ideas: hair scrunchie, baseball card

DLT ("Deli" meat, lettuce, and tomato)

- 2 slices of turkey or chicken GFCF preservative-free organic lunch meats (by Boar's Head, Applegate, or Shelton)
- 2 slices of GFCF bread, toasted
- 1 tablespoon (14 g) GFCF mayonnaise
- Lettuce and tomato

Spread the mayonnaise on a slice of bread. Cover with 2 slices of GFCF lunch meat and top with lettuce and a slice of tomato. Cut into 4 squares and wrap in wax paper.

GFCF Potato Salad

- 3 pounds (1.4 kg) potatoes, cooked until just tender, cubed, cooled
- 5 or 6 hard-cooked eggs, cooled, coarsely chopped, optional
- $^1/_4$ (40 g) to $^1/_2$ cup (80 g) chopped red onion
- $^1/_4$ (25 g) to $^1/_2$ cup (50 g) chopped celery, optional

For the dressing:

- $^3/_4$ cup (175 g) GFCF mayonnaise
- 1 (14 g) to 2 (28 g) tablespoons prepared GFCF mustard
- Salt and pepper to taste

Prepare the dressing, combining the mayonnaise, mustard, and salt and pepper to taste. Combine potatoes, egg, onions, and celery and stir in the dressing.

YIELD: *6 to 8 servings*

Lunch #3: Chicken Salad and Deviled Eggs

- **Chicken Salad ($^1/_3$ to $^1/_2$ cup) (70 to 100 g)**
- **Deviled Eggs (two halves)**
- **Carrot sticks wrapped in wax paper and served with applesauce**

Snack, if needed: GFCF chips & hummus

Toy surprise ideas: mini toy car, hair clip

Chicken Salad

- 3 cups (420 g) cooked chicken, diced
- 2 ribs celery, thinly sliced
- 1 cup (150 g) seedless green grapes, halved
- $^3/_4$ cup (175 g) GFCF mayonnaise
- 2 tablespoons (12 g) finely minced green onions
- 1 teaspoon (5 ml) lemon juice
- $^1/_4$ teaspoon ground ginger
- Salt and pepper, to taste

Combine chicken, celery, and grapes in a large bowl; set aside. In a small bowl, whisk together remaining ingredients. Then, combine with chicken mixture, using as much or as little as necessary to moisten as desired. You may add a little more mayonnaise if you like a creamier salad. Chill and stir again before serving.

YIELD: 4 to 6 servings

Deviled Eggs

- 6 hard-boiled eggs, cooled, shelled, cut in half, yolks removed and set aside
- $1^1/_2$ tablespoons (21 g) GFCF mayonnaise
- 1 teaspoon (4 g) prepared mustard
- $^1/_2$ teaspoon salt
- 2 tablespoons (30 g) sweet pickle relish, or to taste
- Paprika

Mash yolks and combine with mayonnaise, mustard, salt, and relish. Refill centers of the egg whites with the mixture. Garnish with ground paprika.

YIELD: 6 servings (2 halves per person)

Lunch #4: Chicken, Apple Salad, Veggie Muffins

- **Baked or grilled chicken leftovers from dinner, approximately 1/2 chicken breast**
- **Apple Salad, packed in a cold thermos**
- **1 to 2 Magical Veggie Muffins**

Snack, if needed: Carrots and Bean Dip

Toy surprise ideas: hand stamp or mood ring

Apple Salad

- 2 large Red Delicious apples, unpeeled, cored, and cut into 1-inch (2.5 cm) chunks
- $^2/_3$ cup (135 g) crushed and drained pineapple or fresh minced pineapple (reserve juice for dressing)
- $^1/_3$ cup (40 g) diced celery
- 2 tablespoons (20 g) raisins

For the Dressing:

- 3 tablespoons (45 g) soy yogurt
- 2 teaspoons GFCF mayonnaise
- 1 tablespoon (15 ml) pineapple juice
- $^1/_8$ teaspoon cinnamon

In a medium bowl, combine the salad ingredients. In a small bowl, whisk the dressing ingredients together and pour the dressing over the salad. Toss to combine.

YIELD: 2 servings

Magical Veggie Muffins

- 1 box (14.8 ounces, or 425 g) store-bought GFCF cake mix
- 1 cup (245 g) puréed vegetables (Use one or more of the following: carrots, squash, peas, or green beans.)
- $^1/_2$ cup (120 g) applesauce
- 1 cup (175 g) GFCF chocolate chips, optional

In a large bowl, prepare cake mix batter according to package directions. Add puréed vegetables and applesauce and mix to combine. Stir in chocolate chips (if using).

Lightly grease a muffin tin or line with paper liners. Spoon the batter into the muffin cups, filling each about two-thirds full. Bake at 375°F (190°C, or gas mark 5) for 25 to 30 minutes, or until a toothpick inserted in the center of a muffin comes out clean. (Do not overcook, as this will result in dry muffins.)

Once cooled, store the muffins in an airtight container or freeze for later use.

YIELD: *24 muffins*

Lunch #5: Sensory Sensible Pot Pie Muffins and Dip

- **1 to 2 Sensory Sensible Protein Muffins**
- **Hummus dip (with carrots or GFCF crackers)**
- **Applesauce or other fruit**

Toy surprise ideas: festive pencil/pen

Snack, if needed: Organic apple chips

Sensory Sensible Pot Pie Muffins

- 1 box (14.8 ounces, or 425 g) store-bought GFCF muffin or quick bread mix
- 1 cup (245 g) puréed vegetables (Use one or more of the following: carrots, squash, peas, or green beans.)
- $^1/_2$ cup (120 g) applesauce
- $^1/_2$ cup (120 g) puréed chicken*

In a large bowl, prepare cake mix batter according to package directions. Add puréed vegetables, applesauce, and chicken and mix to combine.

Lightly grease a muffin tin or line with paper liners. Spoon the batter into the muffin cups, filling each about two-thirds full. Bake at 375°F (190°C, or gas mark 5) for 25 to 30 minutes, or until a toothpick inserted in the center of a muffin comes out clean. (Do not overcook, as this will result in dry muffins.)

Once cooled, store the muffins in an airtight container or freeze for later use.

*To purée chicken, combine cooked, chopped chicken with a bit of chicken broth or water (or even white grape juice) in a blender, and blend until desired consistency is reached.

YIELD: *24 muffins*

CHAPTER 14

Beverages and Healthy Shakes

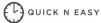 QUICK N EASY

Wonderful Water

It is the only beverage that is essential for human life on Earth.

gluten   milk   soy   egg   corn   nuts

- Water (filtered, bottled, carbonated)

This should be the first and last beverage of every day.

Drink half the body weight in ounces of water.

Drink most between meals, sipped throughout the day.

Drink $1/2$ to 1 glass with meals.

Enjoy.

YIELD: *Unlimited*

 QUICK N EASY

Rice Milk #1

It is best to use warm water and warm rice.

gluten   milk   soy   egg   corn   nuts

Low Oxalate: *Use white rice instead of brown rice.*
Low Phenol
Low Salicylate

- 4 cups (940 ml) hot/warm water
- 1 cup (160 g) cooked rice (white or brown)
- 1 teaspoon (5 ml) vanilla

Process all ingredients in a blender until smooth. Let the milk set for about 30 minutes. Pour the milk steadily into another container (an old honey jar can be used), leaving most of the sediment in the first container. It can be stored in the refrigerator for up to five days.

YIELD: *About 4-4$1/2$ cups (940 ml-1 L)*

Calories (kcal): 63; **Total fat:** trace; **Cholesterol:** 0mg; **Carbohydrate:** 13g; **Dietary fiber:** trace; **Protein:** 1g; **Sodium:** 8mg; **Potassium:** 18mg; **Calcium:** 10mg; **Iron:** trace; **Zinc:** trace; **Vitamin A:** 0IU.

Rice Milk #2

gluten   milk   soy   egg   corn   nuts

Modified for Low Salicylate

- 4 cups (940 ml) boiling water
- 2 cups (370 g) rice (white or brown)
- Oil (high-oleic safflower, avocado)—for texture (optional) (Avoid avocado for low salicylate diet.)
- Pure vanilla flavor to taste (optional)
- Salt to taste (optional)

Rinse rice to clean. Pour 4 cups (940 ml) boiling water over rice and let soak for 1 to 2 hours. Blend 1 cup (185 g) soaked rice with 2^1/$_2$ cups (590 ml) water (can be cold water.) Blend rice to a slurry (textured liquid), pour into a pot, and repeat with rest of rice. Bring to a boil and then reduce heat and simmer for 20 minutes.

Line a colander with a nylon tricot or a few layers of cheesecloth. Put a bowl under colander. Pour rice mix in colander; another 1 cup (235 ml) water (or less or more) can be poured over the rice to get out more milk. Press with the back of a spoon, twist nylon, and squeeze out as much milk as possible. This milk is very plain and can be flavored with oil, vanilla, salt, etc.

YIELD: *4 cups (940 ml)*

Calories (kcal): 351; **Total fat:** 2g; **Cholesterol:** 0mg; **Carbohydrate:** 74g; **Dietary fiber:** 1g; **Protein:** 7g; **Sodium:** 78mg; **Potassium:** 106mg; **Calcium:** 31mg; **Iron:** 4mg; **Zinc:** 1mg; **Vitamin A:** 0IU.

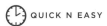 QUICK N EASY

Dana's Drink

gluten   milk   soy   egg   corn   nuts

My favorite flavoring juice is white grape juice. This drink is named by my neighbors because I always serve it as a "soft drink" when we have parties, and it was the official drink of the Garret Park Swim Team for years.

SCD Legal

- 1 (liter) bottle seltzer (not soda water)
- 4–6 tablespoons (2–3 ounces [55–85 g]) 100% frozen fruit juice concentrate, thawed (avoid any juice that is not 100% fruit juice)

  Best juice choices:
  - Organic white grape juice plus squeeze of lemon and lime
  - Orange juice

Pour a small amount of seltzer out of the bottle and slowly add the thawed fruit juice concentrate. Do this slowly so the contents don't fizz out of the bottle. Use just enough to flavor the drink. Leave this in the refrigerator so your family can enjoy this natural soda. Serve over ice, in a pitcher, or in a punch bowl.

When weaning children off sodas, it may be helpful to make the drink slightly sweeter at first.

To make a party punch that is nonalcoholic sangria, add a variety of juices and cut-up fruits. This is a definite crowd-pleaser.

YIELD: *1 liter*

Calories (kcal): 97; **Total fat:** 0g; **Cholesterol:** 0mg; **Carbohydrate:** 22g; **Dietary fiber:** 0g; **Protein:** 1g; **Sodium:** 25mg; **Potassium:** 277mg; **Calcium:** 35mg; **Iron:** 0mg; **Zinc:** 0mg; **Vitamin A:** 0IU.

Agave-Sweetened Fruit Drink or Spritzer

gluten   milk   soy   egg   corn   nuts

An extract of the wild agave cactus from Mexico, agave nectar is a sweetener similar to honey. It has less of an effect on blood glucose compared to sugar. And it is quite versatile and works well in baked goods, puddings, and beverages. Less agave nectar is needed compared to sugar, but that is a matter of taste. Approximately ³/4 cup (255 g) of agave is equal to 1 cup (200 g) of sugar.

Low Phenol, Low Salicylate, Low Oxalate

- ¹/2 medium lemon, squeezed or 2 tablespoons (30 ml) of mango, papaya, or pear juice for low phenol, low salicylate, low oxalate options
- 1 cup (235 ml) water or seltzer water (unflavored GFCF)
- 2 teaspoons agave nectar (to taste)
- Ice cubes

Squeeze fresh lemon into glass of water. Add agave nectar and ice cubes. Stir and enjoy.

YIELD: *1 tall glass (about 12 ounces [355 ml])*

Calories (kcal): 46; **Total fat:** trace; **Cholesterol:** 0mg; **Carbohydrate:** 14g; **Dietary fiber:** trace; **Protein:** trace; **Sodium:** 8mg; **Potassium:** 42mg; **Calcium:** 12mg; **Iron:** trace; **Zinc:** trace; **Vitamin A:** 9IU.

Blueberry Blend

gluten   milk   soy   egg   corn   nuts

This purple-blue shake is inspired by Lisa Barnes in The Petit Appetit Cookbook. *Blueberries contain a number of vitamins, including A, C, and E, as well as anti-oxidants that improve immunity. It is better to serve the blueberries blended as a shake as they can be a choking hazard to young children. This also hides the milder-tasting supplements.*

SCD Legal

- 1¹/2 cups (235 g) frozen blueberries
- ¹/4 cup (60 g) vanilla non-GMO soy or rice yogurt
- ¹/4 cup (60 ml) coconut milk
- 1 cup (235 ml) unfiltered pasteurized organic apple juice

Combine all ingredients in a blender and process until smooth. Strain through a mesh strainer for the smoothest texture.

YIELD: *About 3 servings of 1 cup (235 ml) each*

Calories (kcal): 134; **Total fat:** 6g; **Cholesterol:** 0mg; **Carbohydrate:** 21g; **Dietary fiber:** 3g; **Protein:** 2g; **Sodium:** 6mg; **Potassium:** 193mg; **Calcium:** 15mg; **Iron:** 1mg; **Zinc:** trace; **Vitamin A:** 64IU.

Melon Mango Smoothie or Cold Soup

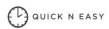

gluten　　milk　　soy　　egg　　corn　　nuts

According to Lisa Barnes (The Petit Appetit Cookbook) this makes a great breakfast soup. Packed with vitamins A and C and calcium, this soup makes a great alternative to a plain piece of fruit or a morning shake. Mangoes are grown throughout the tropics and are often called "the peach of the tropics." This recipe will hide some of the milder-tasting supplements.

SCD Legal, Modified for Low Phenol

- ¹/₂ large cantaloupe
- ¹/₂ large mango
- ³/₄ cup (175 g) plain soy yogurt or ¹/₂ cup (120 ml) rice milk or coconut milk (For SCD, use homemade SCD yogurt. For low phenol, avoid soy yogurt.)

Cut cantaloupe in half and remove seeds. Cut flesh away from skin and cut into 1-inch (2.5 cm) cubes. Peel mango and remove flesh from pit. Cut into 1-inch (2.5 cm) cubes. Put cantaloupe and mango into food processor or blender and process until smooth, about 20 seconds. Pour mixture into a large glass or plastic bowl. Stir yogurt or rice milk into mixture. Cover and chill for 1 hour before serving.

YIELD: *About 3 servings of 1 cup (235 ml) each*

Calories (kcal): 84; **Total fat:** 2g; **Cholesterol:** 0mg; **Carbohydrate:** 15g; **Dietary fiber:** 2g; **Protein:** 3g; **Sodium:** 9mg; **Potassium:** 338mg; **Calcium:** 14mg; **Iron:** trace; **Zinc:** trace; **Vitamin A:** 4310IU.

Great Grape Slush

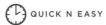

gluten　　milk　　soy　　egg　　corn　　nuts

From Lisa Barnes, The Petit Appetit Cookbook

This is a healthy improvement over the brightly colored slushies with fake flavors and colorings from the fast-food and convenience stores. You can add ice cubes for older children, which will increase the yield.

SCD Legal

- ³/₄ cup (112.5 g) frozen organic seedless purple grapes
- 1 organic apple (150 g), peeled, cored, and chopped
- ¹/₂ cup (120 ml) organic unfiltered apple juice

Add all ingredients to a blender and blend until slushy.

NOTE: *Spread individual grapes on a pan and freeze. Then transfer to a freezer bag or container to have available for kids to eat alone as a frosty snack, or to make this tasty slush.*

YIELD: *1¹/₂ cups (355 ml)*

Calories (kcal): 185; **Total fat:** 1g; **Cholesterol:** 0mg; **Carbohydrate:** 48g; **Dietary fiber:** 4g; **Protein:** 1g; **Sodium:** 5mg; **Potassium:** 444mg; **Calcium:** 28mg; **Iron:** 1mg; **Zinc:** trace; **Vitamin A:** 146IU.

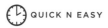

QUICK N EASY

Fruity Good Shakes

gluten   milk   soy   egg   corn   nuts

There are so many varieties of this recipe that there is bound to be one suitable to each child. Children with sensory issues will appreciate the smooth texture, without any lumps or pieces. The addition of coconut milk provides taste, variety, and healing nutritional qualities. According to Sally Fallon and Mary Enig, Ph.D. (Nourishing Traditions), the principal fatty acid in coconut milk is lauric acid, which is antiviral, antifungal, and antimicrobial. This is another good food source for hiding nutritional supplements.

Modified for SCD, Modified for Low Phenol, Modified for Low Oxalate

Low SCD: *Milks: Coconut milk; Fruits: Banana, berries, grapes, mango, melon, papaya, peach, pear, and pineapple*

Low Oxalate and Low Phenol: *Milks: White rice milk or coconut milk; Fruits: Mango, melon, papaya, peach, pear, and pineapple*

- 1¼ cups (295 ml) rice milk or non-milk toddler formula
- ½ glass crushed ice
- 1 tablespoon (3 g) protein powder
- 1 tablespoon (15 ml) coconut milk (optional)
- **FOR BANANA SHAKE:** Add 1 sliced banana
- **FOR PEAR SHAKE:** Add 1 cored and chopped pear
- **FOR BERRY SHAKE:** Add 1 handful strawberries, raspberries, blackberries, or blueberries, or a combination
- **FOR PEACH SHAKE:** Add 1 pitted and chopped ripe peach or nectarine

Blend the milk, crushed ice, rice powder, and coconut milk (if desired) in a blender. Add the fruit or fruits. Blend the mixture at high speed until smooth and thick (no lumps or pieces).

Pour into glasses and serve immediately.

YIELD: *2 to 3 child-size servings*

Calories (kcal): 75; **Total fat:** 2g; **Cholesterol:** 0mg; **Carbohydrate:** 13g; **Dietary fiber:** trace; **Protein:** 1g; **Sodium:** 8mg; **Potassium:** 35mg; **Calcium:** 9mg; **Iron:** trace; **Zinc:** trace; **Vitamin A:** 0IU.

QUICK N EASY

Connor's PB Blast Shake

     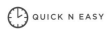
gluten   milk   soy   egg   corn   nuts

Lori Skalitzky offers this delicious recipe, which also is perfect for hiding
supplements, especially those with a strong taste.

Modified for SCD

- ¹/₄ cup (60 ml) organic milk substitute (For SCD, use nut milks.)

- 2 tablespoons (32 g) creamy GFCF peanut butter

- 1 tablespoon (15 ml) 100% maple syrup or 1 tablespoon (20 g) honey (For SCD, use honey.)

- 3–4 scoops vanilla-flavored ice cream substitute (For SCD, use ice cream substitute that is almond or cashew based.)

In a blender, mix the milk substitute, peanut butter, and maple syrup or honey at medium speed until smooth. Add the ice cream substitute and pulse until combined.

YIELD: *1¹/₂ to 2 cups (355 to 475 ml)*

Calories (kcal): 789; **Total fat:** 46g; **Cholesterol:** 116mg; **Carbohydrate:** 85g; **Dietary fiber:** 2g; **Protein:** 18g; **Sodium:** 366mg; **Potassium:** 786mg; **Calcium:** 373mg; **Iron:** 1mg; **Zinc:** 3mg; **Vitamin A:** 1080IU.

> "Our son, Connor, who is now five and a half years old, has been gluten-free and casein-free now for over three years. He is also mostly soy-free, though not 100 percent. Connor was minimally verbal before we started the diet—he said some words but didn't even put two words together for a statement yet. We took him off of milk products first and began to see some improvement; he seemed much more with it. But the most mind-boggling thing for us was when we took him off of gluten. Three days later, our boy was singing full versions of songs, something he had never done before. And now, after many years on the diet and many other interventions, many people tell us that other than a few self-stimming behaviors, he looks just like any other five-year-old around."
>
> **—Lori Skalitzky,** *mother of Connor, a five-year-old with autism*

Creamy Custard Drink

gluten milk soy egg corn nuts

Adapted from Welby Griffin

This thick, creamy beverage is perfect for those who don't like to eat eggs otherwise. It is also a great place to sneak in all sorts of vitamins and supplements.

- ⅓ cup (43 g) cornstarch
- ½ cup (50 g) sugar
- 1 quart (950 ml) rice milk
- 6 large eggs
- 2 teaspoons GFCF vanilla extract

In a large sauce pan, whisk together cornstarch and sugar to eliminate any lumps. Add rice milk and cook over medium-high heat until warm and slightly thickened, but not boiling.

Meanwhile, beat eggs together in a medium bowl. Slowly pour half of warmed milk mixture into the eggs, stirring constantly. Then transfer the egg mixture into the remaining milk mixture in the pan, stirring well to combine. Cook the mixture over medium heat, stirring constantly, until it reaches 175°F. Add the vanilla and allow to cool to room temperature before transferring the custard to the refrigerator to chill completely. Store in a covered container up to 3 days.

NOTE: *If custard becomes too thick or lumpy, pulse in a blender a few times until smooth, while adjusting the consistency by adding more rice milk.*

VARIATION: *Add up to one-half pound of boiled, mashed carrots to the custard after cooking. You may want to add a teaspoon more vanilla or a pinch of nutmeg for flavor, and some extra rice milk to adjust the consistency.*

YIELD: *4 to 6 servings*

Calories (kcal): 250; **Total fat:** 6g; **Cholesterol:** 229mg; **Carbohydrate:** 43g; **Dietary fiber:** trace; **Protein:** 7g; **Sodium:** 128mg; **Potassium:** 116mg; **Calcium:** 40mg; **Iron:** 1mg; **Zinc:** 1mg; **Vitamin A:** 247IU.

QUICK N EASY

Popeye Smoothie I

gluten milk soy egg corn nuts

This smoothie recipe is another way to get a vegetable into kids. It's hard to believe, but you can't taste the spinach in this smoothie. However, the smoothie is bright green, so would need to be hidden in a covered cup, like a sippy cup.

- 2 cups (60 g) baby spinach
- $^1/_2$ banana, very ripe
- 1 cup (235 ml) water
- 4 to 6 ice cubes (about 4 ounces, or 112 g)

Combine all the ingredients in a blender. Blend on high until smooth. Serve immediately.

YIELD: *2 servings*

Calories (kcal): 34; **Total fat:** trace; **Cholesterol:** 0mg; **Carbohydrate:** 8g; **Dietary fiber:** 2g; **Protein:** 1g; **Sodium:** 28mg; **Potassium:** 284mg; **Calcium:** 34mg; **Iron:** 1mg; **Zinc:** trace; **Vitamin A:** 2018IU.

 QUICK N EASY

Popeye Smoothie II

gluten milk soy egg corn nuts

Another variation on the spinach smoothie where, again, you would never know the spinach is in there! Feel free to leave the peel on the apple, but be sure to wash it well.

- 2 cups (60 g) baby spinach
- 1 kiwi, peeled and chopped
- 1 sweet apple, cored and sliced
- 1 to 2 teaspoons lime juice
- $^1/_2$ cup (120 ml) water
- 4 to 6 ice cubes (about 4 ounces, or 112 g)

Combine all the ingredients in a blender. Blend on high until smooth. Serve immediately.

YIELD: *2 servings*

Calories (kcal): 72; **Total fat:** 1g; **Cholesterol:** 0mg; **Carbohydrate:** 18g; **Dietary fiber:** 4g; **Protein:** 1g; **Sodium:** 27mg; **Potassium:** 378mg; **Calcium:** 46mg; **Iron:** 1mg; **Zinc:** trace; **Vitamin A:** 2118IU.

Dairy-Free Delicious Hot Cocoa

gluten milk soy egg corn nuts

SCD Legal, Modified for Low Salicylate

GFCF Chocolate Syrup

- ¹/₂ cup (40 g) GFCF unsweetened cocoa powder (Use organic cocoa powder for low salicylate diet.)
- ³/₄ cup (255 g) agave nectar (Use stevia for low salicylate diet.)
- ¹/₄ cup (60 ml) water
- ¹/₂ teaspoon organic vanilla extract— low salicylate
- Pinch salt

Combine cocoa powder, agave nectar, and water in a small saucepan, and bring to a boil. Add vanilla and salt and cool to room temperature. Store in an airtight container in the refrigerator for up to 5 days.

YIELD: *1 cup, 8 servings*

Hot Cocoa

SCD Legal, Modified for Low Salicylate

- 2 tablespoons (30 ml) GFCF chocolate syrup (Use organic cocoa powder for low salicylate diet.)
- ³/₄ cup (180 ml) soy, almond, or other dairy-free milk of choice (Avoid almond milk for low salicylate.)

Heat milk in a saucepan or in the microwave until very hot but not boiling. Whisk syrup into milk to combine. Serve.

YIELD: *1 serving*

Calories (kcal): 157; **Total fat:** 4g; **Cholesterol:** 0mg; **Carbohydrate:** 28g; **Dietary fiber:** 6g; **Protein:** 6g; **Sodium:** 23mg; **Potassium:** 341mg; **Calcium:** 14mg; **Iron:** 2mg; **Zinc:** 1mg; **Vitamin A:** 60IU.

Nut Milk and Nut Yogurt

gluten milk soy egg corn nuts

SCD Legal

From Karyn Seroussi and Lisa Lewis from The Encyclopedia of Dietary Interventions *(Autism Network for Dietary Intervention) and Julie Matthews in* Cooking To Heal *(Nourishing Hope).*

Nut milk and nut yogurt are alternatives to dairy-based milk and yogurt. They can be made from a variety of nuts, and you can experiment with adding your favorite sweetener and flavorings. Nut yogurt contains far more beneficial bacteria than you can get from a capsule and has a mild pleasant flavor.

Nut Milk

- 2 cups (270 g) nuts (macadamia nuts, raw almonds, and/or walnuts) soaked overnight (8 to 12 hours)
- 4 cups (946 ml) cold water
- 2 tablespoons (40 g) honey or 2 pitted dates (optional)

Combine drained, soaked nuts, and honey or pitted dates (if using) in a blender with cold water, at low speed, and then increase speed to high for 10 to 15 seconds. Then strain (see note below) and serve.

NOTE: *A "nut milk bag" makes it easy to squeeze out the liquid when making nut milk and nut yogurt. You can order one at www.purejoyplanet.com.*

TIP: *You may also sweeten the milk with rice syrup, vegetable glycerin, or stevia; or flavor it with some natural vanilla extract. Some nuts have a slight sweetness on their own, and the addition of fruit for a smoothie may add all the flavor and sweetening needed. The residual nuts can be saved and used in muffins or cookies or* as a "breading" or filler in meatballs or loaves. If unsweetened, or sweetened with honey, nut milk is perfect for monosaccharide diets such as the SCD. Avoid rice syrup, glycerin, and stevia if on SCD.

YIELD: *4 cups (940 ml) nut milk*

Using honey: Calories (kcal): 450; **Total fat:** 37g; **Cholesterol:** 0mg; **Carbohydrate:** 23g; **Dietary fiber:** 8g; **Protein:** 14g; **Sodium:** 8mg; **Potassium:** 525mg; **Calcium:** 189mg; **Iron:** 3mg; **Zinc:** 2mg; **Vitamin A:** 0IU.

Using dates: Calories (kcal): 430; **Total fat:** 37g; **Cholesterol:** 0mg; **Carbohydrate:** 18g; **Dietary fiber:** 8g; **Protein:** 14g; **Sodium:** 8mg; **Potassium:** 547mg; **Calcium:** 190mg; **Iron:** 3mg; **Zinc:** 2mg; **Vitamin A:** 2IU.

Nut Yogurt

- 2 cups (270 g) nuts (macadamia are best), soaked overnight (8 to 12 hours)
- 4 cups (940 ml) hot water
- $1/8$ teaspoon yogurt starter (GI ProStart from GI ProHealth)

Combine drained, soaked nuts and water in a blender, at low speed, and then increase speed to high for 10 to 15 seconds. (Julie suggests the milk then be heated to 160°F [71°C] to prevent the yogurt from separating.) Strain through a fine sieve or nut bag and cool to between 105°F and 110°F (40.5°C and 43°C), then whisk in yogurt starter. Place in a yogurt maker (at 95°F to 105°F [35 to 40.5°C]) for at least 8 hours (if using individual containers, leave the lids off during fermentation to avoid condensation). Place in refrigerator for at least 5 hours. It will separate somewhat, but do not throw away the liquid—it is rich in probiotics. You can drink it, or stir it back in to make a yogurt smoothie. Additional straining of the yogurt is optional and will result in a thicker yogurt.

TIP: *You may add any one or a combination of the following to the yogurt:*

- *Cinnamon*
- *Natural GFCF vanilla extract*
- *Cut-up fruit, stirred into the yogurt*

YIELD: *4 cups*

Calories (kcal): 470; **Total fat:** 49g; **Cholesterol:** 0mg; **Carbohydrate:** 9g; **Dietary fiber:** 6g; **Protein:** 6g; **Sodium:** 10mg; **Potassium:** 247mg; **Calcium:** 52mg; **Iron:** 2mg; **Zinc:** 1mg; **Vitamin A:** 0IU.

CHAPTER 15

Condiments, Dressings, and Sauces

"Condiments are like old friends—
highly thought of, but often taken for granted."

—Marilyn Kaytor

"Condiments: The Tastemakers," Look Magazine, 1963

Butter Substitute

gluten milk soy egg corn nuts

Low Phenol, Low Oxalate

- 6 tablespoons (85 g) Omega Nutrition coconut oil (room temperature)
- 2 tablespoons (30 ml) flax oil
- 2 tablespoons (30 ml) sunflower oil or avocado oil

Place ingredients in a blender and mix until integrated. Do not overmix. Place in an opaque container with a lid to protect the delicate oils from the light. Butter itself is acceptable to use on SCD.

YIELD: *10 tablespoons (140 g)*

Calories (kcal): 119; **Total fat:** 14g; **Cholesterol:** 0mg; **Carbohydrate:** 0g; **Dietary fiber:** 0g; **Protein:** 0g; **Sodium:** trace; **Potassium:** 0mg; **Calcium:** trace; **Iron:** trace; **Zinc:** 0mg; **Vitamin A:** 0IU.

Good Mayonnaise

gluten milk soy egg corn nuts

- 1 egg
- $1/2$ teaspoon dry mustard
- $1/2$ teaspoon sugar
- $1/4$ teaspoon paprika
- 2 tablespoons (30 ml) white wine vinegar
  (or Ener-G yeast-free vinegar powder, reconstituted)
- $1/2$ teaspoon arrowroot (this amount is low in oxalate)
- 1 cup (235 ml) oil (avocado or safflower), divided

Use a blender and combine all of the ingredients except $1/2$ cup (120 ml) of the oil. After all the other ingredients are blended, slowly add the remaining oil and blend until the mixture is smooth and thick. If a blender is not available, use a hand whisk (and a lot of elbow grease).

YIELD: *1$1/2$ cups (360 g)*

Calories (kcal): 201; **Total fat:** 223g; **Cholesterol:** 187mg; **Carbohydrate:** 6g; **Dietary fiber:** trace; **Protein:** 6g; **Sodium:** 56mg; **Potassium:** 104mg; **Calcium:** 27mg; **Iron:** 1mg; **Zinc:** 1mg; **Vitamin A:** 631IU.

QUICK N EASY

Dana's Simple Dressing

    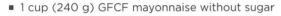

gluten milk soy egg corn nuts

- 1 cup (240 g) GFCF mayonnaise without sugar
- 1/2 cup (120 g) GFCF ketchup

Combine mayonnaise and ketchup without sugar in a small bowl until blended.

YIELD: *1 1/2 cups (360 g)*

Calories (kcal): 170; **Total fat:** 187g; **Cholesterol:** 77mg; **Carbohydrate:** 33g; **Dietary fiber:** 2g; **Protein:** 4g; **Sodium:** 2674mg; **Potassium:** 652mg; **Calcium:** 62mg; **Iron:** 2mg; **Zinc:** 1mg; **Vitamin A:** 1835IU.

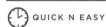 QUICK N EASY

Simple Thousand Island Dressing

gluten milk soy egg corn nuts

- 1 1/2 cups (360g) Dana's Simple Dressing (above)
- 1/4 cup (60 g) GFCF sweet pickle relish
- 1 hard-boiled medium egg, chopped
- 1 tablespoon (10 g) chopped or minced onion (optional)

Combine all ingredients until blended.

YIELD: *2 cups (480 g)*

Calories (kcal): 1862; **Total fat:** 193g; **Cholesterol:** 289mg; **Carbohydrate:** 56g; **Dietary fiber:** 3g; **Protein:** 11g; **Sodium:** 3231mg; **Potassium:** 746mg; **Calcium:** 91mg; **Iron:** 3mg; **Zinc:** 1mg; **Vitamin A:** 2210IU.

 QUICK N EASY

Simple Russian Dressing

     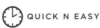

gluten milk soy egg corn nuts

- 1 cup (240 g) GFCF mayonnaise
- 1/4 cup (60 g) GFCF ketchup
- 1/4 cup (60 g) GFCF chili sauce
- 1/4 cup (60 g) GFCF sweet pickle relish
- 1 hard-boiled medium egg, chopped
- 1 tablespoon (10 g) chopped or minced onion (optional)

Place all ingredients in a medium bowl; mix until blended.

YIELD: *2 cups (480 g)*

Calories (kcal): 1812; **Total fat:** 193g; **Cholesterol:** 289mg; **Carbohydrate:** 42g; **Dietary fiber:** 4g; **Protein:** 10g; **Sodium:** 2534mg; **Potassium:** 796mg; **Calcium:** 83mg; **Iron:** 3mg; **Zinc:** 1mg; **Vitamin A:** 6082IU.

Tangy Vinaigrette

gluten   milk   soy   egg   corn   nuts

Jeannie Fritz Godbout offers this quick version.

- ¹/₂ cup (120 ml) balsamic vinegar
- ¹/₄ cup (60 g) GFCF regular or Dijon mustard

Blend ingredients well in a blender (medium-high speed).

YIELD: *3/4 cup (175 ml)*

Calories (kcal): 64; **Total fat:** 3g; **Cholesterol:** 0mg; **Carbohydrate:** 12g; **Dietary fiber:** 2g; **Protein:** 3g; **Sodium:** 753mg; **Potassium:** 211mg; **Calcium:** 58mg; **Iron:** 2mg; **Zinc:** 1mg; **Vitamin A:** 0IU

Really Quick N Easy Raspberry Vinaigrette

gluten   milk   soy   egg   corn   nuts

- 1 cup (235 ml) GFCF oil-and-vinegar dressing—Italian or Balsamic
- ¹/₈ cup (60 g) raspberries (fresh or defrosted frozen)

Place ingredients in a blender. Blend on medium.

YIELD: *1 ¹/₈ cups (260 ml)*

Calories (kcal): 1130; **Total fat:** 125g; **Cholesterol:** 0mg; **Carbohydrate:** 8g; **Dietary fiber:** 1g; **Protein:** trace; **Sodium:** 1mg; **Potassium:** 43mg; **Calcium:** 3mg; **Iron:** trace; **Zinc:** trace; **Vitamin A:** 21IU

Herb-Mustard Vinaigrette

gluten   milk   soy   egg   corn   nuts

This Joyce Mulcahy dressing is adapted from a Southern Living *recipe.*

- 1 (4-ounce [115 g]) jar pear baby food
- 3 tablespoons (45 ml) white grape juice (100%) concentrate (Avoid concentrate if on SCD and use 100% juice with no sugar added.)
- 3 tablespoons (45 ml) GFCF white wine vinegar
- 1 teaspoon GFCF Dijon mustard
- ¹/₄ teaspoon GFCF hot sauce (optional)
- 2 teaspoons fresh tarragon
- 2 teaspoons fresh basil
- 1 tablespoon (15 ml) olive oil (or avocado oil)
- Salt and pepper to taste

Combine all ingredients except olive oil, salt, and pepper. Whisk in olive oil or avocado oil. Salt and pepper to taste.

YIELD: *1 cup (235 ml)*

Calories (kcal): 217; **Total fat:** 14g; **Cholesterol:** 0mg; **Carbohydrate:** 25g; **Dietary fiber:** 6g; **Protein:** 1g; **Sodium:** 368mg; **Potassium:** 315mg; **Calcium:** 86mg; **Iron:** 2mg; **Zinc:** trace; **Vitamin A:** 335IU

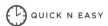

Sweet and Tangy Vinaigrette

gluten   milk   soy   egg   corn   nuts

Expanding on the Tangy Vinaigrette (page 173), we offer the following sweet version. We also added olive oil, especially for those who need more of the good fats and oils.

- $^1/_2$ cup (120 ml) balsamic vinegar
- $^1/_4$ cup (60 g) GFCF regular or Dijon mustard
- $^1/_4$ cup (85 g) honey
- 2 tablespoons (28 ml) light olive oil or avocado oil for low oxalate

Blend ingredients well in a blender (medium-high speed).

YIELD: *1 $^1/_8$ cups (260 ml)*

Calories (kcal): 560; **Total fat:** 30g; **Cholesterol:** 0mg; **Carbohydrate:** 82g; **Dietary fiber:** 2g; **Protein:** 3g; **Sodium:** 756mg; **Potassium:** 255mg; **Calcium:** 64mg; **Iron:** 2mg; **Zinc:** 1mg; **Vitamin A:** 0IU.

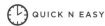

Lemon Tahini Salad Dressing

gluten   milk   soy   egg   corn   nuts

Provided by Seven Oaks Restaurant. This dressing can be used on more than just salad. Try it over a baked potato, in a pasta salad, or over steamed vegetables. It also makes a great dip.

- $^1/_4$ green pepper
- $^1/_4$ large Spanish onion (yellow)
- 1 stalk celery
- $^3/_4$ cup (180 g) tahini
- $1^1/_2$ cups (355 ml) olive oil
- $^1/_2$ cup (120 ml) lemon juice (bottled)
- $^1/_4$ cup (60 ml) tamari
- 1 teaspoon minced garlic (jarred)
- $^1/_4$ teaspoon black pepper

In food processor, add the first three ingredients and process. Then add the rest of the ingredients and process again.

YIELD: *3 cups (710 ml)*

Calories (kcal): 4071; **Total fat:** 424g; **Cholesterol:** 0mg; **Carbohydrate:** 61 g; **Dietary fiber:** 20g; **Protein:** 40g; **Sodium:** 4267mg; **Potassium:** 1297mg; **Calcium:** 824mg; **Iron:** 18mg; **Zinc:** 9mg; **Vitamin A:** 388IU.

Sunflower Seed Healthy Spread

gluten milk soy egg corn nuts

This mild-tasting spread is loaded with vitamins. It can be used on crackers and bread or as a dip with chips or veggies.

- 1 cup (135 g) sunflower seeds, ground
- 1/2 cup (55 g) nutritional yeast or ground flaxseed
- 1/4 cup (35 g) brown rice flour
- Basil, to taste
- Thyme, to taste
- 1 tablespoon (8 g) non-GMO soy protein powder or pea protein powder
- 2 cloves garlic
- 1 carrot, shredded
- 1 onion, chopped
- 1 stalk celery, chopped
- 1/4–1/2 cup (60–120 ml) olive oil or avocado oil
- 2 tablespoons (30 ml) lemon juice
- 2 tablespoons (30 ml) tamari
- 1 cup (235 ml) hot water

Blend the first seven ingredients in a food processor (with 1/4 cup [60 ml] oil), then add vegetables and blend, then add liquids and blend. If too thick, add more oil. If too thin, may adjust with brown rice flour. Bake 55 minutes at 350°F (180°C, or gas mark 4) in a 9 x 9-inch (23 x 23 cm) pan. (Should be about 1-inch [2.5 cm] thick in pan.)

YIELD: *3 cups (675 g)*

Calories (kcal): 234; **Total fat:** 186g; **Cholesterol:** 0mg; **Carbohydrate:** 121g; **Dietary fiber:** 50g; **Protein:** 81g; **Sodium:** 2139mg; **Potassium:** 3837mg; **Calcium:** 334mg; **Iron:** 29mg; **Zinc:** 15mg; **Vitamin A:** 20416IU.

Cranberry Sauce

gluten   milk   soy   egg   corn   nuts

Yes, there is a way to have this holiday favorite without all the corn syrup, and it tastes better, too.

SCD Legal

- 4 cups (380 g) fresh cranberries (2 bags)
- 2$\frac{1}{2}$ cups (590 ml) water, divided
- 3-4 packets organic gelatin powder (Vital Proteins)
- 1$\frac{3}{4}$ cups (595 g) clover honey

Sort through berries, discarding the really light ones and any spoiled fruit. Freeze any amount exceeding 4 cups (380 g). Wash berries and place in a saucepan. Add 2 cups (475 ml) water and place on medium heat, uncovered. Once the berries begin boiling, cover and reduce the heat to continue to simmer. Simmer for 10 minutes.

Meanwhile, pour $\frac{1}{2}$ cup (120 ml) water in large bowl. Sprinkle 3 to 4 packets of gelatin over water—3 will give softer set; if a firmer set is desired, use 4 packets. Do not stir the gelatin; just let it sit a few minutes.

Using a strainer, pour berry mixture into the strainer above the bowl of gelatin. Push the juice and pulp through with a spoon, stirring inside the strainer. Work it through, as the skins will stay behind even with aggressive stirring. Scrape the outside of the strainer into the bowl with a spatula to get all of the pulp. Set aside strainer and skins.

Stir to dissolve gelatin. Add honey, starting with 1$\frac{1}{2}$ cups (510 g) and adding 1 tablespoon (20 g) at a time until it reaches desired sweetness. Place in a serving dish. Cover and refrigerate. It will take several hours to set.

YIELD: *2 cups (550 g)*

Calories (kcal): 230; **Total fat:** 1g; **Cholesterol:** 0mg; **Carbohydrate:** 613g; **Dietary fiber:** 17g; **Protein:** 10g; **Sodium:** 272mg; **Potassium:** 584mg; **Calcium:** 85mg; **Iron:** 3mg; **Zinc:** 2mg; **Vitamin A:** 175IU.

Sassy Salsas

gluten milk soy egg corn nuts

There are numerous wonderful recipes for salsa. This is one of our favorites because the basic recipe is as delicious as the three additional versions. Salsas are versatile and can be used for more purposes than as a snack with corn chips. They are excellent used on top of potatoes, fish, pasta, or eggs.

SCD Legal

- 1^1/$_4$ cups (about 8 ounces [225 g]) seeded and chopped firm, ripe tomatoes
- 1 minced fresh jalapeño pepper to taste (optional)
- ^{1}/$_3$ cup (55 g) minced red onion
- ^{1}/$_4$ cup (15 g) chopped fresh cilantro
- 2 tablespoons (30 ml) fresh lime or lemon juice
- ^{1}/$_2$ teaspoon minced garlic (optional)
- ^{1}/$_2$ teaspoon salt
- ^{1}/$_2$ teaspoon black pepper

Variations: (all SCD Legal)

- **AVOCADO SASSY SALSA:** Add 1 cup (225 g) peeled, chopped avocado
- **BEAN SASSY SALSA:** Add 1 cup (225 g) black beans, rinsed, well drained
- **MANGO SASSY SALSA:** Add 1 cup (175 g) peeled, chopped mango

Mix tomatoes, peppers, onion, and cilantro in a bowl. Add lime or lemon juice and garlic. Mix together gently. Add salt and pepper to taste.

For variations, add either avocado, black beans, or mango and mix gently. A combination of beans and avocado is also delicious.

NOTES: *The recipe can be made from very mild to very hot, depending on how much jalapeño pepper is used. Use no jalapeno if you like it very mild; use up to 2 tablespoons (20 g) minced jalapeño pepper for a hotter salsa.*

Salsa stores well for up to three days in the refrigerator. It can also be frozen.

YIELD: *2^1/$_2$ cups (500 g)*

Calories (kcal): 82; **Total fat:** 1g; **Cholesterol:** 0mg; **Carbohydrate:** 19g; **Dietary fiber:** 4g; **Protein:** 3g; **Sodium:** 1091mg; **Potassium:** 660mg; **Calcium:** 42mg; **Iron:** 2mg; **Zinc:** trace; **Vitamin A:** 1674IU.

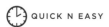 QUICK N EASY

Really Easy Salsa Dip

gluten   milk   soy   egg   corn   nuts

SCD Legal

- 1 jar (16 ounces, or 455 g) GFCF organic Thick and Chunky Salsa (Simple Truth)
- 1 teaspoon chopped fresh cilantro

Mix the cilantro in the salsa and serve.

NOTE: *For a tasty fruit twist on this popular recipe, add 1/4 cup (80 g) GFCF natural fruit spread—mixed berry, grape, or apricot (Whole Foods, Cascadian Farms, Harvest Moon).*

YIELD: *2 cups (480 g)*

Calories (kcal): 127; **Total fat:** 1g; **Cholesterol:** 0mg; **Carbohydrate:** 28g; **Dietary fiber:** 7g; **Protein:** 6g; **Sodium:** 1969mg; **Potassium:** 968mg; **Calcium:** 136mg; **Iron:** 4mg; **Zinc:** 1mg; **Vitamin A:** 2752IU.

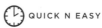 QUICK N EASY

Easy Bean Salsa Dip

gluten   milk   soy   egg   corn   nuts

SCD Legal

- 1 can (16 ounces, or 455 g) GFCF organic traditional refried black beans (Eden or Amy's)
- 2 cups (480 g) Really Easy Salsa Dip (at left)

Spread refried beans on a plate—approximately 1/2 inch (1.25 cm) deep.

Spread Really Easy Salsa Dip over the refried beans. Serve with GFCF corn chips or taco chips. (Avoid corn products on SCD.)

YIELD: *4 cups (935 g)*

Calories (kcal): 511; **Total fat:** 5g; **Cholesterol:** 0mg; **Carbohydrate:** 88g; **Dietary fiber:** 32g; **Protein:** 30g; **Sodium:** 3364mg; **Potassium:** 968mg; **Calcium:** 136mg; **Iron:** 4mg; **Zinc:** 1mg; **Vitamin A:** 2752IU.

Sofrito

gluten milk soy egg corn nuts

SCD Legal

- ³/₄ bunch cilantro
- 3 medium Spanish onions
- 1 head garlic
- 1 green pepper, preferably cubanelle, seeded

Wash cilantro. Peel onions and garlic. Put everything in a food processor and pulse until minced but not liquid.

This will keep in the refrigerator for up to 10 days. Freeze in ice cube trays and use to flavor soups and stews and to make taco recipes.

YIELD: *1¹/₂ cups (225 g)*

Calories (kcal): 223; **Total fat:** 1g; **Cholesterol:** 0mg; **Carbohydrate:** 51g; **Dietary fiber:** 11g; **Protein:** 7g; **Sodium:** 20mg; **Potassium:** 1037mg; **Calcium:** 129mg; **Iron:** 2mg; **Zinc:** 1mg; **Vitamin A:** 1014IU.

Thai Peanut Sauce

gluten milk soy egg corn nuts

This a great dipping sauce. Serve alongside broiled or grilled chicken breasts.

- ¹/₂ cup (130 g) smooth organic peanut butter
- ¹/₄ cup (60 ml) warm water
- 2 tablespoons (30 ml) lime juice
- 1 tablespoon (15 g) brown sugar
- 1 tablespoon (15 ml) GFCF tamari sauce
- 1 small garlic clove, minced
- Pinch of cayenne pepper

Whisk peanut butter and water together. Stir in the remaining ingredients, cover, and refrigerate for 20 minutes, until chilled.

TIP: *Use ¹/₂ to 1 cup (120 to 235 ml) of GFCF chicken broth instead of the water, and use as a sauce for stir-fry.*

YIELD: *1 cup (235 ml), or 6 to 8 servings*

Calories (kcal): 103; **Total fat:** 8g; **Cholesterol:** 0mg; **Carbohydrate:** 5g; **Dietary fiber:** 1g; **Protein:** 4g; **Sodium:** 107mg; **Potassium:** 127mg; **Calcium:** 8mg; **Iron:** trace; **Zinc:** trace; **Vitamin A:** trace.

Spinach Hummus

gluten   milk   soy   egg   corn   nuts

Adapted from Lisa Barnes, The Petit Appetit Cookbook

Is your family ho-hum for hummus? Try this variation using spinach. It goes great on a crudités platter, or even just as a snack.

- 1 (14 ounce, or 400 g) can chickpeas, drained and rinsed
- 1 clove garlic
- 1 cup (30 g) packed organic spinach leaves
- 1 tablespoon (15 ml) freshly squeezed lemon juice
- 1/2 teaspoon ground cumin
- 1 teaspoon kosher salt
- 1/2 teaspoon freshly ground black pepper
- 1/4 cup (60 ml) extra virgin olive oil

In a blender or food processor, combine chickpeas and garlic and purée until smooth. Add spinach, lemon juice, cumin, salt, and pepper, and blend thoroughly. With motor running, gradually add olive oil and process until smooth and creamy. Taste and adjust seasoning as needed.

YIELD: *About 1 1/2 cups, or 10 servings*

Calories (kcal): 77; **Total fat:** 6g; **Cholesterol:** 0mg; **Carbohydrate:** 6g; **Dietary fiber:** 1g; **Protein:** 1g; **Sodium:** 284mg; **Potassium:** 62mg; **Calcium:** 14mg; **Iron:** 1mg; **Zinc:** trace; **Vitamin A:** 209IU.

White Bean and Walnut Spread

gluten   milk   soy   egg   corn   nuts

This is a great spread for GFCF crackers or served with a crudités platter.

- 1 can (15 ounces, or 420 g) cannellini beans
- 1/2 cup (60 g) chopped walnuts, toasted
- 2 tablespoons (30 ml) olive oil
- 3 tablespoons (45 ml) water
- 1 tablespoon (15 ml) lemon juice
- 1 small garlic clove, minced
- 1/2 teaspoon salt
- 1/8 teaspoon ground black pepper (Omit for low phenol/low salicylate diet.)
- 1/4 teaspoon paprika (Omit for low phenol/low salicylate diet.)

Combine all ingredients in a food processor, pulse until smooth, and serve.

YIELD: *8 servings*

Calories (kcal): 255; **Total fat:** 8g; **Cholesterol:** 0mg; **Carbohydrate:** 33g; **Dietary fiber:** 8g; **Protein:** 14g; **Sodium:** 142mg; **Potassium:** 999mg; **Calcium:** 134mg; **Iron:** 6mg; **Zinc:** 2mg; **Vitamin A:** 24IU.

Plenty O' Pesto

gluten   milk   soy   egg   corn   nuts

SCD Legal

Pesto is a versatile condiment and can be made out of any number of combinations of herbs and nuts. It can be used as a sauce for pasta or pizza, a garnish for soup, a topping for grilled or sautéed chicken or fish, or even a flavoring for steamed or mashed vegetables.

- 3 cups (60 g) arugula or basil leaves, or 1 cup (60 g) parsley or cilantro leaves
- 3 cloves garlic
- ¹/₂ cup (75 g) nuts (pecans, walnuts, almonds, unsalted pistachios, or pine nuts)
- ¹/₂ teaspoon salt
- ¹/₄ teaspoon ground black pepper
- ¹/₂ cup (120 ml) extra virgin olive oil
- Water

In a food processor or blender, pulse herbs or greens, garlic, nuts, salt, and pepper until finely chopped. With machine running, slowly add the oil. Add water (if needed), 1 tablespoon (15 ml) at a time, until a smooth paste is formed. Store in an airtight container in the refrigerator for up to 3 days (cover surface of pesto with a thin layer of oil to avoid discoloration).

YIELD: *6 servings*

Calories (kcal): 224; **Total fat:** 24g; **Cholesterol:** 0mg; **Carbohydrate:** 3g; **Dietary fiber:** 1g; **Protein:** 1g; **Sodium:** 178mg; **Potassium:** 82mg; **Calcium:** 21mg; **Iron:** trace; **Zinc:** 1mg; **Vitamin A:** 341IU.

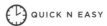 QUICK N EASY

Spinach Pesto

gluten   milk   soy   egg   corn   nuts

SCD Legal

This spinach pesto is a great way to quickly flavor foods and add a nice boost of vegetables. Try it with pasta, meat, fish, or rice.

- 6 cups (180 g) fresh baby spinach, washed and dried
- ¹/₂ cup (75 g) pine nuts, almonds, or walnuts
- 3 large cloves garlic, chopped
- ¹/₂ to ³/₄ cup (120 to 175 ml) extra virgin olive oil (or ¹/₂ cup oil [120 ml] and ¹/₄ cup [60 ml] water as needed to thin pesto)
- 2 teaspoons dried basil
- Salt and ground pepper to taste

Process all ingredients and ¹/₂ teaspoon salt in a food processor until smooth, starting with ¹/₂ cup olive oil and adding more oil (or water) as needed until desired consistency is reached. Season with salt and pepper to taste, and enjoy! Store in air-tight container in refrigerator for up to 1 week.

YIELD: *8 servings*

Calories (kcal): 235; **Total fat:** 25g; **Cholesterol:** 0mg; **Carbohydrate:** 3g; **Dietary fiber:** 1g; **Protein:** 3g; **Sodium:** 18mg; **Potassium:** 194mg; **Calcium:** 34mg; **Iron:** 2mg; **Zinc:** trace; **Vitamin A:** 1549IU.

CHAPTER 16

Breads, Muffins, Waffles, and Pancakes

"OUR DAUGHTER WAS ADDICTED TO WHITE PASTA AND cereal. We didn't know how to break the cycle. Once we reduced sugar, increased protein, and eliminated dairy and gluten from her diet, the whole picture changed. We began to offer healthier replacement foods like greens, protein-rich foods, and alternative grains. Now, at dinnertime she normally cleans her plate. We see her eating vegetables like green beans, spinach, zucchini, and broccoli in greater variety and greater quantities. She stays energetic throughout the day and does not have the highs and lows she once did. She seems to understand that our new way of eating is healthier and makes her feel better."

—MARIE, *mother*

Introduction

Using prepared organic flours or mixes helps make a recipe Quick N Easy.

Pancakes, waffles, breads, muffins, and buns are wonderful places to sneak in better nutrition by substituting some of the liquid ingredients with cooked and puréed vegetables. If your child refuses to eat anything green, select vegetables whose colors will not be obvious (cauliflower, carrot, sweet potato, and squash). If color is not a problem, expand to the greens. Puréed fruits can also be included.

The amount of protein can be increased by adding one or more of the following: extra egg whites, nut flours, or rice protein powder (add 1/8 to 1/4 cup [15 to 30 g] as a replacement for an equal amount of flour). Favorites include almond flour (avoid almond flour on low phenol/low salicylate/low oxalate diet) and hazelnut flour. See the resource product listing in the appendix.

In pancakes, there is room for hiding supplements in what we call the Trojan Horse Technique.

What Can Be Hidden in a Muffin?

- Eggs (added protein, amino acids)
- Nuts (added protein) (See chapters for allowed nuts on specific diets.)
- Dried fruit, molasses (added iron) (See chapters for allowed fruits on specific diets.)
- Flax (linseed) (added omega-3s, fiber)
- Protein powder (if heat stable)
- Calcium powder

Bette Hagman's All-Purpose Flour Substitute

gluten milk soy egg corn nuts

This formula is found in the many Gluten-Free Gourmet books by Bette Hagman. This combination has become the standard mix for replacing all-purpose flour.

Modified for Low Salicylate

- 2 parts white rice flour
- $^2/_3$ part potato starch flour (Use arrowroot for low salicylate diet.)
- $^1/_3$ part tapioca flour

Combine all ingredients. Blend with a whisk and store, ready for use any time a recipe calls for all-purpose flour.

Calories (kcal): 4890; **Total fat:** 15g; **Cholesterol:** 0mg; **Carbohydrate:** 1101g; **Dietary fiber:** 40g; **Protein:** 78g; **Sodium:** 103mg; **Potassium:** 5496mg; **Calcium:** 191mg; **Iron:** 55mg; **Zinc:** 12mg; **Vitamin A:** 0IU.

White Bread—Bread Machine

gluten milk soy egg corn nuts

The kids will never know it's healthy!

Modified for Low Salicylate

- 1 cup (235 ml) water
- 3 tablespoons (45 ml) oil
- 1 teaspoon salt
- 1 cup (140 g) brown rice flour
- $^3/_4$ cup (105 g) garbanzo bean flour
- $^1/_2$ cup (80 g) potato starch (Use arrowroot powder for low salicylate diet.)
- $^1/_4$ cup (30 g) tapioca starch
- 4 egg whites
- 2 teaspoons xanthan gum
- 1 teaspoon yeast

Place ingredients in a bread machine in the order listed. Select setting and start. Store in freezer and slice and toast as needed.

YIELD: *1 loaf (12 slices)*

Calories (kcal): 134; **Total fat:** 4g; **Cholesterol:** 0mg; **Carbohydrate:** 21g; **Dietary fiber:** 1g; **Protein:** 4g; **Sodium:** 201 mg; **Potassium:** 109mg; **Calcium:** 6mg; **Iron:** 1mg; **Zinc:** 1mg; **Vitamin A:** 2IU.

QUICK N EASY

Banana Bread

gluten milk soy egg corn nuts

- $^1/_2$ cup (120 ml) sunflower or safflower oil
- 2 large eggs
- 1 teaspoon vanilla extract
- $^1/_2$ cup (115 g) dairy-free vanilla pudding mixed with 1 teaspoon xanthan gum
- 1 ripe banana, mashed
- 1 package (15 ounces, or 420 g) Old Fashioned Cake and Cookie Mix from Gluten Free Pantry or 1 package (21 ounces, or 588 g) Miss Roben's Yellow Cake Mix

Grease a loaf pan. Preheat oven to 350°F (180°C, or gas mark 4). Mix the first five ingredients. Fold in cake mix. Pour into 6-cup (1.4 L) loaf pan. Bake 50 minutes or until middle is cooked.

YIELD: *1 loaf (12 slices)*

Calories (kcal): 187; **Total fat:** 10g; **Cholesterol:** 32mg; **Carbohydrate:** 22g; **Dietary fiber:** trace; **Protein:** 2g; **Sodium:** 112mg; **Potassium:** 63mg; **Calcium:** 16mg; **Iron:** trace; **Zinc:** trace; **Vitamin A:** 75IU.

 QUICK N EASY

Pecan Bread

gluten milk soy egg corn nuts

This recipe was adapted from the book Breaking the Vicious Cycle: Intestinal Health Through Diet, *by Elaine Gottschall.*

SCD Legal

- $2^1/_2$ cups (300 g) pecan meal
- $^1/_4$ teaspoon salt
- $^1/_2$ teaspoon baking soda
- $^1/_4$ teaspoon cinnamon
- 4 eggs
- $^1/_2$ cup (170 g) honey
- 1 tablespoon (15 ml) olive oil

Mix the dry ingredients, set aside. Break eggs into a separate bowl and whisk in honey. Add dry ingredients to egg mixture and stir. Add olive oil and mix thoroughly. Pour into 8 x 4-inch (20 x 10 cm) loaf pan that is completely lined (even up the sides) with kitchen parchment paper. Bake at 350°F (180°C, or gas mark 4) for 45 minutes. Once removed from the oven, allow the bread to cool for 5 minutes. Then lift the loaf out of the pan by the ends of the paper and gently roll it out of the parchment onto a cooling rack.

NOTE: *The parchment paper will wrinkle when used to line the pan and the loaf will not necessarily be symmetrical, but without it the bread sticks too much to the baking pan.*

YIELD: *1 loaf (12 slices)*

Calories (kcal): 161; **Total fat:** 3g; **Cholesterol:** 62mg; **Carbohydrate:** 25g; **Dietary fiber:** 2g; **Protein:** 10g; **Sodium:** 116mg; **Potassium:** 112mg; **Calcium:** 17mg; **Iron:** 1mg; **Zinc:** 2mg; **Vitamin A:** 125IU.

All-Purpose Buns

gluten milk soy egg corn nuts

Modified for Low Phenol, Modified for Low Salicylate

- 2 teaspoons yeast
- 1¹/₂ cups (355 ml) water
- 1¹/₄ cups (175 g) brown rice flour
- ³/₄ cup (105 g) garbanzo bean flour
- ³/₄ cup (120 g) potato starch (Use arrowroot for low phenol and low salicylate diets.)
- ¹/₃ cup (40 g) tapioca starch
- 1 tablespoon (8 g) xanthan gum
- ¹/₂ tablespoon (9 g) salt
- 6 egg whites
- ¹/₄ cup (60 ml) oil (safflower, avocado) (Use safflower for the low salicylate diet.)

Mix yeast and water and let sit until foamy. Place remaining ingredients in a mixer bowl and add yeast mixture. Blend on low speed to incorporate, then on medium-high speed for 2 minutes. The dough will be sticky. Lightly oil bun pans or cookie sheets and top with parchment paper. Use an ice cream scoop to transfer dough. Cover and let the dough rise for 1 hour. Bake in a 350°F (180°C, gas mark 4) oven for 30 to 35 minutes. Store in freezer until needed.

YIELD: *12 buns*

Calories (kcal): 173; **Total fat:** 5g; **Cholesterol:** 0mg; **Carbohydrate:** 27g; **Dietary fiber:** 2g; **Protein:** 4g; **Sodium:** 300mg; **Potassium:** 133mg; **Calcium:** 8mg; **Iron:** 1mg; **Zinc:** 1mg; **Vitamin A:** 2IU.

Yeast-Free Sweet Potato Buns

gluten milk soy egg corn nuts

Tracey Smith provides a tasty recipe that is perfect for children who love breads and dislike vegetables.

- 1¹/₄ cups (175 g) garbanzo bean flour
- 1¹/₄ cups (150 g) quinoa flour
- 1¹/₄ cups (175 g) brown rice flour
- 1 cup (120 g) tapioca starch
- 4 teaspoons xanthan gum
- 2 teaspoons salt
- 1 teaspoon baking powder
- 8 egg whites
- ¹/₃ cup (80 ml) oil (safflower, avocado)
- 8 ounces (225 g) puréed sweet potatoes
- 1 cup (235 ml) water

Combine the dry ingredients in a mixer bowl. Add liquid ingredients and mix on low to incorporate. Mix on medium-high speed for 1 to 2 minutes, until a smooth dough forms. Dough will be sticky.

Lightly oil bun pans or cookie sheets and top them with parchment paper. Use an ice cream scoop to transfer dough. Bake in a 350°F (180°C, gas mark 4) oven for 30 to 45 minutes. May be stored in the freezer until needed.

YIELD: *12 buns*

Calories (kcal): 248; **Total fat:** 8g; **Cholesterol:** 0mg; **Carbohydrate:** 40g; **Dietary fiber:** 2g; **Protein:** 6g; **Sodium:** 439mg; **Potassium:** 221 mg; **Calcium:** 40mg; **Iron:** 2mg; **Zinc:** 1mg; **Vitamin A:** 967IU.

Better-Than-Bisquick Pancakes

gluten milk soy egg corn nuts

- 2 cups (240 g) quinoa flour
- 2 tablespoons (10 g) baking powder
- $1/4$ teaspoon baking soda
- 2 tablespoons (30 ml) light-flavored oil, such as sunflower or safflower
- $1/2$ cup (75 g) raw cashews
- 2 cups (475 ml) warm water
- 1 teaspoon (5 ml) vanilla extract
- 1 teaspoon (5 ml) lemon juice or $1/4$ teaspoon ascorbic acid crystals dissolved in 2 tablespoons (30 ml) warm water
- 1 teaspoon (5 ml) maple syrup

In a mixing bowl, whisk together quinoa flour, baking powder, and baking soda. In a blender, grind nuts to a fine powder, pausing to scrape under the blades 2 to 3 times. Add water, vanilla extract, lemon juice, and maple syrup to blender and blend 3 to 4 minutes. Pour liquid over dry ingredients and whisk a few times, eliminating lumps. If batter is too thick, add water as necessary.

Pour a scant $1/4$ cup (60 g) batter onto hot non-stick griddle (heated until water dances on it) for each pancake. Serve with fruit sauce or applesauce. (Use peeled pears for low phenol/low salicylate diet.)

VARIATIONS: *Add 1–2 tablespoons (10–20 g) flaxseed to blender with the cashews. For a heartier, buckwheat sourdough pancake, replace up to 1 cup (120 g) quinoa flour with buckwheat flour.*

YIELD: *12 to 14 pancakes*

Calories (kcal): 161; **Total fat:** 7g; **Cholesterol:** 0mg; **Carbohydrate:** 22g; **Dietary fiber:** 2g; **Protein:** 5g; **Sodium:** 278mg; **Potassium:** 240mg; **Calcium:** 156mg; **Iron:** 3mg; **Zinc:** 1mg; **Vitamin A:** trace

Cinnamon Pancakes

gluten milk soy egg corn nuts

- 2 cups (280 g) sorghum or rice flour
- $2/3$ cup (100 g) potato starch
- $1/3$ cup (40 g) tapioca flour
- 3 tablespoons (40 g) sugar
- 2 teaspoons xanthan gum
- 1 tablespoon (5 g) baking powder
- 1 teaspoon cinnamon
- $1/8$ teaspoon salt
- 2 cups (475 ml) water
- 1 cup (235 ml) milk substitute (rice, almond, coconut)
- 3 eggs
- 3 tablespoons (45 ml) oil
- $1/2$ teaspoon vanilla extract

Combine the dry ingredients and set aside. In a separate bowl, mix wet ingredients. Add the dry ingredients to the wet ingredients and cook on a griddle until done.

VARIATION: *Fold $1/2$ cup (75 g) fresh or frozen (thawed) blueberries into the batter.*

YIELD: *12 to 14 pancakes*

Calories (kcal): 200; **Total fat:** 5g; **Cholesterol:** 47mg; **Carbohydrate:** 36g; **Dietary fiber:** 1g; **Protein:** 3g; **Sodium:** 160mg; **Potassium:** 36mg; **Calcium:** 80mg; **Iron:** trace; **Zinc:** trace; **Vitamin A:** 70IU.

Honey Vanilla Pancake Recipe

gluten milk soy egg corn nuts

These really cook up well the next day too. They are light and fluffy.

- 1 large egg
- $^3/_4$ cup (175 ml) milk substitute (rice, non-GMO soy, almond, or coconut)
- 1 tablespoon (20 g) honey
- $^1/_2$ teaspoon vanilla extract
- 1 cup (140 g) GF flour
- $^1/_4$ teaspoon xanthan gum
- $^1/_4$ teaspoon salt
- 1 tablespoon (5 g) baking powder

Combine egg, milk substitute, honey, and vanilla extract in a bowl. In a separate bowl, combine flour, xanthan gum, salt, and baking powder. Add the dry mixture to the wet mixture and blend well. Cook on a hot, greased griddle, using about $^1/_4$ cup of batter for each pancake. Cook until brown on one side and around edge; turn and brown the other side.

VARIATION: *Fold $^1/_2$ cup (75 g) fresh or frozen (thawed) blueberries into the batter.*

YIELD: *4 to 6 pancakes*

Calories (kcal): 161; **Total fat:** 1g; **Cholesterol:** 47mg; **Carbohydrate:** 32g; **Dietary fiber:** 1g; **Protein:** 5g; **Sodium:** 915mg; **Potassium:** 54mg; **Calcium:** 218mg; **Iron:** 2mg; **Zinc:** trace; **Vitamin A:** 70IU.

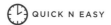 QUICK N EASY

Pecan Meal Pancakes

gluten milk soy egg corn nuts

This recipe was adapted from the book Breaking the Vicious Cycle: Intestinal Health Through Diet, *by Elaine Gottschall.*

SCD Legal

- $2^1/_2$ cups (300 g) pecan meal
- $^1/_2$ teaspoon baking soda
- $^1/_4$ teaspoon salt
- $^1/_3$ cup (115 g) honey (clover)
- 7 large eggs or 8 medium eggs
- 1 teaspoon (5 ml) organic vanilla extract

Combine the dry ingredients in a bowl, and set aside. In a separate bowl, whisk honey into eggs, then add vanilla extract. Whisk the dry mixture into the wet mixture.

Spray a nonstick, electric frying pan with olive oil to lightly coat, and set the temperature to 200°F (95°C). It is best to let the pan preheat; otherwise, the first pan of pancakes may get too dark.

NOTE: *A nonstick electric frying pan is highly recommended for this recipe. Honey causes the pancakes to stick, and pecan meal can cause them to brown quickly. A thermostat-controlled temperature will help to prevent headaches.*

YIELD: *15 to 18 pancakes*

Calories (kcal): 127; **Total fat:** 3g; **Cholesterol:** 100mg; **Carbohydrate:** 17g; **Dietary fiber:** 1g; **Protein:** 10g; **Sodium:** 108mg; **Potassium:** 102mg; **Calcium:** 19mg; **Iron:** 1mg; **Zinc:** 1mg; **Vitamin A:** 174IU.

GFCF "No Yolking Around" Pancakes

gluten　milk　soy　egg　corn　nuts

For those allergic to eggs, this adaptation of Lisa Barnes's recipe in The Petit Appetit Cookbook *is an excellent option.*

- 1 cup (140 g) GF flour (hazelnut or almond)
- $\frac{1}{2}$ tablespoon (6 g) cane sugar
- 2 teaspoons baking powder
- $\frac{1}{4}$ teaspoon salt
- $\frac{1}{2}$ teaspoon baking soda
- $\frac{1}{2}$ teaspoon ground cinnamon
- 1 cup (235 ml) organic milk substitute (almond or coconut)
- 1 tablespoon (15 g) applesauce or pear sauce
- 2 tablespoons (30 ml) safflower, almond, or avocado oil

In a medium mixing bowl, stir together flour, sugar, baking powder, salt, baking soda, and cinnamon. In a separate bowl, whisk together milk, applesauce, and oil. Add milk mixture to flour mixture all at once. Stir with a rubber spatula until just blended. If batter is too thick, thin with milk substitute.

Heat a large nonstick skillet or griddle over medium heat. Lightly grease skillet with cooking spray.

VARIATION: *Puréed vegetables (carrots, sweet potato) can replace some of the liquid (1 to 2 tablespoons [15 to 30 ml]). Add fruits, fruit spread, or fruit purées on top.*

YIELD: *About 8 (5-inch, or 13-cm) pancakes*

Calories (kcal): 115; **Total fat:** 4g; **Cholesterol:** 0mg; **Carbohydrate:** 19g; **Dietary fiber:** 1g; **Protein:** 1g; **Sodium:** 268mg; **Potassium:** 19mg; **Calcium:** 73mg; **Iron:** trace; **Zinc:** trace; **Vitamin A:** trace

Wonderful Waffles

gluten　milk　soy　egg　corn　nuts

This recipe was modified from a recipe that came with the waffle maker itself. Our waffle maker is nonstick and calls for 2/3 cup (80 g) batter per waffle. Modify this recipe to suit your waffle maker's size and shape.

- 1 cup (140 g) GF flour blend of choice
- 3 teaspoons baking powder
- $\frac{1}{4}$ teaspoon salt
- 1 tablespoon (13 g) sugar
- $\frac{1}{2}$ teaspoon guar gum or xanthan gum
- 3 eggs, separated
- 1 cup (235 ml) milk substitute (rice, almond, or cashew)
- $\frac{1}{4}$ cup (60 ml) canola oil
- 1 teaspoon (5 ml) vanilla extract

Preheat a waffle maker and spray with nonstick spray. Whisk together the flour blend, baking powder, salt, sugar, and guar or xanthan gum in a large bowl. Separate the eggs—the whites go into a large mixing bowl and the yolks go into the flour mixture. Add the milk substitute to the flour mixture and whisk well. Beat the egg whites until stiff. Meanwhile, add the oil and vanilla extract to the batter and mix well. Pour the batter over the stiff egg whites and whisk. Pour $\frac{2}{3}$ cup (80 g) of batter onto the waffle maker and cook for 7 minutes each.

YIELD: *4 to 6 waffles*

Calories (kcal): 347; **Total fat:** 18g; **Cholesterol:** 140mg; **Carbohydrate:** 40g; **Dietary fiber:** 1g; **Protein:** 7g; **Sodium:** 543mg; **Potassium:** 75mg; **Calcium:** 226mg; **Iron:** 1mg; **Zinc:** 1mg; **Vitamin A:** 210IU.

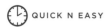

High-Protein Waffles

gluten   milk   soy   egg   corn   nuts

This high-protein waffle mix can sneak in some mineral supplements.

Low Phenol, Low Salicylate

- 1³/₄ cups (245 g) brown rice flour
- 2³/₄ cups (330 g) quinoa flour
- ³/₄ cup (90 g) tapioca starch
- ¹/₂ tablespoon baking soda
- ¹/₂ tablespoon salt
- 6 eggs
- ¹/₃ cup (80 ml) oil (sunflower or safflower)
- 3¹/₂ cups (830 ml) rice or cashew milk

Combine all ingredients with a mixer on low-medium speed for 2 minutes. Lightly oil waffle iron. Pour batter onto waffle iron and cook.

VARIATION: *For a sweeter waffle, replace some of the rice milk with pear juice.*

YIELD: *20 waffles*

Calories (kcal): 200; **Total fat:** 7g; **Cholesterol:** 56mg; **Carbohydrate:** 29g; **Dietary fiber:** 2g; **Protein:** 6g; **Sodium:** 172mg; **Potassium:** 232mg; **Calcium:** 24mg; **Iron:** 3mg; **Zinc:** 1mg; **Vitamin A:** 84IU.

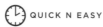

Crispy Breakfast Bars

gluten   milk   soy   egg   corn   nuts

A versatile treat—try it for breakfast, a snack, or as an energy boost.

- 7 cups (98 g) crispy, GF puffed whole-grain cereal
- ³/₄ cup (90 g) dried cranberries
- ³/₄ cup (90 g) dried blueberries
- ¹/₂ cup (65 g) sunflower seeds (optional)
- 1 teaspoon cinnamon
- ³/₄ cup (255 g) brown rice syrup or honey
- ³/₄ cup (190 g) almond or cashew butter
- 2 tablespoons (28 g) butter substitute

Stir together cereal, dried fruits, seeds (if using), and cinnamon in large bowl. Place syrup, almond (or cashew) butter, and butter substitute in a large, microwave-safe measuring cup. Microwave 1¹/₂ minutes on high, or until the butter substitute has melted. Stir well and pour over cereal mixture. Stir to coat.

Dampen your hands with cold water. Press cereal mixture firmly into a 9-inch (23 cm) square baking pan, rewetting hands if necessary to keep mixture from sticking. Freeze 30 minutes. Cut into 15 bars, and store in refrigerator.

YIELD: *15 bars*

Calories (kcal): 232; **Total fat:** 12g; **Cholesterol:** 0mg; **Carbohydrate:** 31g; **Dietary fiber:** 2g; **Protein:** 4g; **Sodium:** 2mg; **Potassium:** 145mg; **Calcium:** 43mg; **Iron:** 1mg; **Zinc:** 1mg; **Vitamin A:** 3IU.

Gluten-Free Zucchini Bread

gluten milk soy egg corn nuts

Another great way to turn veggies into a treat!

- 3 cups (420 g) GF flour blend, plus extra for dusting pans
- $^1/_4$ teaspoon baking powder
- 1 teaspoon baking soda
- $2^1/_4$ teaspoons xanthan gum
- 1 teaspoon salt
- 1 tablespoon (7 g) ground cinnamon (Use nutmeg for low phenol/low salicylate diet.)
- 2 large eggs
- $2^1/_2$ cups (500 g) sugar
- 1 cup (235 ml) safflower oil
- 1 tablespoon (15 ml) vanilla extract
- 2 cups (240 g) grated zucchini
- 1 cup (120 g) finely chopped nuts, such as walnuts or pecans (Use pecans for low phenol/low salicylate diet.)

Preheat oven to 350°F (180°C, gas mark 4). Spray 2 loaf pans and lightly dust with GF flour blend, knocking out excess. Mix the dry ingredients in medium bowl and set aside.

Whisk eggs together in large mixing bowl; add sugar, oil, and vanilla extract, and continue whisking until light and frothy. Stir in zucchini. Add dry ingredients and stir to combine, and then fold in nuts. Divide batter evenly into pans and bake for 1 hour, or until toothpick inserted into the center comes out clean. Cool for 5 minutes, and then carefully remove loaves from pans. Cool completely on wire rack before serving.

YIELD: *2 loaves, or 24 slices*

Calories (kcal): 303; **Total fat:** 12g; **Cholesterol:** 18mg; **Carbohydrate:** 44g; **Dietary fiber:** 4g; **Protein:** 5g; **Sodium:** 163mg; **Potassium:** 84mg; **Calcium:** 15mg; **Iron:** trace; **Zinc:** trace; **Vitamin A:** 103IU.

Pumpkin Bread

gluten   milk   soy   egg   corn   nuts

This bread freezes really well, if it lasts that long!

- 3$^1/_2$ cups (490 g) GF flour blend of choice
- $^1/_2$ teaspoon xanthan gum (corn-free)
- 3 cups (600 g) sugar
- 2 teaspoons cinnamon
- 2 teaspoons nutmeg
- 1$^1/_2$ teaspoons salt
- 2 teaspoons baking soda
- 1 cup (235 ml) canola oil
- $^2/_3$ cup (160 ml) water
- 1 can (15 ounces, or 420 g) pumpkin purée
- 2 eggs, beaten
- 6–12 ounces (170–340 g) GFCF semisweet chocolate chips (optional)

Preheat oven to 350°F (180°C, gas mark 4). Combine flour blend, xanthan gum, sugar, cinnamon, nutmeg, salt, and baking soda in a large bowl. In a separate bowl, combine oil, water, pumpkin, and eggs. Combine the dry and wet mixtures thoroughly. Add the chocolate chips, if using.

Divide the batter equally among three 8 x 4-inch (20 x 10 cm) loaf pans or two 12-compartment muffin pans that have been sprayed with nonstick spray. Bake loaves for 45 to 50 minutes; bake muffins for 40 minutes. When toothpick in the center comes out clean, the loaves/muffins are done. Cool completely before cutting and serving.

YIELD: *3 loaves or 24 muffins*

Calories (kcal): 342; **Total fat:** 14g; **Cholesterol:** 16mg; **Carbohydrate:** 54g; **Dietary fiber:** 2g; **Protein:** 3g; **Sodium:** 246mg; **Potassium:** 112mg; **Calcium:** 17mg; **Iron:** 1mg; **Zinc:** 1mg; **Vitamin A:** 3962IU.

Cornmeal Carrot Muffins

gluten   milk   soy   egg   corn   nuts

The hearty dose of carrots sweetens these muffins while keeping them healthy; the cornmeal adds a nice crunch.

- 1 cup (140 g) GF flour blend
- $^3/_4$ cup (105 g) coarsely ground cornmeal
- 1 teaspoon baking soda
- 1 teaspoon baking powder
- $^1/_2$ teaspoon salt
- $^1/_2$ cup (115 g) brown sugar
- 2 large eggs
- $^1/_2$ cup (120 ml) avocado, sunflower, or safflower oil
- $^1/_2$ cup (120 ml) rice milk
- 1$^1/_2$ cups (165 g) grated carrots

Preheat oven to 350°F (180°C, gas mark 4). Line a 12-cup muffin tin with paper or foil liners. Combine the flour blend, cornmeal, baking soda, baking powder, and salt in a medium bowl and set aside. Whisk the eggs and the brown sugar in a large bowl until frothy. Add the oil and milk and whisk to combine. Stir in the carrots and then the dry mixture, and mix just until no flour clumps remain. Divide the batter evenly between the muffin cups and bake 20 to 25 minutes. Cool 5 minutes, then transfer muffins to wire rack to cool completely. Serve.

YIELD: *12 muffins*

Calories (kcal): 224; **Total fat:** 10g; **Cholesterol:** 36mg; **Carbohydrate:** 30g; **Dietary fiber:** 3g; **Protein:** 4g; **Sodium:** 388mg; **Potassium:** 98mg; **Calcium:** 39mg; **Iron:** 1mg; **Zinc:** trace; **Vitamin A:** 4366IU.

Maya's Favorite Lemon Poppy Seed Muffins

gluten   milk   soy   egg   corn   nuts

From Joanne Bregman (Maya's mother)

- 1³/₄ cups (245 g) GF flour blend
- 3 tablespoons (30 g) MLO Natural Brown Rice Protein Powder
- 2 teaspoons baking powder
- ¹/₂ teaspoon salt
- 1 tablespoon (8 g) poppy seeds
- 2 large eggs
- ²/₃ cup (230 g) agave nectar or honey
- ³/₄ cup (175 ml) rice milk
- ¹/₄ cup (60 ml) safflower oil
- 1 tablespoon (15 ml) lemon juice
- 1 teaspoon lemon extract

Preheat oven to 375°F (190°C, gas mark 5). Grease and flour a 12-cup muffin tin. Mix all dry ingredients in a large bowl and set aside. Whisk eggs, agave nectar, rice milk, oil, lemon juice, and lemon extract together. Add to dry ingredients and mix until just combined. Divide batter evenly between the muffin cups. Bake 20 minutes, until wooden toothpick inserted into the centers comes out clean; cool on wire rack.

YIELD: *12 muffins*

Calories (kcal): 237; **Total fat:** 6g; **Cholesterol:** 37mg; **Carbohydrate:** 41g; **Dietary fiber:** 4g; **Protein:** 6g; **Sodium:** 199mg; **Potassium:** 22mg; **Calcium:** 68mg; **Iron:** 1mg; **Zinc:** trace; **Vitamin A:** 41IU.

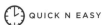 QUICK N EASY

Joe's "Veggies in Disguise" Nutritious Muffins

gluten   milk   soy   egg   corn   nuts

Another great trick for getting a picky eater to eat some veggies!

- 1 cup (120 g) carrots, finely chopped
- 1 cup (120 g) zucchini, finely chopped
- 1 cup (175 g) GFCF chocolate chips, finely chopped
- 1 cup (125 g) walnuts or pecans, finely chopped
- 1 store-bought GFCF cake mix, prepared according to package directions, but not baked

Add carrots, zucchini, chocolate chips, and nuts to prepared cake batter; stir to combine.

Transfer the mixture to a muffin pan, filling each cup about two-thirds of the way. Bake at 375°F (190°C, or gas mark 5) for 20 minutes or until a toothpick inserted in the center of a muffin comes out clean. Do not overcook, as this will result in dry muffins. Once cooled, these muffins can be frozen to be eaten later.

NOTE: *This clever recipe can also incorporate extra protein by adding ¹/₈ to ¹/₄ cup puréed chicken.*

YIELD: *12 muffins*

Calories (kcal): 285; **Total fat:** 15g; **Cholesterol:** 0mg; **Carbohydrate:** 38g; **Dietary fiber:** 2g; **Protein:** 5g; **Sodium:** 204mg; **Potassium:** 218mg; **Calcium:** 74mg; **Iron:** 1mg; **Zinc:** 1mg; **Vitamin A:** 3084IU.

Socca to Me

gluten milk soy egg corn nuts

Socca is a flatbread made from chickpea flour hailing from Southern France. It can be found at the bustling markets in Nice, where it is cooked on giant cast-iron pans in wood-fired ovens. Not only is it surprisingly easy to re-create at home, but it is naturally gluten-free, and delicious plain, or as a base for a variety of toppings.

- 1 cup (140 g) chickpea flour (or chickpea-fava flour blend)
- 1/2 teaspoon salt
- 1/4–1/2 teaspoon freshly ground black pepper (optional)
- 1 cup (235 ml) water
- 3 tablespoons (45 ml) olive oil

Whisk chickpea flour, salt, and pepper (if using) into a medium bowl. Slowly add water, whisking to eliminate lumps. Stir in 2 tablespoons olive oil. Cover and set aside for 1 hour (batter should be about the consistency of heavy cream).

   Preheat oven to 475°F (240°C, gas mark 9). Heat remaining oil in 10-inch nonstick skillet over medium-high heat, swirling the pan to coat until oil is shimmering. Pour batter into the pan, swirling to coat evenly. Place pan in hot oven and cook until batter is lightly browned on top, 12 to 18 minutes. Slide pancake into cutting board, cut into quarters, and serve immediately.

NOTE: *This recipe can easily be doubled and cooked in 2 batches. If you don't have a skillet with an oven-proof handle, a cast-iron skillet can be used instead. If using toppings, they can be added halfway through the baking time or after the socca comes out of the oven.*

TIP: *If there is any socca left over, crumble it up with your fingers, toast the crumbs, and use in any recipe that calls for breadcrumbs.*

YIELD: *4 servings*

Calories (kcal): 175; **Total fat:** 12g; **Cholesterol:** 0mg; **Carbohydrate:** 13g; **Dietary fiber:** 3g; **Protein:** 5g; **Sodium:** 283mg; **Potassium:** 198mg; **Calcium:** 14mg; **Iron:** 1mg; **Zinc:** 1mg; **Vitamin A:** 10IU.

"Joe's issue with gluten and casein is not one where he exhibits sudden behavior changes if he ingests a small amount; the issues gradually appear if the gluten and casein are consumed over a period of time. The same is true for red food coloring and nitrates. So, while it may look as though he does not have any allergic reaction to those foods, experience has taught us better and we keep a gluten-free/casein-free/red-food-coloring-free/nitrate-free house!"

—Pauline McFadden

Quinoa Cake

gluten   milk   soy   egg   corn   nuts

Adapted from Karina's Kitchen (http://glutenfreegoddess.blogspot.com/)
This makes a great breakfast treat or afternoon snack.

- 1¹/₂ cups (250 g) quinoa flakes
- ¹/₂ cup (70 g) sorghum flour
- ¹/₂ cup (60 g) tapioca starch
- ³/₄ cup (90 g) almond meal flour
- 1 teaspoon baking soda
- ¹/₂ teaspoon salt
- 1 teaspoon xanthan or guar gum
- 2 teaspoons ground cinnamon
- 2 large eggs (or the equivalent of egg replacer)
- ¹/₄ cup (60 ml) olive oil
- ¹/₄ cup (60 g) unsweetened applesauce
- ¹/₂ cup (170 g) agave nectar
- ¹/₂ cup (115 g) brown sugar
- ¹/₄ cup (85 g) molasses
- 2 teaspoons GFCF organic vanilla extract
- 1 cup (110 g) grated carrots
- ¹/₂ cup (42 g) unsweetened grated coconut

Preheat oven to 350°F (180°C, gas mark 4). Grease a 9 x 13-inch
(23 x 33 cm) baking pan and then line with parchment paper.

In a medium bowl, combine the first 8 ingredients and set aside. Whisk
the eggs together with the olive oil, applesauce, agave nectar, brown
sugar, molasses, and vanilla extract. Add the dry ingredients and beat well
to combine. Add carrots and coconut and stir until evenly combined. Pour
batter into prepared pan and bake for 25 to 35 minutes, until cake is set
in the center. Allow cake to cool on a wire rack completely before slicing.

NOTE: *Individual pieces of this cake can be wrapped in parchment or*
waxed paper and then stored in a zipper lock plastic bag or container and
frozen for future use.

YIELD: *16 pieces*

Calories (kcal): 251; **Total fat:** 9g; **Cholesterol:** 27mg; **Carbohydrate:** 40g; **Dietary fiber:** 3g; **Protein:** 5g;
Sodium: 174mg; **Potassium:** 257mg; **Calcium:** 45mg; **Iron:** 2mg; **Zinc:** 1mg; **Vitamin A:** 2177IU.

Maya's Waffles

gluten   milk   soy   egg   corn   nuts

Another great high-protein waffle recipe.

- ²/₃ cup (95 g) GF flour blend (see note) (Use buckwheat, rice, or millet for low phenol/low salicylate diet.)
- ¹/₃ cup (30 g) brown rice or soy protein powder (Make sure to use a brand that stays stable when cooked.)
- 2 teaspoons baking powder
- ¹/₄ teaspoon salt
- 2 large eggs
- 1 tablespoon (20 g) organic agave nectar or honey
- ¹/₄ cup (60 ml) sunflower or safflower oil
- ²/₃ cup (160 ml) non-casein milk (Use cashew milk or rice milk, for low phenol/low salicylate diet.)

Stir together all ingredients and cook in waffle maker according to manufacturer's instructions.

YIELD: *2 to 4 servings*

TIP: *You can double the recipe to make extra waffles, and then freeze the leftovers. When you are ready to eat them, simply defrost slightly and toast.*

NOTE: *You can use Bette Hagman's All-Purpose Flour Substitute or this alternative offered by Joanne Bregman:*

- *¹/₂ cup (70 g) brown or white rice flour*
- *³/₄ cup (105 g) sorghum flour*
- *¹/₂ cup (60 g) buckwheat flour*
- *¹/₄ cup (30 g) tapioca starch*

Combine all ingredients and blend with a whisk.

YIELD: *2 cups*

Calories (kcal): 361; **Total fat:** 17g; **Cholesterol:** 106mg; **Carbohydrate:** 36g; **Dietary fiber:** 4g; **Protein:** 16g; **Sodium:** 441mg; **Potassium:** 34mg; **Calcium:** 184mg; **Iron:** 2mg; **Zinc:** trace; **Vitamin A:** 122IU.

CHAPTER 17

Main Dishes and One-Dish Meals

Breakfast Sausage

gluten   milk   soy   egg   corn   nuts

Sometimes it is difficult to come up with a varied source of protein for breakfast. This version avoids the usual additives found in commercial sausages. The recipe can also be made with turkey. Note among the ingredients is the addition of palm oil. This non-hydrogenated all-vegetable shortening is available from Spectrum Naturals.

SCD Legal, Modified for Low Phenol, Modified for Low Oxalate

- 1 pound (455 g) ground pork or ground turkey
- 1 egg lightly beaten (optional)
- 1 teaspoon coarse Kosher salt
- $^1/_2$ teaspoon ground sage
- $^1/_4$ teaspoon ground savory (eliminate for low phenol)
- $^1/_8$ teaspoon ground nutmeg (sage for low phenol, low oxalate)
- $^1/_8$ teaspoon ground ginger (cinnamon for low phenol, low oxalate)
- $^1/_4$ teaspoon black pepper (white pepper for low phenol, low oxalate)
- 3 shakes cayenne pepper (almost $^1/_8$ teaspoon)
- 2 shakes dried thyme (about $^1/_{16}$ teaspoon)
- $1^1/_2$ tablespoons palm oil (or avocado or coconut oil)
- $^3/_4$ teaspoon honey (clover)

Place ground pork in a large bowl, add egg (if using) and mix in well. Combine salt and seasonings. Sprinkle a little of the seasonings over the meat and work in by pushing down with a closed fist, dividing the meat, stacking it, and then pushing down again. Sprinkle a little more of the seasonings and repeat. Do this until the seasonings are worked throughout. Spread the palm oil over the meat and work in. Drizzle honey over the meat and work in.

Shape into nine patties and fry at a lower temperature than normally expected for sausage. If using an electric frying pan, set the temperature to just under 250°F (120°C, or gas mark $^1/_2$), as the honey will cause the sausage to brown quickly. Cover in between turnings. Turn frequently and watch closely. Cook for approximately 10–15 minutes.

YIELD: *9 patties*

Calories (kcal): 141; **Total fat:** 11g; **Cholesterol:** 57mg; **Carbohydrate:** trace; **Dietary fiber:** trace; **Protein:** 9g; **Sodium:** 243mg; **Potassium:** 153mg; **Calcium:** 12mg; **Iron:** 1mg; **Zinc:** 1mg; **Vitamin A:** 50IU.

Crustless Spinach Quiche

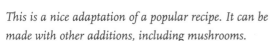

gluten milk soy egg corn nuts

This is a nice adaptation of a popular recipe. It can be made with other additions, including mushrooms.

- 2 cups (500 g) non-GMO silken tofu
- 2 eggs
- $\frac{1}{8}$ teaspoon garlic powder or minced garlic
- 1 small onion, coarsely chopped
- $\frac{1}{8}$ teaspoon turmeric
- $\frac{1}{2}$ teaspoon cumin
- $\frac{1}{8}$ teaspoon nutmeg
- 2 tablespoons (15 g) prepared GFCF mustard
- 1 cup (235 ml) vegetable broth
- 1 teaspoon dried parsley
- Salt and pepper to taste
- 1 pound (455 g) spinach or greens, rinsed, finely chopped, steamed, and drained, or use 1 package (16 ounces, or 455 g) frozen chopped spinach, steamed and drained
- Dash paprika

VARIATIONS

- **OPTION:** 1 jar (2.5 ounces, or 70 g) sliced mushrooms, drained, or 5 tablespoons (22 g) sliced white mushrooms
- **OPTION:** 9-inch (23 cm) prepared or purchased GFCF pie crust

Coat a 9-inch (23 cm) pie plate with vegetable cooking spray (olive oil). (If using pie crust, omit cooking spray and line pie plate with crust.) Set aside.

Preheat oven to 450°F (230°C, or gas mark 8). Place tofu, eggs, garlic, onion, spices, mustard, vegetable broth, and parsley in a blender or food processor and blend on medium speed until smooth. Season with salt and pepper to taste.

In a large bowl, combine mixture with greens. Spoon mixture into greased pie plate. Sprinkle paprika on top.

Bake at 450°F (230°C, or gas mark 8) for 1 hour or until golden brown and a knife inserted in center comes out clean.

YIELD: *8 servings*

Calories (kcal): 106; **Total fat:** 5g; **Cholesterol:** 47mg; **Carbohydrate:** 8g; **Dietary fiber:** 3g; **Protein:** 9g; **Sodium:** 314mg; **Potassium:** 486mg; **Calcium:** 139mg; **Iron:** 6mg; **Zinc:** 1mg; **Vitamin A:** 4494IU.

Scrambled Veggie Eggs

gluten   milk   soy   egg   corn   nuts

SCD Legal

- 8 large eggs (organic)
- 1 tablespoon (15 ml) water
- ¼ cup (55 g) puréed mashed cauliflower
- Salt and pepper to taste
- 1 scallion, thinly sliced
- 1 tablespoon (3 g) chopped fresh basil (optional)
- 2 tablespoons (28 g) Earth Balance Spread or ghee

In a medium bowl, lightly mix eggs with water. Stir in cauliflower, salt, pepper, scallion, and basil (optional).

In a large skillet, melt the spread or ghee. Scramble egg mixture on low heat until done.

NOTE: *To make mashed cauliflower, use the recipe in chapter 19 or purée the following in a blender:*

- *½ cup (65 g) well-steamed/cooked, drained, and dried cauliflower*
- *1 tablespoon (15 ml) or more rice or coconut milk (enough to "wet" the cauliflower)*

YIELD: *8 servings*

Calories (kcal): 97; **Total fat:** 8g; **Cholesterol:** 196mg; **Carbohydrate:** 1g; **Dietary fiber:** trace; **Protein:** 6g; **Sodium:** 58mg; **Potassium:** 70mg; **Calcium:** 24mg; **Iron:** 1mg; **Zinc:** trace; **Vitamin A:** 428IU.

Ground Vegetable Omelet

gluten   milk   soy   egg   corn   nuts

Vegetables that work well in this omelet are broccoli, onions, zucchini, garlic, bell peppers, and carrots.

SCD Legal

- 1 cup (200 g) leftover cooked, chopped vegetables
- 2 to 3 large eggs
- Sea salt
- Pinch cayenne pepper
- 2 tablespoons (30 ml) olive oil

Purée the vegetables in a food processor or blender until smooth. Beat the eggs lightly in a medium bowl and season with salt and cayenne pepper. Mix the vegetables into the eggs.

Heat the oil in a skillet over medium heat. Pour the egg-vegetable mixture into skillet, cover, and cook until egg is completely set.

YIELD: *2 servings*

Calories (kcal): 267; **Total fat:** 21g; **Cholesterol:** 323mg; **Carbohydrate:** 9g; **Dietary fiber:** 3g; **Protein:** 10g; **Sodium:** 145mg; **Potassium:** 265mg; **Calcium:** 61mg; **Iron:** 2mg; **Zinc:** 1mg; **Vitamin A:** 1930IU.

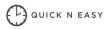 QUICK N EASY

Mexican Breakfast Pizza

gluten milk soy egg corn nuts

Adapted from Karen Joy (http://onlysometimesclever.wordpress.com)

While she admits this is a fairly high-fat recipe, because of its redeeming qualities (it is easy to make and loved by all four of her children), Karen deems it a keeper.

For the Pizza

- 8 ounces (225 g) nitrate-free bacon, diced
- 8 large eggs
- 10 corn tortillas

Optional Garnishes

- Tofutti cheese (contains soy)
- Salsa (contains phenol)
- Diced fresh tomato (contains phenol)
- Sliced scallions
- Chopped cilantro (low oxalate)

In a 12-inch (30 cm) nonstick skillet, cook the bacon over medium-high heat, stirring frequently, until golden and crispy. Transfer bacon with a slotted spoon to a paper towel–lined plate (leaving $1/4$ cup [60 ml] bacon fat in the skillet).

Whisk the eggs in a medium bowl to combine. Arrange the corn tortillas in the skillet to completely cover the bottom (they will be overlapping). Pour the eggs evenly over the tortillas and sprinkle the bacon on top. Cover and cook over medium heat until eggs are cooked through. Slide pizza from the pan onto a large cutting board, cut into six wedges and serve.

NOTE: *If you opt for tofutti cheese, try adding it to the eggs after the bacon so that it melts onto the pizza.*

YIELD: *6 servings*

Calories (kcal): 372; **Total fat:** 25g; **Cholesterol:** 308mg; **Carbohydrate:** 21g; **Dietary fiber:** 2g; **Protein:** 16g; **Sodium:** 434mg; **Potassium:** 89mg; **Calcium:** 35mg; **Iron:** 1mg; **Zinc:** 1mg; **Vitamin A:** 325IU.

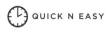 QUICK N EASY

Easy Lettuce Wraps

gluten   milk   soy   egg   corn   nuts

Adapted to SCD, Low Phenol and/or Low Oxalate Based on Vegetable Choices

Tender lettuce leaves stand in for bread in these easy, quick roll-up sandwiches. This is a good way to be clever about including new kinds of vegetables (remember to start with a small amount well mixed in with vegetable favorites). If the diet is low in protein, this is a tasty way to include more.

- 8 whole Boston (or butter) or Bibb lettuce leaves, washed and dried
- 2 cups filling of choice, such as chopped vegetables (based on your specific diet), slices of chicken, chicken salad, or tuna-type salad (salmon is a healthier choice)
- 1/3 cup GFCF dressing or spread of choice (optional)

Fill each lettuce leaf with 1/4 cup filling. Sprinkle with a couple of teaspoons of dressing if using, and then roll it up like a burrito!

TIP: *Expand the variety of fillings and give more taste by adding chopped apples or cut-up grapes. Offer a selection of your child's favorite fillings, and then let them fill and roll themselves!*

YIELD: *4 servings*

Calories (kcal): 319; **Total fat:** 28g; **Cholesterol:** 84mg; **Carbohydrate:** trace; **Dietary fiber:** trace; **Protein:** 15g; **Sodium:** 180mg; **Potassium:** 208mg; **Calcium:** 13mg; **Iron:** 1mg; **Zinc:** 1mg; **Vitamin A:** 873IU.

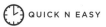 QUICK N EASY

Roll-Up Sandwiches

gluten   milk   soy   egg   corn   nuts

Low Phenol

- 1 large GFCF tortilla (rice or corn) of choice
- 1/3 cup (77 g) GFCF cream cheese
- 2 to 3 slices GFCF (non-deli, organic) luncheon meat of choice

Spread cream cheese evenly over tortilla, and then lay meat slices on top. Roll tortilla up into a tight log, and then slice into 2-inch (5 cm) rounds and serve.

YIELD: *1 to 2 servings*

Calories (kcal): 226; **Total fat:** 17g; **Cholesterol:** 54mg; **Carbohydrate:** 15g; **Dietary fiber:** 1g; **Protein:** 7g; **Sodium:** 459mg; **Potassium:** 48mg; **Calcium:** 26mg; **Iron:** trace; **Zinc:** 0mg; **Vitamin A:** 263IU.

Deviled Eggs

gluten milk soy egg corn nuts

Julie Matthews, CNC, author of Nourishing Hope for Autism, *includes this easy and tasty recipe in her* Cooking to Heal *book. The eggs can be garnished with fresh chives or even salmon roe.*

SCD Legal, Low Oxalate, Modified for Low Phenol

- 12 eggs (pasture-raised)
- ¹/₃ cup (75 g) GFCFSF mayonnaise (page 171)
- 1–2 teaspoons GFCFSF Dijon mustard
- Sprinkle of salt and pepper (limit)
- Garnish options: fresh chives or salmon roe, chopped olives (avoid for low phenol)

Cook the eggs by hard-boiling them. To do so, fill a pot halfway with water and bring to a gentle boil. Carefully lower eggs one at a time in the water. Set a timer for 13 minutes and start timing once you start putting the eggs in the water. Turn up the heat until the water is boiling again and then adjust the heat down to a gentle boil. Move the eggs around in the pan so that the yolk does not settle to one side. Continue cooking until the timer chimes. Do not overcook so that the yolks will not be greenish and sulfur-smelling.

Drain the water and rinse the eggs in cold water until the pot and water are cool. Peel the eggs. Slice them in half lengthwise, reserving the yolks in a bowl. Blend the yolks, mayonnaise, Dijon, salt, and pepper in a food processor. Scoop the egg yolk mixture into the egg white halves. Garnish with one or more of the options and serve chilled.

YIELD: *24 egg halves*

Per half: Calories (kcal): 60; Total fat: 5g; **Cholesterol:** 95mg; **Carbohydrate:** 0g; **Dietary fiber:** 0g; **Protein:** 3g; **Sodium:** 65mg; **Potassium:** 35mg; **Calcium:** 14mg; **Iron:** trace; **Zinc:** trace; **Vitamin A:** 137IU.

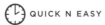 QUICK N EASY

Christina's Delicious Deviled Eggs

gluten milk soy egg corn nuts

This version of deviled eggs provides an additional twist by including the sweet pickle relish and paprika.

Low Oxalate, Low Phenol

- 12 eggs (pasture-raised and hard-boiled as described in Julie Matthews's Deviled Eggs recipe)
- 2 to 3 tablespoons (28 to 42 g) GFCFSF mayonnaise (page 171)
- 2 teaspoons GFCFSF mustard or to taste
- 1 teaspoon salt
- 4 tablespoons (60 g) sweet pickle relish or to taste (avoid for low salicylate)
- 2 pinches of paprika (avoid for low phenol)

Follow Julie Matthews's Deviled Eggs instructions for preparing the eggs (boiling, draining, cooling, peeling, and halving).

To the reserved yolks in the bowl, add the rest of the ingredients and mix to combine. If needed for more moisture, add more mayonnaise. Combine the remaining ingredients and add to the yolks.

Using a baking parchment, cut a triangle, folding it into a cone shape. Secure at the top with a staple. Add the egg yolk mix and squeeze into the egg white halves.

YIELD: *24 egg halves*

Per half: Calories (kcal): 53; Total fat: 4g; **Cholesterol:** 107mg; **Carbohydrate:** 1g; **Dietary fiber:** trace; **Protein:** 3g; **Sodium:** 166mg; **Potassium:** 34mg; **Calcium:** 14mg; **Iron:** trace; **Zinc:** trace; **Vitamin A:** 126IU.

Poultry Recipes

Variety is the best way to achieve good nutrition. When it comes to protein, don't focus on only chicken. Expand to turkey, Cornish game hens, and duck.

Avoid commercial chicken nuggets, which are made with hydrogenated oils and are deep fried. Make them at home or purchase organic GFCF chicken nuggets.

Chicken fat is not to be avoided. Almost 50% of the chicken fat is monounsaturated (just like good fatty acids in olive oil). Eat both white and dark poultry meat. Dark meat is richer in nutrients, including fat-soluble vitamins.

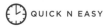 QUICK N EASY

Easy Chicken

gluten   milk   soy   egg   corn   nuts

The chicken fat has the healing fatty acids. Keep the skin on the chicken.

SCD Legal, Low Oxalate

- 4 bone-in chicken thighs or 2 breasts—with skin
- Honey (clover)

Preheat the oven to 350°F (180°C, gas mark 4).

Spread a thin layer of honey in the bottom of a casserole dish. Place chicken pieces meaty-side down on top of the honey. Squirt a little more honey on top. Cover and put in oven.

Approximately 90 minutes later, remove chicken from casserole dish with tongs.

This is great as a snack, or pull the chicken off the bone for use in salad or taco salad.

YIELD: *4 servings*

Calories (kcal): 231; **Total fat:** 14g; **Cholesterol:** 79mg; **Carbohydrate:** 9g; **Dietary fiber:** trace; **Protein:** 16g; **Sodium:** 72mg; **Potassium:** 186mg; **Calcium:** 10mg; **Iron:** 1mg; **Zinc:** 2mg; **Vitamin A:** 136IU.

Chicken Nuggets

gluten   milk   soy   egg   corn   nuts

- 1¹/₂ cups (22 g) GF organic rice cereal
- 4 tablespoons (30 g) tapioca flour
- 1 cup (160 g) potato flour
- ¹/₂ cup (35 g) shredded coconut
- 2 tablespoons (36 g) sea salt
- 2 organic chicken breasts (deboned)
- 2 eggs
- 1¹/₂ cups (355 ml) rice milk
- ¹/₂ cup (120 ml) oil (sunflower, safflower, almond, avocado, or peanut), or more as needed

Use a rolling pin to crush cereal in a resealable plastic bag. Mix dry ingredients with crushed cereal.

Cut chicken into desired sizes, wash and pat dry.

Mix eggs with rice milk, dip chicken pieces into liquid mixture, and then toss in closed resealable plastic bag and coat with mixture. Cook in oil until golden brown.

YIELD: *12 to 16 nuggets*

Calories (kcal): 401; Total fat: 23g; Cholesterol: 112mg; Carbohydrate: 19g; Dietary fiber: 1g; Protein: 29g; Sodium: 1071mg; Potassium: 542mg; Calcium: 24mg; Iron: 4mg; Zinc: 1mg; Vitamin A: 234IU.

Roasted Apple Chicken

gluten   milk   soy   egg   corn   nuts

SCD Legal

- 1 roasting chicken (4–5 pounds, or 1.9–2.3 kg), with skin
- ¹/₂ lemon
- Salt and pepper to taste
- 1 small onion, quartered
- 1 apple, peeled and quartered
- ¹/₄ teaspoon dried rosemary
- ¹/₄ teaspoon dried thyme
- 2 sprigs fresh parsley
- ¹/₂ cup (120 ml) organic chicken broth (recipe page 294)
- ¹/₂ cup (120 ml) apple juice (Avoid concentrated juice if on SCD and use 100% juice with no sugar added.)
- ¹/₄ cup (55 g) ghee, melted

Preheat oven to 350°F (180°C, gas mark 4).

Rub inside of chicken with lemon half, sprinkle with salt and pepper.

Add the onion quarters, apple quarters, dried herbs, and parsley to chicken cavity. Pour chicken broth and apple juice in bottom of the pan. Place chicken in a shallow roasting pan and roast at 350°F (180°C, gas mark 4) for 80 to 100 minutes (20 minutes per pound). Baste with melted ghee and juices from the pan several times. Season with salt and pepper. The chicken's internal temperature should register 175°F (79°C), and the skin should be golden. Remove to a heated platter and keep warm in the oven until ready to serve. Make a sauce with pan juices, if desired.

YIELD: *6 servings*

Calories (kcal): 602; Total fat: 45g; Cholesterol: 186mg; Carbohydrate: 9g; Dietary fiber: 2g; Protein: 40g; Sodium: 230mg; Potassium: 655mg; Calcium: 61mg; Iron: 4mg; Zinc: 3mg; Vitamin A: 1690IU.

Chicken Fingers with Honey Mustard Dipping Sauce

gluten   milk   soy   egg   corn   nuts

Most kids love the idea of dipping their food into a sauce. This sweet and savory sauce is a tasty motivator. The chicken fingers can be made in batches and frozen for future meals.

<u>SCD Legal</u>

Chicken

- 1½ to 2 pounds (680 to 910 g) of pasture-raised chicken breasts without the skin

Breading

- 2 cups (240 g) almond or cashew flour
- 2 tablespoons (3 g) dried parsley
- 1½ tablespoons (9 g) organic Italian seasoning
- 1 teaspoon garlic powder
- 2 teaspoons sea salt
- ¼ teaspoon pepper

Honey Mustard Dipping Sauce

1 tablespoon (15 g) SCD legal Dijon mustard

2 tablespoons (40 g) honey (clover)

Cut or pound the chicken to desired size, approximately 3 inches (7.5 cm) long and ½ to ¾ inch (1.3 to 2 cm) wide. Rinse the chicken and pat dry until damp.

Place a portion of the breading in a shallow bowl and coat each piece of chicken. (Reserve and refrigerate any unused breading mixture to thicken and flavor soups.)

Heat avocado oil in a pan on medium heat and add the chicken. Brown each side of the chicken until cooked thoroughly.

Remove the cooked chicken to a paper towel–lined plate to collect excess oil. Serve warm with Honey Mustard Dipping Sauce.

YIELD: *6 to 8 servings*

Calories (kcal): 280; **Total fat:** 13g; **Cholesterol:** 85mg; **Carbohydrate:** 9g; **Dietary fiber:** 2g; **Protein:** 29g; **Sodium:** 500mg; **Potassium:** 506mg; **Calcium:** 1mg; **Iron:** 1mg; **Zinc:** 1mg; **Vitamin A:** 39IU.

Stir-Fry Lemon Chicken

gluten   milk   soy   egg   corn   nuts

One of the secrets to attractive stir-fry dishes is to vary the shapes and colors of the vegetables chosen. For example, cut the carrots into $^1/4$-inch (6 mm) ridged diagonals; the red or green bell peppers into long, $^1/4$-inch (6 mm) -wide slices; and the green onions into 1-inch (2.5 cm) diagonals. Depending on taste and texture issues, this recipe can be modified.

- 1 pound (455 g) boneless, skinless chicken, cut into 1-inch (2.5 cm) pieces
- $^1/4$ cup (60 ml) GFCF tamari non-GMO soy sauce
- $^1/4$ cup (60 ml) fresh lemon juice
- $^1/4$ cup (60 ml) water
- 1 tablespoon (5 g) grated lemon zest
- 1 teaspoon honey or agave nectar
- 2 teaspoons crushed red pepper flakes
- 2 garlic cloves, minced
- $^1/2$ teaspoon ground ginger
- 1 tablespoon (15 ml) olive oil
- 3 scallions, diagonally cut into 1-inch (2.5 cm) pieces
- 2 medium carrots, diagonally cut into $^1/2$-inch (1.3 cm) pieces
- $^1/2$ cup (45 g) red bell pepper, cut into $^1/4$-inch (6 mm) strips (optional)
- 2 teaspoons cornstarch or arrowroot or tapioca starch
- 2 cups (320 g) hot cooked basmati, brown, or white rice
- Additional scallions and lemon peel strips, for garnish (optional)

Place chicken in a shallow glass dish and set aside. Combine soy sauce, lemon juice, water, lemon zest, honey, crushed red pepper, garlic, and ginger. Pour half of marinade over chicken and reserve remaining half. Marinate chicken in the refrigerator for 30 minutes.

Drain chicken and discard marinade.

In heavy skillet over medium heat, sauté chicken in olive oil until lightly browned. Transfer meat to a plate and cover with foil.

In same skillet, sauté scallions, carrots, and red bell pepper until crisp-tender. Whisk cornstarch into reserved marinade. Stir into vegetables and stir-fry until thickened. Return chicken to skillet; bring to serving temperature.

Serve immediately over cooked rice. Garnish with additional chopped scallions and lemon peel strips, if desired.

YIELD: *4 Servings*

Calories (kcal): 370; **Total fat:** 15g; **Cholesterol:** 70mg; **Carbohydrate:** 38g; **Dietary fiber:** 3g; **Protein:** 20g; **Sodium:** 1078mg; **Potassium:** 436mg; **Calcium:** 49mg; **Iron:** 2mg; **Zinc:** 2mg; **Vitamin A:** 11889IU.

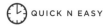 QUICK N EASY

Chicken Continental

gluten   milk   soy   egg   corn   nuts

This recipe is easy and elegant. It makes a tasty purée for those who have texture issues.

Modified for SCD

- 1 pound (455 g) raw chicken, cut into strips
- 1 can (4 ounces, or 115 g) mushrooms, drained
- 1 garlic clove, crushed
- 2 tablespoons (30 ml) olive oil
- 2 cups (475 ml) organic chicken broth (see recipe on page 294)
- 1 package (9 ounces, or 255 g) frozen French-style green beans, defrosted
- 1 teaspoon salt
- $^1/_2$ teaspoon tarragon
- 1 teaspoon pepper
- 1$^3/_4$ cups (166 g) quick-cooking rice or 1$^3/_4$ cups (289 g) cooked brown, basmati, or wild rice (For SCD, use cauliflower rice.)

Sauté chicken, mushrooms, and garlic in oil until chicken is light brown.

Add broth, beans, salt, tarragon, and pepper. Bring to a boil.

Stir in rice. Remove from heat. Cover and let sit for 5 minutes.

YIELD: *4 servings*

Calories (kcal): 391; **Total fat:** 21g; **Cholesterol:** 75mg; **Carbohydrate:** 30g; **Dietary fiber:** 3g; **Protein:** 21g; **Sodium:** 1096mg; **Potassium:** 468mg; **Calcium:** 61mg; **Iron:** 3mg; **Zinc:** 2mg; **Vitamin A:** 1014IU.

Nut-Coated Chicken

gluten   milk   soy   egg   corn   nuts

SCD Legal

- 1¹/₂ pounds (680 g) pasteurized, organic chicken breast
- 2 tablespoons (30 ml) olive oil
- Pecan Meal Coating (recipe follows)

Remove any fat from the chicken breast. Rinse with water and pat dry. Either pound meat to an even thickness or slice into each ¹/₂ breast from the thicker side to the thinner side, not cutting quite all the way through, so that it opens up like a butterfly. Then coat with olive oil.

Dip chicken breast in the pecan meal to coat completely. Cover baking sheet with kitchen parchment paper. Lay chicken, spaced apart, onto baking sheet. Bake at 425°F (220°C, or gas mark 7) for 22 to 25 minutes.

For chicken fingers, use chicken tenders or cut the chicken breast into smaller pieces. For chicken tenders, the cooking time remains the same as above, as they are still somewhat thick. However, if cutting the chicken smaller, reduce the cooking time to 18 to 20 minutes.

YIELD: *4 Servings*

Calories (kcal): 302; **Total fat:** 19g; **Cholesterol:** 87mg; **Carbohydrate:** 2g; **Dietary fiber:** trace; **Protein:** 29g; **Sodium:** 220mg; **Potassium:** 323mg; **Calcium:** 22mg; **Iron:** 1mg; **Zinc:** 1mg; **Vitamin A:** 113IU.

Pecan Meal Coating

Pecan meal can be purchased seasonally from Sunnyland Farms, Inc., Albany, Georgia ([800]-999-2488). It can also be made at home by blending pecans in a blender. However, it is difficult to get the nuts ground as finely as in the purchased meal, so be aware that recipes may need adjusting, either by adding more nut meal or by reducing some of the liquid ingredients.

- 1 cup (120 g) pecan meal
- ¹/₄ teaspoon salt
- 1 tablespoon (9 g) onion powder
- ¹/₂–1 teaspoon garlic powder

Combine all ingredients.

Chicken Purée

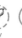

gluten   milk   soy   egg   corn   nuts

This can be used to improve protein in many types of foods, from muffins and pancakes to tomato sauce and GFCF pizza. (Avoid tomatoes on low phenol/low salicylate/low oxalate diets.)

SCD Legal, Modified for Low Phenol, Modified for Low Salicylate, Modified for Low Oxalate

- 1 (^{3}/$_4$–1 pound, or 340–455 g) organic boneless chicken breast
- 1/2 envelope (1/2 tablespoon, or 3.5 g) organic unflavored gelatin (Vital Proteins)
- ^{1}/$_4$ cup (60 ml) organic chicken broth (or recipe, page 294)

POACHING METHOD: Heat ^{1}/$_2$ inch (1.25 cm) of water in a medium skillet over medium-high heat until simmering. Add chicken breast. Water should not cover chicken, but come up about halfway. Simmer chicken until opaque and cooked through, 3 to 4 minutes per side.

OVEN METHOD: Preheat oven to 400°F (200°C, or gas mark 6). Place chicken breast on a greased baking rack over a baking pan. Bake chicken 12 minutes on each side, or until cooked through.

Add ^{1}/$_2$ envelope unflavored gelatin to chicken broth or cooking liquid (if using poaching method) and stir well.

Coarsely chop chicken and transfer to a food processor. Process chicken for about 1 minute. While processor is running, slowly add ^{1}/$_4$ cup (60 ml) of the liquid-gelatin mixture and continue to process until a paste forms. Add more liquid as needed to reach desired consistency.

VARIATIONS:

For a creamier texture, add tofu. (Do not use tofu for SCD.)
For sweetness, add ^{1}/$_2$ cup (125 g) puréed apples or pears.
Add ^{1}/$_2$ cup (125 g) puréed vegetables. (Acorn squash or carrots work best.)

Quick N Easy Version

Use organic puréed infant foods.

YIELD: *Four ^{1}/$_2$-cup (105 g) servings*

Calories (kcal): 140; **Total fat:** 2g; **Cholesterol:** 66mg; **Carbohydrate:** 2g; **Dietary fiber:** 0g; **Protein:** 27g; **Sodium:** 130mg; **Potassium:** 284mg; **Calcium:** 14mg; **Iron:** 1mg; **Zinc:** 1mg; **Vitamin A:** 32IU.

Fruity Rice Chicken or Turkey

gluten　milk　soy　egg　corn　nuts

This recipe is a one-dish meal for children who have sensory issues and do not like "lumps and bumps" in their food.

Modified for SCD

- 1 tablespoon (15 ml) olive oil
- 1 small onion, chopped
- 3 tablespoons (45 g) applesauce or pear sauce
- 2 dried apricots or more applesauce or pear sauce for SCD
- 3 tablespoons (42 g) chicken breast or turkey breast
- 3 plum tomatoes, skinned, seeded, and chopped, or 2 tablespoons (32 g) tomato purée
- 2 tablespoons (20 g) golden raisins
- $^3/_4$ teaspoon finely chopped fresh rosemary
- 3 pinches each ground coriander and cinnamon
- $^3/_4$ teaspoon finely chopped garlic (optional)
- $^3/_4$ cup (175 ml) water
- $^3/_4$ cup (175 ml) organic chicken broth (or recipe, page 294)
- 3 tablespoons (30 g) cooked basmati rice
  (For SCD, use cauliflower rice.)

Heat the oil in a small pan over medium heat. Add the onion and fry until soft, about 2 minutes.

Mix in the fruits, chicken, tomatoes or tomato purée, and raisins.

Add the rosemary, spices, garlic, water, and broth. Bring to a boil, then reduce the heat, cover, and simmer for about 20 minutes, stirring occasionally to prevent sticking.

Add the cooked rice (or cauliflower rice for SCD) to the pan and stir.

Purée all ingredients in a blender. Add extra water if a thinner consistency is preferred, or more cooked rice if a thicker consistency is better.

YIELD: *About 2 to 3 child-size servings*

Calories (kcal): 352; **Total fat:** 7g; **Cholesterol:** 7mg; **Carbohydrate:** 72g; **Dietary fiber:** 10g; **Protein:** 8g; **Sodium:** 217mg; **Potassium:** 1537mg; **Calcium:** 64mg; **Iron:** 5mg; **Zinc:** 1mg; **Vitamin A:** 6680IU.

Spanish Chicken

gluten milk soy egg corn nuts

Look for the Goya seasonings in the international aisle of your supermarket.

- 3 pounds (1.35 kg) organic chicken pieces, such as thighs, drumsticks, or bone-in chicken breasts
- $^3/_4$ cup (150 g) sofrito (Use Quick N Easy recipe on page 179, or Goya brand, found in the freezer section of most grocery stores.)
- $^1/_2$ small can (8 ounces, or 225 g) tomato sauce
- 2 tablespoons (12 g) Goya Adobo all-purpose seasoning w/ pepper
- 1 packet Sazón Goya w/ Coriander & Annatto
- 1 medium potato, peeled and cut into cubes
- 3 bay leaves

Put chicken into a pressure cooker, and then add just enough water to cover. Add sofrito, tomato sauce, seasonings, potatoes, and bay leaves. Cook according to your pressure cooker's instructions for cooking chicken (our pressure cooker cooks chicken for 9 minutes after steady steam). Serve chicken and its juices over choice of rice.

YIELD: *4 servings*

Calories (kcal): 615; **Total fat:** 37g; **Cholesterol:** 195mg; **Carbohydrate:** 12g; **Dietary fiber:** 2g; **Protein:** 56g; **Sodium:** 1080mg; **Potassium:** 104mg; **Calcium:** 47mg; **Iron:** 3mg; **Zinc:** 5mg; **Vitamin A:** 837IU.

Thai Ginger Chicken

gluten milk soy egg corn nuts

- $^1/_4$ cup (50 ml) avocado or safflower oil
- 1 tablespoon (10 g) minced garlic
- 2 tablespoons (12 g) minced ginger
- 12 ounces (340 g) ground organic chicken
- 2 medium red bell peppers, diced
- 2 scallions, chopped
- 1 tablespoon (15 ml) GFCF tamari
- 2 teaspoons white grape juice or apple juice
- $^1/_2$ teaspoon sugar
- $^1/_4$ teaspoon salt
- $^1/_3$ cup (20 g) basil leaves (whole, torn, or chopped)

Heat the oil in a wok or large skillet over high heat. Add the garlic and ginger and quickly fry for 30 seconds. Add the ground chicken and cook for 1 minute. Add the peppers, scallions, tamari, juice, sugar, and salt and cook for 2 minutes. Stir in the basil and serve with rice.

YIELD: *2 to 4 servings*

Calories (kcal): 338; **Total fat:** 22g; **Cholesterol:** 80mg; **Carbohydrate:** 8g; **Dietary fiber:** 1g; **Protein:** 27g; **Sodium:** 449mg; **Potassium:** 375mg; **Calcium:** 33mg; **Iron:** 2mg; **Zinc:** 2mg; **Vitamin A:** 510IU.

Yellow Chicken and Rice

gluten milk soy egg corn nuts

This dish is named for the vibrant color given by the annatto seeds in the Goya mix, found in the international aisle of the supermarket. Goya Sofrito can be found in the freezer section, or use the Quick N Easy Sofrito recipe, page 179.

Modified for SCD

- 2 boneless, skinless organic chicken breasts
- 1 tablespoon (15 ml) olive oil
- $^3/_4$ cup (150 g) sofrito
- 1 package Sazón Goya with Coriander & Annatto
- 1$^1/_2$ cups (293 g) medium grain rice (For SCD, use cauliflower rice.)
- 1 teaspoon salt, plus more to taste

In medium sauce pan, bring 3 cups (710 ml) water to a boil over high heat. Add chicken and cook for 5 minutes, or until chicken is no longer pink in the center. Remove chicken and cut into thin strips; reserve cooking water. In large pot, heat oil over medium heat. Add Goya Sofrito, Sazón Goya, and chicken and cook for 3 minutes. Add rice and stir to combine, and then add reserved chicken-water and 1 teaspoon salt. Bring to a boil, then cover, reduce heat, and simmer for 20 minutes, stirring occasionally, until rice is tender. Off heat, let mixture sit for 5 minutes, season to taste, and then serve.

YIELD: *4 servings*

Calories (kcal): 516; **Total fat:** 12g; **Cholesterol:** 68mg; **Carbohydrate:** 61g; **Dietary fiber:** 2g; **Protein:** 37g; **Sodium:** 544mg; **Potassium:** 535mg; **Calcium:** 41mg; **Iron:** 4mg; **Zinc:** 2mg; **Vitamin A:** 33IU.

Chicken Fried Rice

gluten milk soy egg corn nuts

This is a great recipe to use up leftover rice.

- 2 tablespoons (30 ml) avocado or safflower oil
- $^1/_2$ pound (225 g) organic boneless, skinless chicken breast, cut into small pieces
- 1 medium onion, chopped
- 2 cloves garlic, minced
- 2 eggs, lightly beaten
- 4 cups (750 g) cooked rice
- 1 tomato, seeded and diced
- 1 tablespoon (15 ml) GFCF tamari
- 1 teaspoon sugar
- $^1/_2$ teaspoon ground black pepper
- 2 scallions, sliced thin

Heat the oil in large skillet over high heat. Add chicken and cook 1 minute. Add the onion and cook another 2 minutes, until chicken is lightly browned and cooked through. Add the garlic and eggs and stir constantly until eggs are cooked. Add the rice, tomato, tamari, sugar, and pepper, stir to combine, and cook for 2 minutes to heat through. Sprinkle with the scallions and serve.

YIELD: *4 servings*

Calories (kcal): 431; **Total fat:** 11g; **Cholesterol:** 139mg; **Carbohydrate:** 59g; **Dietary fiber:** 2g; **Protein:** 23g; **Sodium:** 315mg; **Potassium:** 392mg; **Calcium:** 56mg; **Iron:** 2mg; **Zinc:** 2mg; **Vitamin A:** 359IU.

Easy Chicken Kebobs

gluten   milk   soy   egg   corn   nuts

This very simple marinade adds flavor to and livens up a basic chicken kebob.

- 1 pound (455 g) boneless, skinless organic chicken breasts
- 2 tablespoons (30 ml) GFCF tamari
- 2 tablespoons (30 ml) avocado or safflower oil
- 1 teaspoon ground black pepper

Cut the chicken into 1-inch (2.5 cm) cubes and place in a shallow dish. Mix the tamari, oil, and pepper with 1 tablespoon (15 ml) water and pour over the chicken; cover and refrigerate for at least 1 hour.

Thread the chicken cubes onto metal skewers and grill over medium heat for 20 minutes, turning and basting occasionally with the leftover marinade, until cooked through (be sure to discard any marinade that will not be cooked). Serve immediately.

YIELD: *3 to 4 servings*

Calories (kcal): 195; **Total fat:** 8g; **Cholesterol:** 66mg; **Carbohydrate:** 1g; **Dietary fiber:** trace; **Protein:** 27g; **Sodium:** 551mg; **Potassium:** 297mg; **Calcium:** 15mg; **Iron:** 1mg; **Zinc:** 1mg; **Vitamin A:** 33IU.

Crispy Chicken Nuggets

gluten   milk   soy   egg   corn   nuts

This recipe is adapted from Martha Holland, who says these are perfect for the child who loves crunchy things.

- ¹/₂ cup (112 g) ghee, melted
- 2 cups (150 g) crushed GFCF potato chips or cassava chips of choice
- 1 large egg
- 2 tablespoons (30 ml) milk substitute (coconut, rice, soy)
- 1 pound (455 g) boneless, skinless chicken breasts, cut into 1-inch (2.5 cm) cubes
- Salt and pepper

Preheat oven to 350°F (180°C, gas mark 4). Brush a baking sheet with 2 tablespoons (28 g) of the melted ghee. Spread the crushed chips in a shallow dish; beat the egg together with the milk substitute in a medium bowl.

Toss the chicken pieces in the egg mixture until thoroughly coated. Then drop each piece separately into the chips, cover them to coat, and then transfer to the greased baking sheet. When all the pieces are coated, drizzle the remaining ghee over the tops and lightly season with salt and pepper. Bake for 15 to 18 minutes, until golden brown. Serve with your favorite GFCF sauce or dressing.

TIP: *The chips can be quickly and easily crushed, either in the food processor, or in a zipper lock baggy with a rolling pin.*

NOTE: *These nuggets freeze well after baking.*

YIELD: *4 servings*

Calories (kcal): 533; **Total fat:** 32g; **Cholesterol:** 194mg; **Carbohydrate:** 34g; **Dietary fiber:** 2g; **Protein:** 28g; **Sodium:** 87mg; **Potassium:** 243mg; **Calcium:** 22mg; **Iron:** 2mg; **Zinc:** 1mg; **Vitamin A:** 1129IU.

Chicken Curry

gluten milk soy egg corn nuts

The bones add a lot of flavor to this braise, but feel free to use boneless chicken instead, or sneak the bones out after the chicken is cooked.

- 3 pounds (1.4 kg) bone-in organic chicken pieces, skin removed (or 2 pounds boneless, skinless chicken)
- ¼ cup (55 g) ghee (or other suitable oil)
- 1 medium onion, finely chopped
- 3 cloves garlic, minced
- 2 tablespoons (16 g) grated ginger
- 1 small jalapeño pepper, seeded and diced
- Cardamom seeds from 2 pods, crushed
- 3 cloves
- 1 cinnamon stick
- 1 bay leaf
- 1 can (14 ounces, 400 g) diced tomatoes, drained
- ½ teaspoon turmeric
- ½ teaspoon chili powder
- 1 tablespoon (6 g) ground coriander
- 1 teaspoon salt
- ½ teaspoon ground black pepper
- 1 pound (455 g) potatoes, peeled and diced
- Water
- ¼ cup (4 g) cilantro leaves, chopped (optional)

Heat the ghee in a large pot or Dutch oven over medium heat. Add the onion and cook for 5 minutes, until golden. Add the garlic, ginger, jalapeño, cardamom, cloves, cinnamon, and bay leaf and cook for 1 minute, until fragrant. Then add the tomatoes and remaining spices and cook for 3 minutes. Add the chicken pieces and cook in the tomato mixture for 5 minutes. Add the potatoes and just enough water to cover and bring to a boil; reduce heat to low and simmer, covered, for 1 hour, until chicken and potatoes are tender. Sprinkle with cilantro if using and serve with basmati or other rice of choice.

YIELD: *4 to 6 servings*

Calories (kcal): 349; **Total fat:** 12g; **Cholesterol:** 111mg; **Carbohydrate:** 24g; **Dietary fiber:** 5g; **Protein:** 38g; **Sodium:** 572mg; **Potassium:** 1062mg; **Calcium:** 105mg; **Iron:** 4mg; **Zinc:** 2mg; **Vitamin A:** 928IU.

Orange Sesame Chicken

gluten milk soy egg corn nuts

This stir-fry is healthier than but just as tasty as the deep-fried version.

- 1 pound (455 g) boneless, skinless, organic chicken breasts
- $^1/_4$ cup (60 ml) GFCF tamari, divided
- 1 tablespoon (8 g) cornstarch, divided
- $^1/_2$ cup (120 ml) orange juice
- $^1/_4$ cup (60 ml) GFCF organic chicken broth (see the recipe on page 294)
- 2 teaspoons sesame oil
- 2 garlic cloves, minced
- 1 tablespoon (6 g) minced fresh ginger
- $^1/_4$ teaspoon hot pepper flakes
- 2 tablespoons (30 ml) avocado or safflower oil, divided
- $^1/_2$ pound (225 g) asparagus, sliced thinly
- 1 small red bell pepper, chopped
- 2 medium carrots, grated
- 2 scallions, thinly sliced
- 2 tablespoons (16 g) toasted sesame seeds

Cut the chicken into $^1/_2$-inch pieces; combine 1 tablespoon (15 ml) tamari and 1 teaspoon cornstarch in a medium bowl and then add the chicken and toss to combine. Let sit for 5 minutes.

For the sauce, whisk the orange juice, broth, remaining tamari and cornstarch, sesame oil, garlic, ginger, and hot pepper flakes and set aside.

Heat 1 tablespoon (15 ml) of oil in a large skillet over high heat. Add the chicken pieces and cook 2 to 3 minutes, stirring occasionally, until lightly browned and cooked through. Transfer to a clean bowl. Heat remaining oil in skillet; add asparagus, pepper, and carrot and cook 3 minutes, until tender. Return chicken to the skillet, add the sauce ingredients and cook for 2 minutes, until thickened. Add scallions and sesame seeds and serve over rice.

YIELD: *4 servings*

Calories (kcal): 300; **Total fat:** 13g; **Cholesterol:** 66mg; **Carbohydrate:** 15g; **Dietary fiber:** 3g; **Protein:** 30g; **Sodium:** 1067mg; **Potassium:** 615mg; **Calcium:** 45mg; **Iron:** 2mg; **Zinc:** 2mg; **Vitamin A:** 105431IU.

Chicken or Steak Fajitas

gluten milk soy egg corn nuts

You can make one or the other, or do a little of both for some variety! Some good condiments to serve alongside this dish are lime wedges, diced avocados or tomatoes, minced cilantro, and plain non-GMO soy yogurt or coconut yogurt.

- 1¹/₂ pounds (680 g) boneless, skinless chicken breasts, sliced into thin strips, or whole flank steak
- Salt and ground black pepper
- 3 tablespoons (45 ml) olive oil
- 1 green bell pepper
- 1 red bell pepper
- 1 red onion
- 2 tablespoons (30 ml) water
- 1 teaspoon chili powder
- ¹/₄ teaspoon cumin
- 1 small garlic clove, minced
- 2 tablespoons (30 ml) lime juice
- 1 tablespoon (15 ml) GFCF Worcestershire sauce
- 1 teaspoon agave nectar (or clover honey)
- 12 small brown rice tortillas

Season the chicken or steak with salt and pepper. Heat 1 tablespoon of oil in large nonstick skillet over medium-high heat. Add meat and brown on both sides, 5 to 10 minutes total (cooking chicken thoroughly, and steak to desired doneness). Transfer meat to a plate and cover to keep warm; let steak rest for 10 minutes before slicing into thin strips.

Add another tablespoon of oil to the pan and heat over medium heat. Add peppers, onion, water, chili powder, cumin, and ¹/₂ teaspoon salt and cook for 5 minutes, until vegetables have softened. Transfer to a serving plate or bowl.

Combine remaining oil, garlic, lime juice, Worcestershire, and agave with a pinch of salt and toss with sliced meat. Warm tortillas in microwave or oven if desired, and serve with meat and vegetables.

YIELD: *4 to 6 servings*

With chicken: Calories (kcal): 484; **Total fat:** 15g; **Cholesterol:** 69mg; **Carbohydrate:** 55g; **Dietary fiber:** 5g; **Protein:** 30g; **Sodium:** 413mg; **Potassium:** 527mg; **Calcium:** 25mg; **Iron:** 1mg; **Zinc:** 1mg; **Vitamin A:** 414IU.

With steak: Calories (kcal): 550; **Total fat:** 24 g; **Cholesterol:** 58mg; **Carbohydrate:** 55g; **Dietary fiber:** 5g; **Protein:** 27g; **Sodium:** 432mg; **Potassium:** 708mg; **Calcium:** 18mg; **Iron:** 3mg; **Zinc:** 4mg; **Vitamin A:** 398IU.

Herb Turkey Burgers

gluten   milk   soy   egg   corn   nuts

These are not the typical dried-out turkey burgers. The addition of mushrooms and onions gives this recipe a tender, juicy texture the family will love. It is also a good way to hide some vegetables as long as they are well minced/blended and the color does not stand out. Start with a small amount (1 tablespoon [16 g]) at first, then increase.

- 1¹/₂ pounds (680 g) organic ground turkey (white and dark meat)
- ¹/₂ cup (3 ounces, or 85 g) finely minced mushrooms
- ¹/₂ small onion, finely minced (about ¹/₂ cup, or 80 g)
- ¹/₈ cup (25 g) minced vegetables (squash, peas, sweet potato)
- 1 teaspoon prepared GFCF barbeque sauce
- 1 teaspoon chopped fresh oregano
- 1 teaspoon ground cumin
- 1 tablespoon (15 ml) balsamic vinegar
- ¹/₂ teaspoon GFCF hot sauce

To serve (optional)
- Toasted buns, pita pockets, or the child's favorite bread
- Spreads and condiments such as GFCF ketchup or mustard

In a medium bowl, combine all ingredients, using a wooden spoon or by hand. Be sure mushrooms and onion are equally distributed throughout mixture. By hand, press meat together to form 8 equal-size patties.

Heat a grill pan or skillet over medium heat. Spray pan with cooking spray, and cook patties for 5 minutes on each side or until cooked through. For cheeseburgers, add a GFCF cheese slice to top of patty after flipping.

No bun is required. Some kids would rather dip their patties right into GFCF ketchup or mustard and don't want a bun.

YIELD: *8 servings of 1 burger each*

Calories (kcal): 132; **Total fat:** 7g; **Cholesterol:** 67mg; **Carbohydrate:** 1g; **Dietary fiber:** trace; **Protein:** 15g; **Sodium:** 88mg; **Potassium:** 234mg; **Calcium:** 16mg; **Iron:** 1mg; **Zinc:** 2mg; **Vitamin A:** 16IU.

Andrew's Turkey Tacos O' Fun

gluten milk soy egg corn nuts

Modified for SCD

- 2 pounds (910 g) ground organic turkey
- 1/4 cup (60 ml) extra virgin olive oil
- 3/4 cup (195 g) Sofrito (see recipe, page 179)
- 2 cans (15 ounces, or 420 g, each) red kidney beans, drained
- 2 cans (8 ounces, or 225 g, each) tomato sauce
- 1 tablespoon (8 g) chili powder, red or green
- 1/4 teaspoon paprika
- Salt to taste

Brown turkey completely in the olive oil on high heat. Add sofrito and lower to medium heat, continuing to mix. Add beans and mix. Add tomato sauce, spices, and salt and mix well.

For SCD tortillas, use almond flour, GFCFSF tortillas by Siete. If SCD is not an issue, use rice or corn tortillas.

VARIATION: *Serve on field greens or romaine lettuce for a taco salad. Optional condiments include onions, tomatoes, gluten-free guacamole, and chopped cilantro.*

YIELD: *6 servings*

Calories (kcal): 828; **Total fat:** 23g; **Cholesterol:** 120mg; **Carbohydrate:** 97g; **Dietary fiber:** 24g; **Protein:** 60g; **Sodium:** 631 mg; **Potassium:** 2672mg; **Calcium:** 162mg; **Iron:** 12mg; **Zinc:** 7mg; **Vitamin A:** 1338IU.

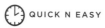 QUICK N EASY

Puréed Beef Broccoli (and Other Options)

gluten   milk   soy   egg   corn   nuts

This recipe can be modified to include a variety of meats and vegetables.

SCD Legal

- 6 ounces (170 g) organic lean ground round or sirloin
- 2 cups (140 g) chopped broccoli florets
- ¹/₂ cup (120 ml) beef or chicken stock (see beef stock recipe on page 295 and chicken stock recipe on page 294)

Brown beef in a skillet over medium-high heat, breaking up any large pieces, about 7 minutes.

Drain off fat and return beef to skillet.

Add broccoli and stock; cover, reduce heat, and simmer until broccoli is very tender, about 15 minutes. Let cool.

Transfer to blender and purée on high speed to desired consistency.

NOTES: *To accommodate those with aversions to green foods, substitute 2 cups (260 g) chopped carrots or sweet potato for the broccoli. (Do not use sweet potato for SCD.)*

Expand this recipe to a more complete whole-dish meal by adding ¹/₂ cup (85 g) cooked brown, white, or basmati rice. If the consistency is too thick, add more stock to thin. (For SCD, use cauliflower rice.)

YIELD: *2 cups (430 g)*

Calories (kcal): 458; **Total fat:** 30g; **Cholesterol:** 117mg; **Carbohydrate:** 10g; **Dietary fiber:** 5g; **Protein:** 37g; **Sodium:** 1222mg; **Potassium:** 1097mg; **Calcium:** 98mg; **Iron:** 6mg; **Zinc:** 8mg; **Vitamin A:** 2715IU.

QUICK N EASY

Beanie Weanies

gluten   milk   soy   egg   corn   nuts

This is another one of Elynn DeMattia's son's favorites—he who would never eat a hot dog in its true form, devours them in this recipe. This dish also makes a great packable school lunch.

- 1 tablespoon (15 ml) safflower or avocado oil
- 2 GFCF organic beef or turkey hot dogs (Organic Prairie, Applegate Organics), sliced into bite-size pieces
- 1 can (14 ounces, or 400 g) organic GFCF baked beans (Amy's)

In a medium skillet, heat the oil over medium heat. Add the hot dog pieces and cook until golden brown on the edges. Add the beans and stir to combine, cooking until heated through, 3 to 4 minutes. Serve.

YIELD: *2 to 3 servings*

Calories (kcal): 241; **Total fat:** 10g; **Cholesterol:** 27mg; **Carbohydrate:** 31g; **Dietary fiber:** 5g; **Protein:** 10g; **Sodium:** 904mg; **Potassium:** 0mg; **Calcium:** 41mg; **Iron:** 2mg; **Zinc:** 0mg; **Vitamin A:** 0IU.

Maple-Glazed Pork Chops

gluten   milk   soy   egg   corn   nuts

Use pure maple syrup for this dish—grade B is better for cooking because it has a stronger flavor.

Low Oxalate, Modified for SCD

- 1 cup (235 ml) GFCF organic chicken broth (see the recipe on page 294)
- $^3/_4$ cup (175 ml) maple syrup (for SCD use clover honey)
- 2 tablespoons (30 ml) cider vinegar
- $^1/_2$ teaspoon dry mustard
- Salt and ground black pepper (optional)
- 1 tablespoon (15 ml) safflower oil
- 4 boneless pork chops, 1-inch (2.5 cm) thick

Whisk together chicken broth, maple syrup, vinegar, dry mustard, and $^1/_4$ teaspoon salt in small bowl and set aside.

Heat the oil in a large skillet over medium-high heat. Season the pork chops with salt and pepper on both sides and carefully add to the hot pan. Cook for 4 minutes, or until browned on one side. Flip chops, add glaze ingredients and reduce heat to medium; cover and cook for 5 to 10 minutes, until pork registers 140°F (60°C) in the center. Remove chops and cover with foil to keep warm. Continue cooking glaze, uncovered, until thickened (adding any accumulated pork juices), 5 to 8 minutes. Pour glaze over chops and serve.

YIELD: *4 servings*

Calories (kcal): 409; **Total fat:** 18g; **Cholesterol:** 62mg; **Carbohydrate:** 40g; **Dietary fiber:** trace; **Protein:** 21g; **Sodium:** 193mg; **Potassium:** 518mg; **Calcium:** 67mg; **Iron:** 1mg; **Zinc:** 2mg; **Vitamin A:** 7IU.

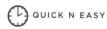 QUICK N EASY

Lighter Beef and Broccoli

gluten   milk   soy   egg   corn   nuts

This is a simple version of a popular dish.

- 1 large bunch broccoli (about 1¹/₂ pounds, or 680 g)
- 1 pound (455 g) beef tenderloin steaks, trimmed, thinly cut into ¹/₈-inch (3 mm) strips
- 3 garlic cloves, crushed with garlic press
- 1 tablespoon (8 g) peeled, grated fresh ginger
- ¹/₄ teaspoon crushed red pepper
- 1 teaspoon (5 ml) olive oil, divided
- ³/₄ cup (175 ml) chicken broth
- 3 tablespoons (45 ml) GFCF non-GMO soy sauce
- 1 tablespoon (8 g) cornstarch
- ¹/₂ teaspoon Asian sesame oil

Cut broccoli florets into 1¹/₂ -inch (3.8 cm) pieces. Peel broccoli stems and cut into ¹/₄-inch (6 mm) diagonal slices.

In a nonstick 12-inch (30 cm) skillet, heat ¹/₂ inch (1.3 cm) water to boiling over medium-high heat. Add broccoli and cook 3 minutes, uncovered, or until tender-crisp. Drain broccoli and set aside. Wipe skillet dry.

In a medium bowl, toss beef with garlic, ginger, and crushed red pepper. Add ¹/₂ teaspoon olive oil to skillet and heat over medium-high heat until hot but not smoking. Add half of beef mixture and cook 2 minutes or until beef just loses its pink color throughout, stirring quickly and frequently. Transfer beef to a plate. Repeat with remaining ¹/₂ teaspoon olive oil and beef mixture.

In a cup, mix broth, soy sauce, cornstarch, and sesame oil until blended. Return cooked beef to skillet. Stir in cornstarch mixture; heat to boiling. Cook 1 minute or until sauce thickens slightly, stirring. Add broccoli and toss to coat.

NOTE: *This can be puréed to suit those with texture issues or those who have difficulty chewing meats.*

YIELD: *4 main-dish servings*

Calories (kcal): 402; **Total fat:** 28g; **Cholesterol:** 80mg; **Carbohydrate:** 12g; **Dietary fiber:** 5g; **Protein:** 26g; **Sodium:** 1010mg; **Potassium:** 904mg; **Calcium:** 89mg; **Iron:** 4mg; **Zinc:** 4mg; **Vitamin A:** 4571IU.

Sweet and Spicy Drumsticks

gluten   milk   soy   egg   corn   nuts

Modified for Low Oxalate

- 8 chicken legs, skin on
- 2 tablespoons (16 g) grated ginger
- 2 cloves garlic, minced
- 2 tablespoons (30 ml) lemon juice
- 4 tablespoons (85 g) honey
- 1 tablespoon (7 g) paprika
- 1 teaspoon chili powder
- 1 tablespoon (8 g) cornstarch or tapioca starch for low oxalate
- $^1/_2$ teaspoon salt

Mash together the ginger, garlic, lemon juice, honey, paprika, chili powder, corn or tapioca starch, and salt with a mortar and pestle or in a bowl to make a smooth paste. Wash and dry the chicken pieces, and then prick them all over with a sharp knife. Combine the paste and the chicken in a large zipper lock bag or in a shallow dish and marinate in the refrigerator for at least 20 minutes.

Preheat oven to 400°F (200°C, gas mark 6). Place the marinated chicken pieces on a wire rack set on top of a baking sheet or roasting pan (line pan with foil for easier cleanup). Cook for 45 minutes, until the meat is cooked through. Serve.

YIELD: *4 to 6 servings*

Calories (kcal): 473; **Total fat:** 27g; **Cholesterol:** 185mg; **Carbohydrate:** 15g; **Dietary fiber:** 1g; **Protein:** 41g; **Sodium:** 359mg; **Potassium:** 502mg; **Calcium:** 30mg; **Iron:** 3mg; **Zinc:** 4mg; **Vitamin A:** 1117IU.

Mexican Egg "Noodles"

gluten   milk   soy   egg   corn   nuts

You'll need a good nonstick skillet to cook the thin omelets used to make the fun egg ribbons in this dish.

- $^1/_4$ cup (60 ml) oil
- 8 eggs, lightly beaten
- 3 cups (780 g) salsa (pages 177)
- 2 tablespoons (4 g) chopped cilantro

Heat 1 tablespoon (15 ml) of the oil over medium heat in a large nonstick skillet. Add one-quarter of the eggs at a time, swirling the pan to coat with an even layer of egg. When the omelet is almost cooked through, flip over with a spatula and cook for an additional minute. Slide omelet onto a cutting board and repeat process to make 3 more omelets, stacking them on top of the first. Slice the stack of omelets into thin noodle-like ribbons.

Heat the salsa in the now-empty skillet until warmed through. Add the egg ribbons and toss to combine. Sprinkle with cilantro and serve.

YIELD: *4 servings*

Calories (kcal): 323; **Total fat:** 24g; **Cholesterol:** 424mg; **Carbohydrate:** 13g; **Dietary fiber:** 3g; **Protein:** 15g; **Sodium:** 983mg; **Potassium:** 550mg; **Calcium:** 111mg; **Iron:** 4mg; **Zinc:** 2mg; **Vitamin A:** 1690IU.

Singapore Noodles

gluten   milk   soy   egg   corn   nuts

This quick and simple noodle dish can pack a good amount of protein.

- ³/₄ pound (340 g) protein of choice (shrimp, chicken, pork, or firm tofu all work well), cut into bite-size pieces
- 1 tablespoon (6.3 g) mild GFCF curry powder
- ¹/₄ cup (60 ml) GFCF tamari
- 8 ounces (225 g) rice vermicelli
- 2 tablespoons (30 ml) safflower or avocado oil, divided
- 2 eggs, lightly beaten
- 3 medium cloves garlic, minced
- 1 tablespoon (6 g) minced ginger
- 1 small onion, chopped
- 1 red bell pepper, seeded and chopped
- 1 cup (235 ml) GFCF chicken broth (see recipe on page XXX)
- 1 tablespoon (20 g) agave nectar or clover honey
- 1 cup (50 g) bean sprouts

Toss the protein with 1 teaspoon curry powder and 1 tablespoon (15 ml) tamari and let marinate at least 10 minutes. Pour enough boiling water over the noodles to cover and let stand 5 minutes; drain noodles and set aside.

In a large skillet or wok, heat 1 tablespoon (15 ml) oil over medium-high heat. Add the protein and marinade and stir-fry until lightly browned and cooked through. Add the eggs and cook, stirring constantly to break up eggs, until cooked through; remove and set aside. Heat remaining oil in the now-empty skillet. Add the garlic, ginger, and remaining curry powder and cook until fragrant, 30 seconds. Add the onion and pepper and cook until softened, 3 minutes. Add the broth, remaining tamari, and agave nectar and stir to combine. Finally, add the reserved protein, noodles, and bean sprouts, tossing to combine ingredients and allow the noodles to absorb the sauce. Serve.

YIELD: *4 servings*

Calories (kcal): 301; **Total fat:** 15g; **Cholesterol:** 107mg; **Carbohydrate:** 29g; **Dietary fiber:** 3g; **Protein:** 14g; **Sodium:** 1130mg; **Potassium:** 288mg; **Calcium:** 123mg; **Iron:** 6mg; **Zinc:** 1mg; **Vitamin A:** 403IU.

Vietnamese Spring Rolls

gluten   milk   soy   egg   corn   nuts

There is no end to what you can stuff these fun rice paper rolls with—a great way to include hidden vegetables. These are just a few suggestions. Assembly can be a family effort, much like making your own tacos. You can also serve these with Thai Peanut Sauce, page 179.

- 2 ounces (55 g) cellophane noodles (also known as glass or bean thread noodles; rice vermicelli can also be used)
- 8 (9-inch, or 23 cm) dried rice paper wrappers
- 1 carrot, shredded
- 1 cucumber, peeled, seeded, and cut into thin strips
- 1 red bell pepper, seeded and thinly sliced
- 4 scallions, sliced into thin strips on the diagonal
- 2 cups (280 g) cooked, shredded organic chicken breasts
- 1/2 cup (10 g) cilantro, basil, or mint leaves, cut into thin strips or left whole

Pour enough boiling water over the cellophane noodles to cover; let soak 5 minutes, or until tender. Drain and rinse under cold water. Cut into 7-inch lengths.

Fill a shallow dish such as a pie plate with warm water. Slide one rice paper wrapper into the water for a few seconds, until pliable. Remove and place on clean plate. Add desired fillings in a line along the center of the wrapper, leaving a 1-inch border on either end (don't overfill). Fold the bottom third of the wrapper up and over the filling, fold in the shorter sides, and then continue to roll until you reach the top (similar to making a burrito). Cut in half on the bias or leave whole.

Lime Chili Sauce

- 1/4 cup (60 ml) fresh squeezed lime juice
- 2 tablespoons (42 g) agave nectar or honey
- 1/4 teaspoon hot pepper flakes
- 1 small clove garlic
- 1 teaspoon grated ginger
- 1/4 teaspoon salt

Combine all ingredients and whisk well to dissolve salt.

NOTE: *These can be made a few hours ahead of time—simply wrap each one in wax paper and refrigerate until needed.*

YIELD: *4 servings*

Calories (kcal): 292; **Total fat:** 9g; **Cholesterol:** 61mg; **Carbohydrate:** 31g; **Dietary fiber:** 3g; **Protein:** 22g; **Sodium:** 224mg; **Potassium:** 654mg; **Calcium:** 92mg; **Iron:** 3mg; **Zinc:** 1mg; **Vitamin A:** 6255IU.

Indian Kebobs with Tomato-Onion Raita

gluten   milk   soy   egg   corn   nuts

If you can't find garam masala, you can substitute a pinch each of ground cardamom, cinnamon, cloves, and black pepper.

Modified for SCD

- 1 pound (455 g) lean ground meat of choice
- 2 tablespoons (16 g) grated ginger
- 1 small jalapeño, seeded and minced (optional)
- Salt
- $1/2$ teaspoon garam masala
- 1 medium onion, finely chopped
- $1/2$ chili powder
- $1/2$ teaspoon ground black pepper
- $1/2$ teaspoon ground cumin
- $1/4$ cup (4 g) cilantro leaves, chopped
- 1 large egg, lightly beaten
- 1 tablespoon (15 ml) avocado or safflower oil

In the bottom of a large bowl, combine the ginger, jalapeño, $1/2$ teaspoon salt, and the garam masala with 1 to 2 tablespoons (15 to 30 ml) water to make a paste. Add the ground meat and the remaining ingredients and combine well. Roll the mixture into small sausage-like balls and thread onto skewers. Grill over medium heat for 20 minutes, basting with a little oil if necessary and turning frequently, until cooked through.

Tomato-Onion Raita

- $1/2$ cup (115 g) non-GMO soy yogurt (For SCD, use a non-soy homemade yogurt.)
- $1/2$ small onion, minced and rinsed under warm water
- 1 tablespoon (2 g) minced cilantro
- 1 tablespoon (8 g) grated ginger
- $1/2$ teaspoon salt
- $1/2$ teaspoon ground cumin, dry toasted
- $1/2$ cup (90 g) seeded and diced tomatoes

Combine the first six ingredients well; add tomatoes just before serving.

YIELD: *4 servings*

Kebobs Only: Calories (kcal): 227; **Total fat:** 13g; **Cholesterol:** 127mg; **Carbohydrate:** 4g; **Dietary fiber:** 1g; **Protein:** 25g; **Sodium:** 102mg; **Potassium:** 97mg; **Calcium:** 18mg; **Iron:** 1mg; **Zinc:** trace; **Vitamin A:** 261IU.

Tomato-Onion Raita: Calories (kcal): 33; **Total fat:** 1g; **Cholesterol:** 0mg; **Carbohydrate:** 6g; **Dietary fiber:** 1g; **Protein:** 1g; **Sodium:** 273mg; **Potassium:** 73mg; **Calcium:** 57mg; **Iron:** trace; **Zinc:** trace; **Vitamin A:** 151IU.

Combined Calories (kcal): 260; **Total fat:** 14g; **Cholesterol:** 127mg; **Carbohydrate:** 10g; **Dietary fiber:** 1g; **Protein:** 26g; **Sodium:** 375mg; **Potassium:** 170mg; **Calcium:** 75mg; **Iron:** 1mg; **Zinc:** trace; **Vitamin A:** 412IU.

Shepherd's Pie

gluten   milk   soy   egg   corn   nuts

Traditionally this comforting dish is made with ground lamb, but lean ground beef is much more kid-friendly.

For Filling

- 1¹/₂ pounds (680 g) lean organic ground beef
- 1 yellow onion, minced
- 1 celery stalk, minced
- 2 teaspoons dried thyme
- ¹/₂ teaspoon salt
- 2 tablespoons (20 g) potato starch
- 1 tablespoon (16 g) tomato paste
- 2 cups (470 ml) GFCF chicken broth
- 1 tablespoon (15 ml) GFCF tamari
- Pinch cayenne pepper
- 1 cup (130 g) frozen peas
- 1 cup (130 g) diced carrots, cooked

For Mashed Potatoes

- 1¹/₂ pounds (680 g) russet potatoes, peeled, boiled, and drained
- 6 tablespoons (85 g) ghee, melted
- ¹/₃ cup (80 ml) soy milk
- ¹/₂ teaspoon salt
- ¹/₄ teaspoon pepper

FOR THE FILLING: In large nonstick skillet over medium heat, cook ground beef, stirring to break up, for 3 minutes or until no longer pink. Transfer to a plate, and drain off all but 1 tablespoon of fat. Add the onion, celery, dried thyme, and salt, and cook for 5 minutes. Add potato starch and tomato paste, stirring to combine, and cook for 1 minute. Add broth, tamari, cayenne, and reserved meat and bring to a simmer. Cover and cook over medium-low heat 6 to 8 minutes, until sauce has thickened. Add peas and carrots and heat through, then transfer mixture to a large baking dish.

FOR THE MASHED POTATOES: Mash potatoes with potato masher or ricer. Add 4 tablespoons melted ghee, non-GMO soy milk, salt, and pepper and gently mix to combine. Spread potatoes in a thin layer over beef mixture, and then brush with remaining ghee. Broil until topping is brown, 3 to 5 minutes. (If you can't keep the baking dish 6 inches away from the broiler, preheat oven to 500°F [250°C, gas mark 10] and cook on the upper-middle rack for 5 to 8 minutes.)

YIELD: *4 to 6 servings*

Calories (kcal): 363; **Total fat:** 25g; **Cholesterol:** 87mg; **Carbohydrate:** 11g; **Dietary fiber:** 3g; **Protein:** 23g; **Sodium:** 669mg; **Potassium:** 479mg; **Calcium:** 38mg; **Iron:** 3mg; **Zinc:** 5mg; **Vitamin A:** 6296IU.

Mexican Meatballs with Vegetable Chili Sauce

gluten   milk   soy   egg   corn   nuts

An interesting twist on the standard meatballs and sauce. Masa harina is the traditional flour used to make tortillas, tamales, and other Mexican dishes. Literally translated from Spanish, it means "dough flour," because the flour is made from dried masa, a dough from specially treated corn.

For the Meatballs

- 8 ounces (225g) lean organic ground beef
- 3 to 4 tablespoons (22.5 to 30 g) masa harina
- 1 large egg, lightly beaten
- 1 small onion, finely chopped
- 1 clove garlic, minced
- 1/2 teaspoon ground cumin
- 1 teaspoon chopped parsley
- 1 tablespoon (6 g) chopped mint
- 1 pinch dried thyme
- 1 pinch ground cloves
- Salt and pepper

For the Sauce

- 2 tablespoons (30 ml) safflower or avocado oil
- 2 tablespoons (15 g) chili powder
- 1 small onion, chopped
- 2 cloves garlic, minced
- 1 can (14 ounces, or 400 g) diced or puréed tomatoes
- 1½ cups (350 ml) GFCF organic chicken stock
- 1/8 teaspoon ground cinnamon
- 2 tablespoons (18 g) raisins or currants
- 2 teaspoons brown sugar
- 2 tablespoons (30 ml) apple cider vinegar
- 1 sweet potato, peeled and chopped
- 1 zucchini, chopped
- 2 carrots, peeled and chopped
- 2 tablespoons (4 g) chopped cilantro

FOR THE MEATBALLS: Mix the meat with the remaining ingredients and season with salt and pepper. Roll into egg-shaped meatballs and set aside in the refrigerator.

FOR THE SAUCE: Heat the oil in a large pot or Dutch oven over medium heat. Add the onion and chili powder and cook 3 minutes, until onion is soft. Add garlic and tomatoes and continue cooking 5 minutes, or until mixture has darkened and reduced slightly. Add the stock, cinnamon, raisins or currants, brown sugar, vinegar, sweet potato, zucchini and carrots, and bring to a boil. Add reserved meatballs, cover, and reduce heat to low. Simmer mixture 20 to 30 minutes, occasionally basting the meatballs with the sauce, until meatballs are cooked through. Add cilantro and serve over rice or with corn tortillas.

YIELD: *4 servings*

Meatballs: Calories (kcal): 202; **Total fat:** 13g; **Cholesterol:** 96mg; **Carbohydrate:** 7g; **Dietary fiber:** 1g; **Protein:** 13g; **Sodium:** 57mg; **Potassium:** 222mg; **Calcium:** 31mg; **Iron:** 2mg; **Zinc:** 3mg; **Vitamin A:** 158IU.

Sauce: Calories (kcal): 188; **Total fat:** 9g; **Cholesterol:** 2mg; **Carbohydrate:** 27g; **Dietary fiber:** 5g; **Protein:** 4g; **Sodium:** 423mg; **Potassium:** 672mg; **Calcium:** 75mg; **Iron:** 2mg; **Zinc:** 1mg; **Vitamin A:** 18747IU.

Combined: Calories (kcal): 391; **Total fat:** 22g; **Cholesterol:** 98mg; **Carbohydrate:** 34g; **Dietary fiber:** 6g; **Protein:** 17g; **Sodium:** 480mg; **Potassium:** 894mg; **Calcium:** 106mg; **Iron:** 4mg; **Zinc:** 3mg; **Vitamin A:** 18904IU.

Yummy Sloppy Joes

gluten　milk　soy　egg　corn　nuts

- 1¹/₂ pounds (680 g) lean organic ground beef
- 1 can (14 ounces, or 400 g) diced tomatoes
- 1¹/₄ cups (300 g) GFCF ketchup
- ¹/₂ cup (125 g) GFCF honey barbeque sauce
- 1 tablespoon (15 ml) GFCF Worcestershire sauce
- ¹/₂ cup (120 ml) water
- ¹/₂ teaspoon ginger
- 2 teaspoons (8 g) sugar or honey
- Salt and pepper to taste
- 6 GFCF hamburger buns

Cook ground beef in a large skillet over medium-high heat, stirring until beef crumbles and is no longer pink. Drain well. Return cooked beef to skillet.

Stir in the rest of the ingredients. Reduce heat and simmer, stirring as the mixture heats and blends. Add more sauce for desired consistency and taste.

Spoon mixture on the buns and serve.

YIELD: *6 servings*

Calories (kcal): 564; **Total fat:** 33g; **Cholesterol:** 96mg; **Carbohydrate:** 43g; **Dietary fiber:** 3g; **Protein:** 24g; **Sodium:** 1112mg; **Potassium:** 765mg; **Calcium:** 89mg; **Iron:** 4mg; **Zinc:** 5mg; **Vitamin A:** 1104IU.

Meatballs

gluten　milk　soy　egg　corn　nuts

This recipe is a good way to hide vegetables for picky eaters. The "hidden" avocado provides a good source of healthy fats. The meatballs freeze well for future meals.

SCD Legal

- 1 medium zucchini
- 2 carrots
- ¹/₂ large onion
- 2 cloves of garlic (minced)
- 1 ripe avocado (or 2 if small)
- ¹/₃ cup (20 g) chopped fresh parsley
- 2 teaspoons salt
- ¹/₄ teaspoon pepper
- 2 tablespoons (12 g) organic Italian seasoning
- 2 pounds (910 kg) organic ground beef, chicken or turkey (A combination works best.)

Preheat oven to 350°F (180°C, or gas mark 4). Shred zucchini, carrots, and onion in a food processor (or grate by hand).

Cook zucchini, carrots, onion, and garlic over medium heat until vegetables are soft. Add chopped parsley, salt, pepper, and Italian seasoning.

Mash the avocado and add to large mixing bowl. Add cooked vegetables and ground meat and mix thoroughly. Using a cookie dough scoop or spoon, form the mixture into balls and place on a parchment-lined baking sheet. Drizzle the meatballs with olive oil and bake for 35–40 minutes.

Serve with SCD marinara sauce, pesto, or ketchup.

YIELD: *6 servings*

Calories (kcal): 330; **Total fat:** 20g; **Cholesterol:** 115mg; **Carbohydrate:** 7g; **Dietary fiber:** 3g; **Protein:** 30g; **Sodium:** 890mg; **Potassium:** 945mg; **Calcium:** 39mg; **Iron:** 3mg; **Zinc:** 5mg; **Vitamin A:** 3792IU.

Meatball Sauce #1— Regular Version

gluten milk soy egg corn nuts

Modified for SCD

- 1 can (8 ounces, or 225 g) tomato sauce
- 1/4 cup (60 g) GFCF ketchup
- 2 tablespoons (20 g) finely chopped onion
- 1 tablespoon (15 ml) vinegar
- 1 tablespoon (15 ml) GFCF organic, sugar-free, soy-free Worcestershire sauce
- 1/2 teaspoon salt
- 1/4 teaspoon black pepper
- 1/4 teaspoon ground organic allspice (home-made with equal amounts cinnamon, cloves, and nutmeg)
- 1/4 cup (60 ml) water
- 1/3 cup (105 g) GFCF natural fruit spread—mixed berry or grape
- 1/4 cup (60 g) puréed vegetables including one or more of the following store-bought Stage 1 or 2 organic baby food or puréed organic fresh or frozen vegetables: carrots, squash, yam, sweet potato, peas, green beans, beets (Do not use yams or sweet potatoes for SCD.)

In a medium saucepan, combine tomato sauce, ketchup, onion, vinegar, Worcestershire, salt, pepper, allspice, water, fruit spread, and puréed vegetables. Bring to a boil, lower heat, and simmer for 15 minutes. Add meatballs and simmer another 15 to 30 minutes. Spear meatballs with wooden picks.

NOTE: *When beginning to add vegetables, start with 1 tablespoon (15 g) and increase as tolerated. Expand the vegetables as each addition is tolerated.*

YIELD: *2 cups (500 g)*

Calories (kcal): 413; **Total fat:** 1g; **Cholesterol:** 0mg; **Carbohydrate:** 107g; **Dietary fiber:** 6g; **Protein:** 5g; **Sodium:** 3342mg; **Potassium:** 1390mg; **Calcium:** 99mg; **Iron:** 4mg; **Zinc:** 1mg; **Vitamin A:** 2863IU.

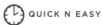 QUICK N EASY

Meatball Sauce #2— Always a Party Favorite!

gluten milk soy egg corn nuts

Modified for SCD

- 1 jar (14 ounces, or 400 g) GFCF organic pasta sauce
- 1/3 cup (105 g) GFCF organic natural fruit spread—mixed berry or grape
- 1/4 cup (60 g) puréed vegetables including one or more of the following store-bought Stage 1 or 2 organic baby food vegetables: carrots, squash, yam, sweet potato, peas, green beans, beets

In a medium saucepan, combine pasta/spaghetti sauce, fruit spread, and puréed vegetables. Bring to a boil, lower heat, and simmer for 15 minutes. Add meatballs and simmer another 15 to 30 minutes. Spear meatballs with wooden picks.

NOTE: *When beginning to add vegetables, start with 1 tablespoon (15 g) and increase as tolerated. Expand the vegetables as each addition is tolerated.*

YIELD: *2 cups (500 g)*

Calories (kcal): 258; **Total fat:** trace; **Cholesterol:** 0mg; **Carbohydrate:** 69g; **Dietary fiber:** 1g; **Protein:** 1g; **Sodium:** 43mg; **Potassium:** 82mg; **Calcium:** 21mg; **Iron:** trace; **Zinc:** trace; **Vitamin A:** 13IU.

Meatballs with Vegetables

gluten　milk　soy　egg　corn　nuts

Modified for SCD

- 1 pound (455 g) organic beef, pork, turkey, or chicken
- 1 cup (240 g) ground vegetables (choose SCD legal, e.g., peas, carrots, onions)
- Salt and pepper to taste (Omit for low phenol/low salicylate diet.)
- Seasoning options: chili pepper, thyme, pepper, oregano

Mix meat, vegetables, and seasonings. Roll into 1¹/₂-inch (3.8 cm) meatballs and bake in a 350°F (180°C, gas mark 4) oven for 20 to 22 minutes (turning once) on a cookie sheet lined with parchment paper. These can also be formed into patties.

YIELD: *About 35 to 40 meatballs or 15 to 20 meat patties*

Calories (kcal): 40; **Total fat:** 3g; **Cholesterol:** 11mg; **Carbohydrate:** 0g; **Dietary fiber:** 0g; **Protein:** 2g; **Sodium:** 9mg; **Potassium:** 30mg; **Calcium:** 1mg; **Iron:** trace; **Zinc:** trace; **Vitamin A:** 0IU.

 QUICK N EASY

Quick N Easy Meatballs

For purchased frozen organic meatballs—check the ingredients to ensure that they are GFCF.

Adjust to diet. SCD vegetables (peas, carrots, green beans, and onions).

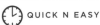 QUICK N EASY

Spaghetti and Meatballs

gluten　milk　soy　egg　corn　nuts

This recipe is a good place to hide puréed or mashed vegetables.

- 1 small yellow onion
- 1 slice gluten-free rice bread
- 2 tablespoons (30 ml) water
- 1 teaspoon salt
- ¹/₂ teaspoon oregano (Use basil for low phenol/low salicylate diet.)
- 1 pound (455 g) ground beef
- 2 jars (26 ounces, or 737 g, each) GFCF organic pasta sauce
- 1 pound (455 g) GF organic spaghetti of choice
- Extra virgin olive oil

Put onion in a food processor and mince. Add bread, water, salt, and oregano and mix again. Pour mixture into a mixing bowl. Knead by hand together with ground beef until thoroughly mixed. Shape into desired meatball size.

Put meatballs into a slow cooker. Add spaghetti sauce and cook for 4 hours. Cook spaghetti according to package directions. Drain and sprinkle with extra-virgin olive oil and toss. Serve with meatball sauce.

OPTIONS: *Add ¹/4 cup (60 g) or more single or mixed vegetables (puréed or mashed) to the spaghetti sauce.*

YIELD: *4 to 6 servings*

Calories (kcal): 1232; **Total fat:** 53g; **Cholesterol:** 97mg; **Carbohydrate:** 149g; **Dietary fiber:** 16g; **Protein:** 41g; **Sodium:** 2481mg; **Potassium:** 1912mg **Calcium:** 152mg; **Iron:** 9mg; **Zinc:** 6mg; **Vitamin A:** 4535IU.

Nutritious, Delicious Meatballs in Sauce

gluten milk soy egg corn nuts

Meatballs are great for appetizers, snacks, or part of a meal. Kids love them for dipping.

The grape spread in the sauce adds a sweet and fruity taste without all the sugar found in jellies. The addition of puréed vegetables to the meatballs and the sauce makes these more nutritious and a perfect way to sneak in more vegetables.

- 1 pound (455 g) lean organic ground beef
- $^1/_2$ cup (15 g) crushed GF organic cornflakes or GF organic cracker crumbs
- $^1/_4$ cup (40 g) finely chopped onion
- 2 tablespoons (30 g) GFCF ketchup
- 2 tablespoons (30 ml) GFCF maple syrup
- 1 teaspoon dried thyme leaves
- 1 teaspoon salt
- $^1/_4$ teaspoon black pepper
- $^1/_4$ teaspoon chili powder
- $^1/_4$ cup (60 g) puréed vegetables (one or more of the following store-bought organic baby food or puréed organic fresh or frozen vegetables: carrots, squash, yam, sweet potato, peas, green beans, beets)

Preheat oven to 400°F (200°C, or gas mark 6). Grease a baking sheet or line with parchment paper.

In a large bowl, combine beef, cornflakes, onion, ketchup, maple syrup, thyme, salt, pepper, chili powder, and puréed vegetables until well mixed. Shape into meatballs (1 tablespoon [15 g] each). Place on prepared baking sheet. Baked for 15 to 20 minutes, until nicely browned.

YIELD: *36 meatballs (1 tablespoon [15 g] each)*

Calories (kcal): 48; **Total fat:** 3g; **Cholesterol:** 11mg; **Carbohydrate:** 2g; **Dietary fiber:** trace; **Protein:** 2g; **Sodium:** 91mg; **Potassium:** 39mg; **Calcium:** 4mg; **Iron:** 1mg; **Zinc:** trace; **Vitamin A:** 47IU.

Spinach Mushroom Lasagna

gluten   milk   soy   egg   corn   nuts

*Adapted from Mary Frances
(www.glutenfreecookingschool.com).*

*Mary Frances used puréed beans as a substitute for
the creamy ricotta filling in this lasagna. Not only is it
gluten-free, casein-free, and soy-free, but it is also a good
source of protein.*

- 4 cups (940 ml) GFCF organic marinara sauce of choice
- ¹/₄ cup (60 ml) olive oil, divided
- 1 pound (455 g) mushrooms, chopped
- 1 large onion, diced
- 4 cloves garlic, minced
- 2 teaspoons salt, divided
- 1 pound (455 g) frozen chopped spinach, thawed and drained
- 1 can (14 ounces, or 400 g) chickpeas
- 1 can (14 ounces, or 400 g) red beans
- Water
- 2 packages GF lasagna noodles

Preheat oven to 375°F (190°C, gas mark 5). Heat 2 tablespoons (30 ml) of the oil in a large skillet over medium heat. Add mushrooms and cook until they have released their liquid. Add the onion, garlic, and 1 teaspoon salt and cook for 10 minutes, stirring occasionally. Add the spinach, reduce heat to low, and simmer until vegetables are heated through.

Drain and rinse the chickpeas and red beans. Pulse in a food processor with remaining 1 teaspoon salt 5 times, and then scrape down the side of the bowl. Add the remaining olive oil and process until smooth. Continue processing and adding 1 tablespoon (15 ml) of water at a time, until the purée is creamy and spreadable.

Spread 1 cup (235 ml) of the marinara sauce into a 9 x 13-inch (23 x 33 cm) baking dish. Add a layer of the dry noodles (about 4) on top. Dab one-third of the bean purée on top of the noodles and spread it out with the back of a spoon or a rubber spatula. Top the bean purée with one-third of the veggie mixture. Repeat 2 more times, ending with a fourth layer of noodles and sauce. Cover the lasagna with aluminum foil and bake for one hour.

YIELD: *8 servings*

Calories (kcal): 228; **Total fat:** 9g; **Cholesterol:** 0mg; **Carbohydrate:** 31g; **Dietary fiber:** 8g; **Protein:** 8g; **Sodium:** 906mg; **Potassium:** 438mg; **Calcium:** 121mg; **Iron:** 3mg; **Zinc:** 1mg; **Vitamin A:** 4223IU.

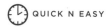

 QUICK N EASY

Quick Macaroni and Cheese

     (gluten) (milk) (soy) (egg) (corn) (nuts)

Daiya cheese is a GFCF cheese that melts better than other brands. Elynn DeMattia tweaks the recipe by adding some salty goodness to the mix.

Low Phenol

- 12 ounces (340 g) brown rice elbow noodles, or GFCF elbow noodles of choice
- 1 1/2 teaspoons salt
- 1 cup (235 ml) GFCF chicken broth
- 1 package (8 ounces, or 225 g) GFCF cheese (Daiya), grated or torn into pieces

Bring 2 quarts (2 liters) of water to a boil in a large pot. Add noodles and salt and cook according to package instructions. Drain noodles and return to pot. Over low heat, add chicken broth and cheese and stir until melted. Serve.

YIELD: *4 servings*

Calories (kcal): 485; **Total fat:** 12g; **Cholesterol:** 1mg; **Carbohydrate:** 69g; **Dietary fiber:** 10g; **Protein:** 27g; **Sodium:** 1484mg; **Potassium:** 0mg; **Calcium:** 5mg; **Iron:** 3mg; **Zinc:** 0mg; **Vitamin A:** 152IU.

Spaghetti and Marinara Sauce

      gluten milk soy egg corn nuts

Adapted from The Book of Yum *(http://www.bookofyum.com)*

- 2 tablespoons (30 ml) extra virgin olive oil
- 1 medium onion, diced
- 4 garlic cloves, minced
- 1/4 medium carrot, grated
- 2 cans (28-ounces, or 784 g, each) peeled whole tomatoes
- 1/4 cup (10 g) chopped fresh basil
- Salt
- 1 pound (455 g) GFCF spaghetti of choice

In a large pot or Dutch oven, heat the oil over medium heat. Add the onion and cook until light golden brown, 8 to 10 minutes. Add the garlic and carrot and cook for 5 minutes, turning heat down if vegetables get too dark. Add tomatoes and their juices and bring mixture to a boil, stirring to break apart the tomatoes. Reduce heat and simmer on low for 30 minutes, until sauce has thickened. Add basil and salt to taste.

Meanwhile, bring a large pot of water to a boil, and cook spaghetti according to package instructions. Serve with sauce.

NOTE: *This sauce makes a great filling for vegetarian Sloppy Joes, served on GFCF hamburger buns.*

YIELD: *4 to 6 servings*

Calories (kcal): 365; **Total fat:** 6g; **Cholesterol:** 0mg; **Carbohydrate:** 76g; **Dietary fiber:** 5g; **Protein:** 5g; **Sodium:** 410mg; **Potassium:** 649mg; **Calcium:** 91mg; **Iron:** 2mg; **Zinc:** trace; **Vitamin A:** 3330IU.

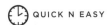 QUICK N EASY

Elynn's Quick Pizza

gluten   milk   soy   egg   corn   nuts

Adapted from Elynn Demattia

*Elynn's son doesn't like any of the GFCF pizza crusts,
so she came up with her own simple solution.*

- 1 large (10-inch, or 25 cm) brown rice tortilla
- $^3/_4$ cup (187.5 g) GFCF spaghetti sauce of choice
- $^1/_2$ cup diced non-GMO soy cheese
- 10 to 12 slices GFCF organic pepperoni

Preheat the oven to 350°F (180°C, gas mark 4). Lightly oil a baking sheet, or line with parchment paper. Place the tortilla on the baking sheet, and spread sauce on top. Sprinkle evenly with cheese, and place the pepperoni slices on top. Bake for 10 to 12 minutes, and then carefully slide the pizza from the baking sheet directly onto the rack for 2 to 3 minutes to crisp up the bottom (this is more easily done when the pizza is left on the parchment paper). Cut into wedges and serve.

YIELD: *2 to 4 servings*

Calories (kcal): 205; **Total fat:** 13g; **Cholesterol:** 21mg; **Carbohydrate:** 12g; **Dietary fiber:** 2g; **Protein:** 11g; **Sodium:** 598mg; **Potassium:** 24mg; **Calcium:** 15mg; **Iron:** 1mg; **Zinc:** 0mg; **Vitamin A:** 150IU.

Pizza with Easy Tomato Sauce

gluten   milk   soy   egg   corn   nuts

Pizza sauce is an excellent way to hide puréed vegetables and meats. Add those that will be least easily detected.

- 1¹/₃ cups (185 g) garbanzo bean flour
- ¹/₂ cup (70 g) brown rice flour
- ¹/₂ cup (60 g) tapioca starch
- 1 tablespoon (8 g) and 1 teaspoon (3 g) xanthan gum
- 1 teaspoon salt
- 1 tablespoon (15 ml) oil
- 1¹/₃ cups (315 ml) water

Blend all the ingredients on low speed, then medium-high speed for 2 minutes. The dough will be sticky. Cover a pizza pan with parchment paper. Roll out dough. Bake in a 425°F (220°C, or gas mark 7) oven for 20 minutes. Add sauce (recipe to follow) and toppings and bake for another 20 minutes.

VARIATIONS: *The same recipe can be used to make pretzels or bread sticks. Cover cookie sheet with parchment paper. Place dough in cookie press. Form pretzels using nozzle with a ¹/4- to ¹/2-inch (0.6 to 1.25 cm) opening. Sprinkle with salt. Bake in 425°F (220°C, or gas mark 7) oven for 20 minutes. A half batch makes 1 tray of pretzels. Best eaten fresh and warm out of the oven.*

YIELD: *1 pizza (serves 6 to 8)*

Calories (kcal): 226; **Total fat:** 4g; **Cholesterol:** 0mg; **Carbohydrate:** 42g; **Dietary fiber:** 5g; **Protein:** 8g; **Sodium:** 1176mg; **Potassium:** 760mg; **Calcium:** 48mg; **Iron:** 3mg; **Zinc:** 1mg; **Vitamin A:** 1435IU.

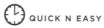 QUICK N EASY

Easy Tomato Sauce

gluten   milk   soy   egg   corn   nuts

Modified for SCD

- 2 cans (6 ounces, or 170 g, each) tomato paste
- 12 ounces (355 ml) water (Use tomato paste cans to measure.)
- 1 teaspoon salt
- 1 teaspoon onion powder
- 1 teaspoon dried basil
- 1 teaspoon dried oregano
- ¹/₈ teaspoon pepper
- ¹/₈ teaspoon garlic powder

Mix all ingredients and simmer 30 minutes.

VARIATIONS: *Add 1 tablespoon (15 g) puréed vegetables to expand nutrition. Add puréed turkey or beef to improve the protein.*

YIELD: *3 cups (750 g)*

Calories (kcal): 25; **Total fat:** 0g; **Cholesterol:** 0mg; **Carbohydrate:** 6g; **Dietary fiber:** 2g; **Protein:** 1g; **Sodium:** 290mg; **Potassium:** 280mg; **Calcium:** 5mg; **Iron:** 1mg; **Zinc:** 0mg; **Vitamin A:** 260IU.

Pizza Sauce and Crust

gluten   milk   soy   egg   corn   nuts

This recipe is tasty, even if it lacks the cheese typically associated with pizza. Having kids participate in making the recipe is not only a fun activity, it may encourage them to be more creative in their tastes. Pizza sauce is a favorite way to add hidden puréed vegetables and meats.

Pizza Sauce (SCD)

- 1 can (8 ounces, or 225 g) tomato sauce
- 1¹/₂ teaspoons sugar or honey
- 1 tablespoon (15 g) puréed vegetables (carrot, peas, squash)
- 1 tablespoon (15 g) puréed meat (chicken, turkey, beef)
- ¹/₂ teaspoon dried oregano leaves
- ¹/₂ teaspoon dried basil leaves
- ¹/₂ teaspoon crushed dried rosemary leaves
- ¹/₂ teaspoon fennel seed
- ¹/₂ teaspoon salt
- ¹/₄ teaspoon garlic powder (avoid for SCD)

Pizza Crust

- 1 tablespoon (12 g) active dry yeast
- ²/₃ cup (95 g) brown rice flour
- ¹/₂ cup (60 g) tapioca flour
- 2 teaspoons xanthan gum
- 1 teaspoon unflavored gelatin powder
- 1 teaspoon Italian seasoning
- ¹/₂ teaspoon sugar or honey
- ¹/₂ teaspoon salt
- ³/₄ cup (175 ml) warm milk (rice or non-GMO soy) (110°F [43°C])
- 1 teaspoon (5 ml) olive oil
- 1 teaspoon (5 ml) cider vinegar
- Rice flour, for sprinkling

Combine all sauce ingredients in a small saucepan. Bring to a boil over medium heat. Reduce heat to low; simmer for 15 minutes while crust is being assembled. Makes about 1 cup (250 g).

Preheat oven to 425°F (220°C, or gas mark 7). Grease a 12-inch (30 cm) pizza pan or baking sheet. In a medium mixer bowl using regular beaters (not dough hooks), blend yeast, flours, xanthan gum, gelatin powder, Italian seasoning, sugar, and salt on low speed. Add warm milk, oil, and vinegar.

Beat on high speed for 2 minutes. The dough will resemble soft bread dough. If dough is too stiff, add water 1 tablespoon (15 ml) at a time. Put mixture on a prepared pan. Liberally sprinkle rice flour onto dough, then press dough into pan, continuing to sprinkle with flour to prevent sticking to the pan. Makes edges thicker to hold the toppings.

Bake pizza crust for 10 minutes. Remove from oven. Top pizza crust with sauce and preferred toppings. Bake for another 20 to 25 minutes or until top is nicely browned.

YIELD: *Serves 6 (1 slice per serving)*

Calories (kcal): 143; **Total fat:** 2g; **Cholesterol:** 2mg; **Carbohydrate:** 30g; **Dietary fiber:** 2g; **Protein:** 3g; **Sodium:** 589mg; **Potassium:** 250mg; **Calcium:** 20mg; **Iron:** 1mg; **Zinc:** 1mg; **Vitamin A:** 409IU.

 QUICK N EASY

Quick N Easy Pizza Sauce & Crust

Use premade organic GFCF pizza sauce and pizza crust.

Veal or Pork Scaloppini

     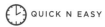

gluten milk soy egg corn nuts

This dish tastes gourmet, yet it's incredibly easy to make.

- 4 veal or pork cutlets (1^1/$_2$ pounds, or 680 g)
- Salt and pepper to taste

Sauce

- 2 tablespoons (30 ml) olive oil or safflower oil
- 2 tablespoons (30 ml) fresh lemon juice
- ^{1}/$_2$ cup (120 ml) chicken broth or white grape juice
- 2 tablespoons (28 g) ghee or ^{1}/$_2$ teaspoon arrowroot mixed in 2 teaspoons (10 ml) water to form a paste
- 2 tablespoons (18 g) GF capers, packed in salt or salt brine, not vinegar (optional)
- 1 tablespoon (1 g) dried parsley or ^{1}/$_4$ cup (15 g) chopped fresh parsley (optional)
- ^{1}/$_8$ teaspoon ground nutmeg (optional)

Season veal (or pork) with salt and pepper. (If using pork cutlets, pound to ^{1}/$_4$-inch (6 mm) thickness.) In a large, heavy skillet, brown meat in batches in the oil about 2 minutes on each side. Remove meat from skillet but keep warm.

To make sauce, increase skillet heat to high and add lemon juice and broth. Continue cooking until reduced by half. Add melted ghee or arrowroot paste and whisk thoroughly. Stir until liquid is reduced and thickens slightly.

To thicken the sauce, add a pinch to ^{1}/$_2$ teaspoon arrowroot. To thin the sauce, add more broth.

VARIATIONS: *Depending on the tastes of the family, add capers, parsley, and nutmeg to the sauce and serve over rice.*

YIELD: *4 servings*

Calories (kcal): 373; **Total fat:** 25g; **Cholesterol:** 157mg; **Carbohydrate:** 1g; **Dietary fiber:** trace; **Protein:** 34g; **Sodium:** 277mg; **Potassium:** 587mg; **Calcium:** 33mg; **Iron:** 2mg; **Zinc:** 5mg; **Vitamin A:** 333IU.

Spicy Pork Tenderloin

gluten   milk   soy   egg   corn   nuts

The ginger in this dish adds just the right flavor, moving it from ordinary to extraordinary.

SCD Legal, Modified for Low Phenol, Modified for Low Oxalate

- 1–3 tablespoons (3–24 g) GFCF chili powder
- 1 teaspoon salt
- 1/4 teaspoon ground ginger (use cinnamon for SCD, Low Phenol, Low Oxalate)
- 1/4 teaspoon thyme
- 1/4 teaspoon white pepper
- 2 organic pork tenderloins (1 pound [455 g] each)

Combine the first five ingredients and rub over tenderloins. Cover and refrigerate 4 hours. Grill over hot heat 15 minutes per side, until juices run clear and a meat thermometer registers 155°F to 160°F (68°C to 71°C).

Delicious served with a side of rice and a green salad. (For SCD, use cauliflower rice.)

YIELD: *8 servings*

Calories (kcal): 74; **Total fat:** 2g; **Cholesterol:** 37mg; **Carbohydrate:** 1g; **Dietary fiber:** 1g; **Protein:** 12g; **Sodium:** 314mg; **Potassium:** 245mg; **Calcium:** 11mg; **Iron:** 1mg; **Zinc:** 1mg; **Vitamin A:** 660IU.

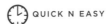 QUICK N EASY

Reddings' Really Delicious Fish

gluten   milk   soy   egg   corn   nuts

SCD Legal, Modified for Low Phenol, Modified for Low Oxalate

Sue and Dick Redding are experienced in the art of preparing and presenting delicious and healthy foods. They offer this easy and quick way to prepare a tasty fish dish.

- 1 pound (455 g) fish (salmon, rockfish, sea bass, white fish)
- 1/2 cup (120 ml) water
- 1–2 tablespoons (8–16 g) GFCF organic seasoning blend for seafood
- Seasoning options for SCD, low phenol, and low oxalate: cayenne, chives, cinnamon, dill, mustard seed, tarragon, thyme, white pepper

Place fish in a 9 x 13-inch (23 x 33 cm) baking dish. If desired, pan can be lined with oil-sprayed aluminum foil.

Add 1/2 cup (120 ml) water to gently poach the fish. Sprinkle fish with seasoning to taste. Bake at 350°F (180°C, gas mark 4), until fish juices run clear and form a white milky curd on top of fish (approximately 30 to 45 minutes, depending on thickness of fish).

VARIATIONS: *In lieu of a seasoning blend, sprinkle salt, pepper, fresh lemon juice, or herbs to taste.*

YIELD: *4 servings*

Calories (kcal): 0; **Total fat:** 0g; **Cholesterol:** 0mg; **Carbohydrate:** 0g; **Dietary fiber:** 0g; **Protein:** 0g; **Sodium:** 1mg; **Potassium:** 0mg; **Calcium:** 1mg; **Iron:** trace; **Zinc:** trace; **Vitamin A:** 0IU.

Favorite Salmon

gluten   milk   soy   egg   corn   nuts

Salmon is an excellent source of low-fat protein, plus the essential omega-3 fatty acids EPA and DHA, which are so important to those with autism spectrum issues, skin conditions, and immune problems. These good fats help with immunity and brain development and function and improve skin health. Avoid farm-raised and buy wild, ocean sockeye salmon, which has a natural orange color from eating the smaller fish that feed on algae rich in EPA and DHA.

Modified for SCD, Modified for Low Phenol, Modified for Low Oxalate

Seasoning Rub Ingredients

- 3 tablespoons (60 g) honey or (45 ml) maple syrup (For SCD, use honey.)
- 1 teaspoon ground cumin (optional)
- 1 teaspoon ground coriander
- 1 teaspoon (5 ml) hot water
- 3/4 teaspoon grated fresh lime peel (optional)
- 3/4 teaspoon salt
- 1/4 teaspoon coarsely ground white pepper

Main Ingredients

- 4 fillets (6 ounces, or 170 g, each) salmon, skin on
- 3 tablespoons (12 g) chopped fresh cilantro

Preheat a grill pan or prepare an outdoor grill for covered, direct grilling over medium heat.

Stir together the seasoning rub until well blended. Rub mixture over fillets.

Place salmon fillets, skin-side up, on hot grill pan or rack and cook 4 minutes. Use a wide spatula to turn salmon over. Cook until opaque throughout (4 to 5 minutes longer.)

Sprinkle salmon with cilantro and serve with lime wedges.

YIELD: *4 servings*

Calories (kcal): 248; **Total fat:** 6g; **Cholesterol:** 88mg; **Carbohydrate:** 13g; **Dietary fiber:** trace; **Protein:** 34g; **Sodium:** 516mg; **Potassium:** 573mg; **Calcium:** 32mg; **Iron:** 2mg; **Zinc:** 1mg; **Vitamin A:** 259IU.

Deviled Crab

gluten   milk   soy   egg   corn   nuts

Fresh lump crabmeat is the best for this dish.

- 3 tablespoons (45 g) ghee or CF no-trans-fatty acid spreads
- 2 teaspoons GF flour mix
- 1 cup (235 ml) non-GMO soy or rice milk, heated
- 1 teaspoon salt
- Dash cayenne pepper
- $^1/_4$ teaspoon GFCF Old Bay seasoning
- 1 teaspoon GFCF Worcestershire sauce
- $^1/_4$ teaspoon GFCF mustard
- 2 egg yolks, slightly beaten
- 2 cups (250 g) lump crabmeat (fresh)
- $^1/_2$ teaspoon lemon juice

Preheat oven to 450°F (230°C, or gas mark 8).

In a medium saucepan, melt the ghee and stir in the flour mix and milk. Add the salt, pepper, Old Bay, Worcestershire sauce, and mustard. Add the egg yolks and cook over medium-high heat, stirring constantly until the mixture starts to thicken. Add the crab and cook until the sauce is thickened and the crab is hot. Remove from heat and stir in the lemon juice.

Spoon the mixture into 4 single-serving baking shells or ramekins. Bake about 20 to 25 minutes until brown.

YIELD: *4 servings*

Calories (kcal): 205; **Total fat:** 15g; **Cholesterol:** 185mg; **Carbohydrate:** 3g; **Dietary fiber:** 1g; **Protein:** 15g; **Sodium:** 752mg; **Potassium:** 325mg; **Calcium:** 79mg; **Iron:** 1mg; **Zinc:** 3mg; **Vitamin A:** 591IU.

 QUICK N EASY

Simple Crab Supreme

gluten   milk   soy   egg   corn   nuts

Modified for SCD

This can be served as a main dish in individual servings or in a casserole. Dana's family loves this best served as an appetizer with GFCF rice crackers or rice almond crackers.

- 2 cups (1 pound, or 455 g) backfin lump crabmeat
- 1 teaspoon GFCF Old Bay seasoning (celery salt, black pepper, crushed red pepper flakes, and paprika)
- 1 teaspoon minced garlic
- $^1/_2$ cup (115 g) GFCF mayonnaise (homemade SCD legal)

Preheat oven to 350°F (180°C, gas mark 4).

Drain the crabmeat and gently sort to remove any shell pieces. Try to leave the crabmeat in lumps.

Mix the seasoning and minced garlic into the mayonnaise.

Add the mayonnaise mix just enough to moisten the crabmeat. Use less or more of the mayonnaise mix as needed.

Place in an ovenproof casserole dish and bake at 350°F (180°C, gas mark 4) for 20 to 30 minutes or until there is a touch of golden brown on top. The crab mixture can also be baked in individual ramekins ($^1/_2$ cup [145 g] each).

YIELD: *4 servings ($^1/_2$ cup [145 g] each)*

Calories (kcal): 257; **Total fat:** 24g; **Cholesterol:** 62mg; **Carbohydrate:** trace; **Dietary fiber:** trace; **Protein:** 13g; **Sodium:** 371 mg; **Potassium:** 234mg; **Calcium:** 66mg; **Iron:** 1mg; **Zinc:** 2mg; **Vitamin A:** 80IU.

Fish Pockets

gluten milk soy egg corn nuts

This is a really healthy way to cook healthy fish! Essentially steaming in its own juices, the fish can be served right in the pocket—a nice sensory experience for some. You can use any fish fillet (skin removed) for this recipe, but reduce the cooking time if they are very thin.

SCD Legal, Modified for Low Oxalate, Modified for Low Phenol

- Olive oil
- 1 piece fresh ginger, 1^1/$_2$ inches (4 cm) long, peeled and cut into thin matchsticks (^{1}/$_2$ to 1 teaspoon cinnamon for low phenol)
- 4 cod fillets, 6 ounces (170 g) each
- Himalayan or Celtic sea salt and white pepper to taste
- 8 sprigs of cilantro

Preheat oven to 425°F (220°C, gas mark 7). Cut 4 pieces of parchment paper, at least 12 x 14-inches (30 x 35 cm). Fold each piece in half to form a 12 x 7-inch (30 x 17.5 cm) piece; unfold.

Brush one side of paper with olive oil. Place one-quarter of the ginger pieces on the oiled side. Pat each piece of fish dry, season with salt and pepper, and place on top of the ginger. Place a couple of sprigs of cilantro on top of each fillet, and then fold over the parchment paper. Seal the 3 open sides well by folding them up over themselves, leaving a small amount of space inside the pocket for steam. Place the 4 pockets in a baking dish, and cook for 15 to 20 minutes (cut into 1 pocket to check doneness of fish), until fish is cooked through, opaque, and flaky. Serve in the pockets, or transfer to a plate (leaving the ginger behind).

TIP: *You can add some simple, quick-cooking vegetables to the pockets as well. Snap peas, thinly sliced carrots, zucchini, and tomatoes all work well, and lemon slices placed over the fish can add a lot of flavor too.*

YIELD: *4 servings*

Calories (kcal): 154; **Total fat:** 1g; **Cholesterol:** 73mg; **Carbohydrate:** 3g; **Dietary fiber:** trace; **Protein:** 31g; **Sodium:** 100mg; **Potassium:** 889mg; **Calcium:** 73mg; **Iron:** 2mg; **Zinc:** 1mg; **Vitamin A:** 765IU.

Lentil Loaf

gluten　milk　soy　egg　corn　nuts

From the Great Sage Restaurant. This is a staple for the vegetarian, GFCF diet. Serve with mashed potatoes and a vegetable for an updated version of a classic meal.

- 3 cups (600 g) lentils
- 4 bay leaves
- 2 tablespoons (30 ml) canola oil
- 1¹/₂ cups (240 g) diced yellow onions
- 1 cup (100 g) walnuts, toasted, cooled, and chopped
- ¹/₂ cup (60 g) finely ground rice white bread (or GF bread crumbs)
- 1 cup (165 g) cooked brown rice
- 1¹/₂ teaspoons sea salt
- ¹/₄ cup (60 ml) GF tamari
- 1¹/₂ tablespoons (15 g) minced garlic
- 2¹/₂ cups (625 g) barbeque sauce, divided
- ¹/₂ cup (120 g) GFCF ketchup
- 1 tablespoon (3 g) dried thyme
- 1 tablespoon (2 g) dried sage
- ¹/₂ teaspoon black pepper

Preheat oven to 350°F (180°C, gas mark 4). Lightly oil two 6-cup (1.4 L) loaf pans and place parchment on the bottom.

For the lentils: Wash lentils in a bowl of water, removing any broken ones that float to the top. Drain and rinse. Place lentils and bay leaves in a large pot and fill with enough water to cover lentils by 2 inches (5 cm). Place over medium heat and bring to a rolling boil.

Reduce heat to low and simmer 45 minutes, or until tender. Stir often and add water as needed, always keeping the water level 2 inches (5 cm) above lentils.

When the lentils are tender, remove from heat and drain well. Spread the lentils out on a baking sheet and chill in the refrigerator for 30 minutes to 1 hour. Remove bay leaves and transfer lentils to a mixer.

For the lentil loaf: In a medium sauté pan, heat oil over medium-high heat. Add onions and sauté until tender and lightly browned, about 10 minutes. Transfer onions to the mixer with the lentils, and add the chopped walnuts, bread crumbs, cooked rice, salt, tamari, garlic, ¹/₂ cup (125 g) barbeque sauce, ketchup, thyme, sage, and black pepper. Mix until all ingredients are well combined and the lentils are somewhat mashed. Turn mixer off and stir from the bottom with a rubber spatula. Combine well.

Transfer the mixture to the oiled loaf pans. Fill within ¹/₂ inch (1.25 cm) from top and smooth with a spatula. Cover the tops with parchment paper. Bake for 35 to 40 minutes or until browned around the edges and firm in the middle. Remove the parchment paper and spread 2 cups (500 g) of barbeque sauce over the loaves. Put back in oven, uncovered, for about 6 minutes or until set. Remove from oven and place on a cooling rack for about 1 hour. If not properly cooled, loaves will fall apart easily. Gently tap out of pans onto their sides. Cut each into 10 slices.

YIELD: *2 small loaves; serves 10 people (10 slices)*

Calories (kcal): 415; **Total fat:** 12g; **Cholesterol:** 0mg; **Carbohydrate:** 58g; **Dietary fiber:** 20g; **Protein:** 23g; **Sodium:** 1390mg; **Potassium:** 839mg; **Calcium:** 86mg; **Iron:** 8mg; **Zinc:** 3mg; **Vitamin A:** 755IU.

Dahl (Vegetarian or with Chicken)

gluten   milk   soy   egg   corn   nuts

This traditional vegetarian dish from India is adapted from Lizzie Vann's Organic Baby & Toddler Cookbook. *The non-vegetarian version uses added chicken, which expands protein. This recipe can be served puréed.*

- 3 tablespoons (45 ml) good-quality safflower, light olive, or avocado oil
- 3 small onions, finely chopped
- $^3/_4$ teaspoon turmeric
- $^1/_2$ tablespoon ground coriander or cumin seeds
- $1^1/_2$ cups (300 g) red lentils, washed and picked over
- 3 carrots, finely chopped
- $3^3/_4$ cups (885 ml) water or 2 cups (475 ml) water and $1^3/_4$ (410 ml) cup chicken broth (store-bought or homemade, see page 294)
- $^1/_3$ cup (25 g) shredded cabbage
- 2 ounces (55 g) cooked organic chicken breast, shredded (optional)

Heat the oil in a pan over medium heat. Add the onion and fry gently until soft, about 5 minutes. Mix in the spices and cook for another 2 minutes.

Add the lentils, carrots, and water and bring to a boil. Reduce the heat and simmer for 20 minutes, until the lentils are soft and the dahl has a smooth consistency. Add the cabbage and chicken (optional) and cook for another 5 minutes, stirring from time to time.

YIELD: *4 servings ($^1/_2$ cup [125 g] each)*

Calories (kcal): 392; **Total fat:** 11g; **Cholesterol:** 0mg; **Carbohydrate:** 55g; **Dietary fiber:** 25g; **Protein:** 22g; **Sodium:** 37mg; **Potassium:** 989mg; **Calcium:** 80mg; **Iron:** 7mg; **Zinc:** 3mg; **Vitamin A:** 15225IU.

Jonathan's Falafel

gluten milk soy egg corn nuts

Leonardo Hosh provides this tasty recipe enjoyed by his son Jonathan. This recipe can work as a side dish as well.

- 2 pounds (910 g) dry garbanzo beans
- 1 bunch parsley (about 1 cup [60 g] finely chopped)
- 1 medium potato
- 1 medium onion
- Garlic salt to taste
- 1/8 teaspoon baking soda
- 1/4 teaspoon salt
- 3 cups (710 ml) canola or vegetable oil for deep-frying

Soak garbanzo beans in water for 2 days; drain and change water several times throughout.

Clean the parsley and potato and peel onion. Rough chop all three and place in a food processor.

Add the beans to the processor and grind until fine and homogeneous in color. Add garlic salt if desired.

Divide the mixture into serving sizes (approximately 1 cup [250 g] portions) and freeze for later use.

To cook, thaw the mixture, add to each 1-cup (250 g) batch: 1/8 teaspoon baking soda and 1/4 teaspoon salt and mix well.

Form into bite-size balls (may use a small ice cream scoop). Heat oil to 375° (185°C), and deep-fry the balls in hot canola or vegetable oil until they turn golden. They are best served immediately after deep-frying.

VARIATION: *Other seasonings can be added if desired:*
- *1 tablespoon (7 g) ground coriander*
- *1 tablespoon (7 g) ground cumin*
- *1 teaspoon cayenne pepper*

YIELD: *12 bite-size balls per cup*

Calories (kcal): 309; **Total fat:** 7g; **Cholesterol:** 0mg; **Carbohydrate:** 49g; **Dietary fiber:** 14g; **Protein:** 15g; **Sodium:** 79mg; **Potassium:** 759mg; **Calcium:** 89mg; **Iron:** 5mg; **Zinc:** 3mg; **Vitamin A:** 311IU.

CHAPTER 18

Rice and Beans

QUICK N EASY

Coconut Jasmine Rice

gluten milk soy egg corn nuts

Both simple to make and elegant to serve, this recipe is a delicious variation from the usual rice dishes.

Low Phenol, Low Oxalate, Modified for SCD

- 1 cup (195 g) jasmine rice (For SCD, use cauliflower rice.)
- 2 cups (475 ml) water
- $1/4$ cup (60 ml) coconut milk
- Sea salt to taste
- $1/4$ teaspoon tarragon

Cook rice in water according to package directions. Stir in coconut milk, salt, and tarragon.

YIELD: *2 servings*

Calories (kcal): 407; **Total fat:** 8g; **Cholesterol:** 0mg; **Carbohydrate:** 76g; **Dietary fiber:** 2g; **Protein:** 7g; **Sodium:** 16mg; **Potassium:** 191mg; **Calcium:** 38mg; **Iron:** 5mg; **Zinc:** 1mg; **Vitamin A:** 8IU.

Brown Rice Pilaf

gluten milk soy egg corn nuts

With the added vegetables, this provides a nice side dish.

- 1 cup (190 g) brown rice (For SCD, use cauliflower rice.)
- 1 tablespoon (15 ml) extra virgin olive oil, divided
- $1/2$ cup (80 g) chopped onion
- $1/4$ cup (25 g) chopped celery
- $1/4$ cup (35 g) chopped carrots
- 1 medium garlic clove, minced
- $1/4$ cup (35 g) raisins
- $1/2$ teaspoon dried sage leaves
- $1/2$ teaspoon dried thyme leaves
- $1/4$ teaspoon black pepper
- $2^{1}/2$ cups (570 ml) chicken stock (store-bought or homemade, [page 294])
- 1 bay leaf

Place rice and half of the oil in a heavy saucepan. Sauté rice over medium heat, stirring frequently, until lightly browned (about 5 minutes). Remove rice from pan. Place remaining oil in a saucepan and sauté onion, celery, and carrots over medium heat until tender, about 5 to 8 minutes.

Add remaining ingredients and bring to a boil. Cover, reduce heat, and simmer mixture for 50 minutes or until liquid is absorbed. Discard bay leaf before serving.

YIELD: *4 servings ($1/2$ cup [85 g] each)*

Calories (kcal): 267; **Total fat:** 6g; **Cholesterol:** 0mg; **Carbohydrate:** 47g; **Dietary fiber:** 2g; **Protein:** 7g; **Sodium:** 490mg; **Potassium:** 410mg; **Calcium:** 42mg; **Iron:** 2mg; **Zinc:** 1mg; **Vitamin A:** 2285IU.

Colorful Celebration Rice

gluten   milk   soy   egg   corn   nuts

This is a clever recipe children will enjoy making.

- 1¹/₂ cups (280 g) uncooked long-grain brown rice (plain or basmati)
- 2¹/₂ cups (570 ml) chicken broth (store-bought or homemade [page 294])
- ¹/₄ cup (35 g) peas, fresh and lightly steamed, or frozen
- ¹/₄ cup (40 g) corn, fresh and uncooked, or frozen
- ¹/₄ cup (18 g) chopped broccoli, steamed or blanched until just tender
- ¹/₄ cup (35 g) diced carrots, steamed or blanched until just tender
- 1 scallion, trimmed of roots, sliced into thin rounds (white and green parts)
- GFCF non-GMO soy sauce
- Sea salt

Combine the rice and chicken broth in a saucepan and bring to a boil. Turn the heat to the lowest simmer, cover the pot, and cook undisturbed for 40 minutes, or until the rice is tender. Remove from the heat and fluff with a fork to let the steam escape, and transfer to a bowl. This can also be cooked in a rice cooker for the same amount of time.

If using frozen peas or corn, place each in a strainer or a colander and run under room-temperature tap water to thaw. Drain thoroughly and cook until tender. Combine the vegetables and rice and reheat if necessary. Let children help with this recipe and serve themselves. Place rice and all vegetables in separate bowls, letting the children create their own mixtures.

Add a few drops of non-GMO soy sauce and sea salt to taste.

VARIATIONS: *Expand the vegetables to include red and green peppers if desired. Increase the amount of vegetables and decrease the rice.*

YIELD: *5 or 6 servings*

Calories (kcal): 245; **Total fat:** 2g; **Cholesterol:** 0mg; **Carbohydrate:** 48g; **Dietary fiber:** 2g; **Protein:** 8g; **Sodium:** 595mg; **Potassium:** 344mg; **Calcium:** 32mg; **Iron:** 2mg; **Zinc:** 1mg; **Vitamin A:** 1956IU.

Coconut Sweet Rice

gluten milk soy egg corn nuts

The cinnamon in this sweet rice variation makes this dish quite tasty.

Modified for SCD

- 1 cup (235 ml) water
- 1 cup (190 g) short-grain brown rice (For SCD, use cauliflower rice.)
- ¹/₂ cup (70 g) raisins or currants
- 1 cinnamon stick
- 1 cup (235 ml) coconut milk
- ¹/₄ teaspoon turmeric

Boil water. Add rice and bring back to a boil. Reduce heat and simmer for 10 minutes. Add raisins or currants, cinnamon stick, coconut milk, and turmeric. Cook an additional 20 minutes or until water has evaporated.

YIELD: *2 servings*

Calories (kcal): 747; **Total fat:** 32g; **Cholesterol:** 0mg; **Carbohydrate:** 113g; **Dietary fiber:** 9g; **Protein:** 11g; **Sodium:** 32mg; **Potassium:** 884mg; **Calcium:** 155mg; **Iron:** 7mg; **Zinc:** 3mg; **Vitamin A:** 21IU.

Rice Fruit Pudding

gluten milk soy egg corn nuts

This is an excellent way to incorporate new fruits. It is best to start with a fruit the child already prefers, then gradually include others.

Modified for Low Phenol, Modified for Low Salicylate, Modified for SCD

- 1 cup (235 ml) water
- ¹/₄ cup (190 g) short-grain white or basmati rice (rinsed) (For SCD, use cauliflower rice.)
- Pinch of salt
- ¹/₄ cup (40 g) fruit—one kind or mixed (cut-up pears, peaches, apricots) (Use a peeled pear for low phenol or low salicylate diets.)
- 2 tablespoons (30 g) non-GMO soy yogurt (For SCD, use a non-soy homemade yogurt.)

Bring the water to a boil in a small pan. Add the rice and simmer gently for 15 minutes, stirring occasionally to prevent sticking.

Add the fruit(s) and simmer for about 5 minutes.

Purée the mixture by pushing through a sieve or by using a blender. Stir in the yogurt, and add more water if a thinner consistency is preferred.

YIELD: *About 2 to 4 servings, depending on the age and appetite of the child*

Calories (kcal): 46; **Total fat:** trace; **Cholesterol:** 0mg; **Carbohydrate:** 9g; **Dietary fiber:** trace; **Protein:** 1g; **Sodium:** 36mg; **Potassium:** 13mg; **Calcium:** 5mg; **Iron:** 1mg; **Zinc:** trace; **Vitamin A:** 0IU.

Red or Black Beans and Rice

gluten   milk   soy   egg   corn   nuts

Arborio rice is particularly tasty with this bean recipe.

Beans

- ¹/₂ cup Sofrito (page 179)
- ¹/₄ cup (60 ml) extra virgin olive oil
- 4 cans (15 ounces, or 420 g, each) organic beans, drained
- ¹/₂ can (3 ounces, or 85 g) tomato paste
- 3 cups (710 ml) chicken broth
- Salt to taste
- 3 bay leaves (only if using black beans)

Sauté Sofrito in oil. Add remaining ingredients. Cook on medium heat for 15 minutes. Reduce heat to low, cover, and simmer for 10 minutes.

Rice

- 2 cups (400 g) Arborio rice
- 2¹/₂ cups (570 ml) water or chicken broth
- Salt to taste
- 2 tablespoons (30 ml) extra virgin olive oil

Mix rice, water or chicken broth, salt, and oil in a medium saucepan. Cook on medium-high until most of the liquid evaporates, about 5 minutes. Reduce heat to low, stir, and cover. Cook until rice is soft.

YIELD: *6 to 8 servings beans and rice*

Calories (kcal): 650; **Total fat:** 18g; **Cholesterol:** 0mg; **Carbohydrate:** 94g; **Dietary fiber:** 18g; **Protein:** 25g; **Sodium:** 1749mg; **Potassium:** 523mg; **Calcium:** 41mg; **Iron:** 4mg; **Zinc:** 1mg; **Vitamin A:** 593IU.

 QUICK N EASY

Spicy Black Beans and Rice

gluten   milk   soy   egg   corn   nuts

This simple version of black beans and rice is ideal for busy parents trying to put dinner on the table quickly.

Modified for SCD

- ¹/₂ cup (80 g) chopped onion
- 4 cloves garlic, minced
- 2 tablespoons (30 ml) olive oil
- 1 can (15 ounces, 420 g) black beans, rinsed and drained
- 1 can (14.5 ounces, 411 g) Mexican-style stewed tomatoes
- ¹/₈–¹/₄ teaspoon ground red pepper
- 2 cups (330 g) hot cooked brown or long-grain rice (For SCD, use cauliflower rice.)

In a medium saucepan, cook onion and garlic in hot oil until tender but not brown. Carefully stir in beans, undrained tomatoes, and ground red pepper. Bring to a boil and reduce heat. Simmer uncovered for 15 minutes.

To serve, mound rice on serving plates and make a well in each mound. Spoon the black bean mixture into the wells. If desired, sprinkle with ¹/₄ cup (40 g) chopped onion.

YIELD: *4 servings*

Calories (kcal): 310; **Total fat:** 8g; **Cholesterol:** 0mg; **Carbohydrate:** 50g; **Dietary fiber:** 8g; **Protein:** 10g; **Sodium:** 357mg; **Potassium:** 324mg; **Calcium:** 54mg; **Iron:** 1mg; **Zinc:** 1mg; **Vitamin A:** 562IU.

Homemade Refried Beans

gluten milk soy egg corn nuts

Note that lard can be used and is much healthier to use than any hydrogenated oil; however, canola or olive oil can also be used.

- 2 cups (500 g) dried pinto beans
- 6 cups (1.4 L) water
- 2 cups (475 ml) chicken broth
- 1 teaspoon salt
- $^1/_4$ teaspoon dried and crumbled oregano (optional)
- $^1/_8$–$^1/_4$ cup (28–55 g) lard (bacon drippings) or (28–60 ml) canola oil or olive oil
- 1 medium onion, peeled and minced or finely chopped
- 1–2 tablespoons (10–20 g) minced garlic (optional)

Go through the beans thoroughly, removing stones or bad beans.

Place beans in a strainer and rinse well under cold water. Put beans, water, and broth into a large pot and bring to a boil. Skim any gray foam from the surface.

Lower the heat to medium and let the beans simmer rapidly for 30 minutes. Add the salt and any other seasoning.

Continue to simmer for another $1^1/_2$ hours or until beans are very soft.

In a large skillet, heat lard or oil over medium heat. Add onion and garlic and sauté until almost golden.

Increase heat to medium-high and add 1 cup (100 g) of the beans and some of their cooking liquid.

Using a potato masher, mash the beans in the pan while they fry. Additional bean-cooking liquid or water may be necessary to keep the beans hydrated and not too dry. The consistency should be smooth, with some small chunks of whole beans mixed in.

Serve in a bowl or use as part of a recipe that calls for refried beans.

NOTE: *If the chunks of beans are a problem for those with texture issues, mash more thoroughly to make the mixture much more uniform in consistency.*

YIELD: *8 servings ($^1/_4$ cup [60 g] each)*

Calories (kcal): 240; **Total fat:** 7g; **Cholesterol:** 6mg; **Carbohydrate:** 33g; **Dietary fiber:** 12g; **Protein:** 12g; **Sodium:** 468mg; **Potassium:** 723mg; **Calcium:** 73mg; **Iron:** 3mg; **Zinc:** 1mg; **Vitamin A:** 6IU.

White Bean Ratatouille

gluten   milk   soy   egg   corn   nuts

This recipe pleases parents and kids alike. The cooked peppers make it sweeter and kid-friendly.

- 3 tablespoons (45 ml) olive oil
- 1 onion, diced
- 6 cloves garlic, minced
- Salt to taste
- Pepper to taste
- Dried oregano to taste
- Red chili flakes (optional)
- 1 red pepper, diced
- 1 yellow or orange pepper, diced
- 1 sprig fresh rosemary, leaves stripped from stem
- 2 fresh sage leaves, chopped
- 1 zucchini, diced
- 1 small to medium eggplant, peeled and diced
- 1 cup (225 g) white beans, cooked or canned
- 15 kalamata olives (optional)
- 6 basil leaves, chopped
- 1 bag (10 ounces, or 280 g) prewashed spinach

Heat oil in a deep skillet. Add onion and garlic and sauté until soft. Add salt, pepper, oregano, chili flakes, peppers, rosemary, and sage and sauté until soft. Add zucchini and eggplant and sauté until soft. Add beans (and olives, if using) and stir. Add basil and spinach and sauté until wilted.

Serve over GFCF pasta or rice. (For SCD, do not use pasta or rice; instead, use cauliflower rice.)

YIELD: *4 to 6 servings*

Calories (kcal): 276; **Total fat:** 15g; **Cholesterol:** 0mg; **Carbohydrate:** 31g; **Dietary fiber:** 10g; **Protein:** 9g; **Sodium:** 290mg; **Potassium:** 1202mg; **Calcium:** 151mg; **Iron:** 5mg; **Zinc:** 1mg; **Vitamin A:** 6841IU.

Happy Hummus

gluten   milk   soy   egg   corn   nuts

This popular and traditional recipe was sent in by several of our parents.
It can be used for dipping or on a sandwich.

- 2 cups (480 g) chickpeas, cooked or canned
- ¹/₃ cup (80 ml) fresh lemon juice
- ¹/₄ cup (65 g) tahini
- 2 cloves garlic, minced or pressed
- 1 tablespoon (15 ml) extra virgin olive oil
- 1 teaspoon paprika or cayenne pepper
- ¹/₄ cup (60 ml) or more water
- Salt to taste

Drain and rinse the chickpeas. Place in a blender or food processor with the lemon juice, tahini, minced garlic, oil, and paprika. Blend well, adding water as needed to form a smooth paste. (Add less water to make a thicker hummus for sandwich spread.) Add salt to taste.

Place hummus in a covered container. It tastes best if it is refrigerated before serving.

Spread on GFCF bread for sandwiches or serve with GFCF crackers or raw vegetables for dipping.

YIELD: *Makes about 3 cups (750 g)*

Calories (kcal): 108; **Total fat:** 52g; **Cholesterol:** 0mg; **Carbohydrate:** 132g; **Dietary fiber:** 28g; **Protein:** 35g; **Sodium:** 1509mg; **Potassium:** 1253mg; **Calcium:** 431 mg; **Iron:** 13mg; **Zinc:** 8mg; **Vitamin A:** 1566IU.

Quinoa Veggie Sauté

gluten   milk   soy   egg   corn   nuts

Adapted from Lisa Barnes, The Petit Appetit Cookbook

Quinoa is an ancient grain with a nutty flavor and light texture, similar to couscous. Quinoa is a valuable source of protein (ounce for ounce it has as much protein as meat), which makes this not only a colorful dish side, but a viable and healthy main course as well. You can find quinoa in a box near the rice or in the bulk section of specialty and organic grocers.

- $^1/_2$ cup (85 g) quinoa
- 2 tablespoons (30 ml) olive oil, divided
- $1^1/_2$ cups (355 ml) water
- $^1/_2$ teaspoon salt
- $^1/_2$ teaspoon black pepper
- $^1/_2$ cup (80 g) chopped onion
- 1 cup (8 ounces, or 120 g) grated zucchini
- 2 tablespoons (19 g) currants
- $^1/_2$ teaspoon ground cumin
- 2 tablespoons (30 ml) fresh lemon juice
- 1 tablespoon (4 g) chopped fresh parsley
- $^1/_2$ teaspoon minced fresh basil

Preheat oven to 375°F (190°C, gas mark 5). In a small saucepan, combine the quinoa in 1 tablespoon olive oil to coat. Add water, salt, and pepper and bring to a boil over medium-high heat. Cover and simmer over low heat for 20 minutes. Quinoa will be translucent when fully cooked. Remove from heat.

Pour remaining tablespoon of olive oil into a large skillet and sauté onion, zucchini, currants, and cumin over medium-high heat for 3 to 5 minutes, or until onions are translucent. Add lemon juice, parsley, basil, and mix to combine. Add quinoa to the pan and mix thoroughly until heated throughout.

YIELD: *4 servings*

Calories (kcal): 168; **Total fat:** 8g; **Cholesterol:** 0mg; **Carbohydrate:** 22g; **Dietary fiber:** 2g; **Protein:** 4g; **Sodium:** 277mg; **Potassium:** 329mg; **Calcium:** 34mg; **Iron:** 3mg; **Zinc:** 1mg; **Vitamin A:** 167IU.

Curried Quinoa Sauté

gluten milk soy egg corn nuts

- ¹/₂ cup (85g) quinoa
- Salt
- 1 tablespoon (15 ml) safflower oil
- 1 medium yellow onion, finely diced
- 1 tablespoon (6.3 g) curry powder
- 1 cup (71 g) chopped broccoli
- 1 cup (100 g) chopped cauliflower
- 1 cup (130 g) frozen peas
- 1 medium red bell pepper, diced
- ¹/₂ cup (120 ml) GFCF chicken broth (see page 294) or water

For the quinoa: Place quinoa, 1 cup (235 ml) water, and ¹/₈ teaspoon salt in medium saucepan. Cover and bring to a boil over high heat, then reduce heat to medium-low and cook for 10 minutes, until quinoa is tender and translucent.

For the sauté: In large sauté pan, heat oil over medium-high heat. Add onion, ¹/₄ teaspoon salt, and curry powder and cook for 3 minutes, or until soft. Add remaining vegetables, and cook for another 3 minutes. Add broth or water, cover pan, and cook for 5 minutes. When vegetables are tender, add quinoa and stir to combine. Serve.

YIELD: *4 servings*

Calories (kcal): 178; **Total fat:** 6g; **Cholesterol:** 1mg; **Carbohydrate:** 27g; **Dietary fiber:** 6g; **Protein:** 7g; **Sodium:** 133mg; **Potassium:** 478mg; **Calcium:** 52mg; **Iron:** 3mg; **Zinc:** 1mg; **Vitamin A:** 809IU.

Edamame Succotash

gluten milk soy egg corn nuts

This is a slight twist in the original Southern dish, but feel free to use the more traditional lima beans in place of the edamame (baby non-GMO soybeans) if you are trying to avoid soy.

- 2 tablespoons (30 ml) safflower or canola oil
- 2 scallions, finely chopped
- 1 clove garlic, minced
- 2 cups (450 g) cooked corn kernels
- 2 cups (340 g) cooked, shelled edamame (non-GMO soybeans)
- ¹/₂ teaspoon salt
- ¹/₄ teaspoon freshly ground black pepper
- 1 cup (150 g) grape or cherry tomatoes, halved or quartered
- ¹/₄ cup (10 g) basil leaves, torn or chopped

Heat oil in a skillet over medium heat; add scallions, garlic, corn, edamame, and salt and pepper and gently cook until heated through, about 5 minutes. Add tomatoes and basil and let cool completely. Serve chilled or at room temperature.

YIELD: *4 servings*

Calories (kcal): 326; **Total fat:** 16g; **Cholesterol:** 0mg; **Carbohydrate:** 33g; **Dietary fiber:** 8g; **Protein:** 19g; **Sodium:** 294mg; **Potassium:** 1028mg; **Calcium:** 16mg; **Iron:** 1mg; **Zinc:** trace; **Vitamin A:** 306IU.

Polenta

gluten   milk   soy   egg   corn   nuts

Polenta is simply cornmeal porridge—naturally gluten-free and a great accompaniment to saucy dishes. It is a traditional staple food throughout much of northern Italy but also popular (under other names) in Switzerland, Austria, Bosnia, Croatia, Cuba, Hungary, Romania, Corsica, Africa, Argentina, Uruguay, Brazil, Peru, Venezuela, Haiti, Mexico, and Turkey.

Low Phenol, Low Oxalate

- 1 quart (1 L) water
- 1 tsp salt
- 1 cup (140 g) coarsely ground cornmeal

In a large pot, bring the water and salt to a boil. Reduce the heat to low and slowly add cornmeal, whisking constantly to avoid lumps. Cover and cook, stirring occasionally, for 30 minutes or until polenta is thick and creamy. Serve immediately.

TIP: *Ways to use polenta*

Polenta can be used instead of mashed potatoes or rice—with roasted chicken, sliced meat, shrimp, fish, or scallops. It can be embellished with your own mix of chopped fresh or dried herbs, garlic, chopped arugula or spinach, roasted red peppers, olives, and more. Dress it up with lots of veggies and pile them on top or mix them in and serve it casserole style.

NOTE: *For fried, sautéed, or grilled polenta, spread hot polenta into a greased 8-inch (20 cm) square baking dish and chill until set. Then cut into pieces and cook as desired. This can be used as the base for appetizers or snacks topped with pesto (has nuts), chopped tomatoes, olives, hummus, or chicken salad.*

YIELD: *4 servings*

Calories (kcal): 126; **Total fat:** 1g; **Cholesterol:** 0mg; **Carbohydrate:** 27g; **Dietary fiber:** 3g; **Protein:** 3g; **Sodium:** 541mg; **Potassium:** 56mg; **Calcium:** 10mg; **Iron:** 1mg; **Zinc:** trace; **Vitamin A:** 142IU.

Baked Grits

gluten   milk   soy   egg   corn   nuts

Crumbled sausage can be substituted for the bacon, and feel free to vary the vegetables. Do not use the quick-cooking grits.

- 6 cups (1.4 L) water
- Salt
- 1½ cups (235 g) stone-ground yellow grits
  (For SCD, use cauliflower rice.)
- ½ pound (225 g) nitrate-free bacon, cut into ½-inch (1.3 cm) pieces
- 1 medium onion, chopped
- 2 cups (170 g) sliced mushrooms
- 1 red bell pepper, cored, seeded, and chopped
- 3 cups (90 g) baby spinach
- 3 scallions, thinly sliced
- 4 large eggs, lightly beaten
- ½ teaspoon ground black pepper

In a large pot, bring water and 1 teaspoon salt to a boil; slowly pour in grits, while stirring constantly. Reduce heat and simmer 30 minutes or until thick, stirring frequently.

Preheat oven to 350°F (180°C, gas mark 4). Grease a 9 x 13-inch (23 x 33 cm) baking pan.

Meanwhile, cook bacon in a large skillet over medium heat until browned and crisp, 5 to 8 minutes. Transfer bacon with a slotted spoon to a paper towel–lined plate. Pour off all but 2 tablespoons (30 ml) fat, add onions and mushrooms and cook until onions have softened and mushroom liquid has evaporated, 5 to 8 minutes. Add bell pepper, spinach, and scallions and cook until tender, 2 to 4 minutes.

When the grits are done, stir in the vegetables, eggs, and black pepper off heat. Pour the mixture into the prepared pan and smooth out the top. Sprinkle the top with the reserved bacon and bake 30 to 40 minutes. Cool on rack 20 minutes before serving.

YIELD: *8 servings*

Calories (kcal): 296; **Total fat:** 16g; **Cholesterol:** 127mg; **Carbohydrate:** 27g; **Dietary fiber:** 2g; **Protein:** 11g; **Sodium:** 304mg; **Potassium:** 263mg; **Calcium:** 37mg; **Iron:** 2mg; **Zinc:** 1mg; **Vitamin A:** 1159IU.

Kasha Pilaf with Mushrooms

gluten milk soy egg corn nuts

Kasha is a traditional Slavic porridge almost always made with toasted buckwheat groats. The mushrooms can be omitted.

- ¹/₄ cup (60 ml) olive oil, divided
- 1 pound (455 g) mushrooms, cleaned and sliced
- 1 small onion
- Salt
- 1 cup (200 g) Kasha, or buckwheat groats, rinsed well
- 2 cups (475 ml) water

Heat 2 tablespoons (30 ml) of the oil in a large skillet over medium heat. Cook mushrooms and ¹/₂ teaspoon salt until mushrooms have released their water; increase heat to medium-high and cook until mushrooms are completely dry and have turned golden brown, 10 to 12 minutes. Set aside.

Heat remaining oil in a saucepan over medium heat. Add the onion and ¹/₂ teaspoon salt and cook until softened, 3 minutes. Add the kasha and sauté until golden and fragrant, 3 minutes. Add the water, and bring to a boil. Cover, reduce heat to low, and simmer for 15 to 20 minutes, until kasha is tender. Gently stir in the mushrooms, season to taste with salt, and serve.

YIELD: *4 servings*

Calories (kcal): 294; **Total fat:** 15g; **Cholesterol:** 0mg; **Carbohydrate:** 37g; **Dietary fiber:** 6g; **Protein:** 7g; **Sodium:** 13mg; **Potassium:** 559mg; **Calcium:** 18mg; **Iron:** 2mg; **Zinc:** 2mg; **Vitamin A:** 0IU.

Vegetable Risotto

gluten milk soy egg corn nuts

Modified for SCD

- $1/4$ cup (60 ml) olive oil, divided
- 3 cups (400 g) grated or finely chopped vegetables (For SCD, use fresh asparagus, carrots, and peas.)
- 3 cups (710 ml) GFCF chicken broth
- 1 small onion, chopped fine
- $1/2$ teaspoon salt
- 1 cup (200 g) Arborio rice
- 1 tablespoon (15 ml) lemon juice
- $1/2$ cup (120 ml) water
- $1/4$ teaspoon ground black pepper
- $1/2$ teaspoon lemon zest

In a large skillet, heat 2 tablespoons (30 ml) of olive oil over medium heat. Add vegetables and sauté until just tender. Reserve.

Heat chicken broth in a small pot until steaming; keep warm. In a large pot, heat the remaining oil over medium heat. Add onion and salt and cook until softened but not browned, 3 minutes. Add rice and cook 3 minutes, until edges of rice are translucent. Add lemon juice and water and cook until completely absorbed. Add the broth, $1/2$ cup (120 ml) at a time until absorbed, stirring occasionally. Next, add the reserved vegetables, pepper, and lemon zest, and cook until broth is absorbed. (If rice is not as tender as you'd like at this point, add 1/2 cup [120 ml] warm water and continue cooking until absorbed.) Serve.

Risotto Cakes

It is worth doubling this recipe so that you have enough left over to make these cakes. The tricks to avoiding heavy breading and a lot of fat for frying is a nonstick skillet and cooking low and slow; this allows the natural starches in the rice to brown and crisp up. The risotto needs to be chilled at least overnight to be firm enough to shape into patties.

Modified for SCD

- 2 cups (330 g) leftover risotto (with or without vegetables added)
- 2 tablespoons (30 ml) olive oil
- Salt to taste

Shape $1/2$ cup risotto into a ball, and then flatten to form a patty (wetting your hands first helps to minimize sticking); repeat with remaining risotto, and sprinkle the cakes with salt. In a nonstick skillet, heat the oil over medium-low heat. Add the cakes and cook for 10 to 15 minutes, until crisp and light golden on the bottom. Flip and repeat for the other side. Serve plain, or topped with your favorite GFCF tomato sauce. (Avoid tomatoes on low phenol/low salicylate diet.)

YIELD: *4 cakes*

Calories (kcal): 442; **Total fat:** 22g; **Cholesterol:** 4mg; **Carbohydrate:** 51g; **Dietary fiber:** 4g; **Protein:** 9g; **Sodium:** 837mg; **Potassium:** 295mg; **Calcium:** 38mg; **Iron:** 1mg; **Zinc:** 1mg; **Vitamin A:** 9895IU.

CHAPTER 19

Vegetables and Side Dishes

Don't skip this chapter!

Some of you are saying "No way! My child gags at vegetables." Well, hang in there. One of these ideas may be your child's breakthrough.

This chapter includes creative ways to include vegetables in the diet for those who like them and those who can't stand them. From eating frozen peas to the Trojan Horse technique of hiding puréed vegetables in other foods, we hope our suggestions will be helpful.

Many parents report that their children ate a wide variety of foods when on baby food but had appetite changes once solid foods were introduced. This may be due to sensory issues, which frequently include aversions or strong dislikes to certain textures and to specific foods, especially vegetables. Most of the children who dislike vegetables are also particular about texture and color. For this reason, it is important to carefully and slowly add anything new.

Mashed Potatoes

gluten milk soy egg corn nuts

This simple and delicious GFCF version of mashed potatoes is destined to become a family favorite.

Low Phenol

- 5 Yukon Gold potatoes, washed and peeled
- $^1/_4$ cup (55 g) GFCF butter substitute or ghee
- $^1/_2$ cup (120 ml) non-GMO soy milk
- $^1/_2$ teaspoon sea salt
- $^1/_2$ teaspoon black peppercorns, ground

Cut potatoes into 2-inch (5 cm) cubes and place in a pot, covering with cold water by 1 inch (2.5 cm). Bring potatoes to a boil, reduce heat, and simmer 10 minutes or until tender. Drain. Place in bowl of an electric mixer. Add butter substitute, non-GMO soy milk, salt, and pepper. Whip until well combined. Adjust seasoning as necessary.

YIELD: *6 or more servings*

Calories (kcal): 167; **Total fat:** 10g; **Cholesterol:** 23mg; **Carbohydrate:** 19g; **Dietary fiber:** 2g; **Protein:** 3g; **Sodium:** 189mg; **Potassium:** 586mg; **Calcium:** 11mg; **Iron:** 1mg; **Zinc:** trace; **Vitamin A:** 347IU.

Pleasing Frozen Peas— Try this!

gluten milk soy egg corn nuts

SCD Legal, Low Phenol, Low Salicylate, Low Oxalate

Frozen peas (regular or baby) are a favorite of many children and adults. They are especially well tolerated by those who favor "crunchy" textures. Many children with sensory issues and aversions to vegetables find eating the individual frozen peas a delight. Serve these as a snack or part of the meal. Of course, organic is better!

Also consider expanding to other frozen vegetables or a medley of frozen vegetables if allowed on your child's diet.

Calories (kcal): 55; **Total fat:** trace; **Cholesterol:** 0mg; **Carbohydrate:** 10g; **Dietary fiber:** 3g; **Protein:** 4g; **Sodium:** 81mg; **Potassium:** 107mg; **Calcium:** 16mg; **Iron:** 1mg; **Zinc:** 1mg; **Vitamin A:** 523IU.

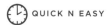 QUICK N EASY

Suzi's Guilt-Free French Fries and Sweet Potato Fries

    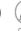
gluten   milk   soy   egg   corn   nuts

"They taste great," says Suzi Gifford. This is a healthy version of a favorite food.

- 2 large unpeeled russet potatoes, or 2 unpeeled sweet potatoes
- 2 egg whites (large egg)
- 1 teaspoon black pepper, freshly ground
- 1–2 teaspoons salt
- Oil spray or 1 tablespoon (15 ml) light olive oil

Cut potatoes into thin strips. In a bowl, whip egg whites until foamy. Add black pepper and salt and mix.

Add potatoes and toss to coat well. Spray a cookie sheet with GFCF oil spray or wipe the surface with oil or use a nonstick cookie sheet or nonstick foil. Spread potatoes on the cookie sheet.

Bake for 30 to 35 minutes at 450°F (230°C, or gas mark 8) or until potatoes are crisp and brown.

VARIATIONS: *Sweet potatoes have excellent nutrition. Combine the two types of potatoes to expand the vegetable choices.*

Add some spice by adding the following to the egg-white foam:
- *1 tablespoon (8 g) chili powder*
- *½ teaspoon cayenne pepper*

Make garlic fries by adding the following to the egg-white foam:
- *1 teaspoon garlic powder*
- *1 teaspoon paprika*

YIELD: *3 to 4 servings*

Calories (kcal): 69; **Total fat:** 3g; **Cholesterol:** 0mg; **Carbohydrate:** 7g; **Dietary fiber:** 1g; **Protein:** 3g; **Sodium:** 563mg; **Potassium:** 234mg; **Calcium:** 9mg; **Iron:** trace; **Zinc:** trace; **Vitamin A:** 1IU.

Potato Pancakes

gluten milk soy egg corn nuts

Not only is this recipe delicious, but also including the garbanzo bean flour in the mix means they're packed with protein.

Low Phenol

- 3 cups (675 g) mashed potatoes
- 1¼ cups (185 g) garbanzo bean flour
- ½ cup (70 g) brown rice flour
- ½ cup (60 g) tapioca starch
- ½ tablespoon xanthan gum
- ½ tablespoon (9 g) salt
- ½ tablespoon baking soda
- 3 tablespoons (45 ml) oil
- 3 tablespoons (45 ml) rice milk

Mix ingredients well in a large bowl. Roll out pancakes between two floured pieces of wax paper. Cook on high heat on a griddle until brown, turning once.

YIELD: *Makes 20 pancakes*

Calories (kcal): 68; **Total fat:** 3g; **Cholesterol:** 1mg; **Carbohydrate:** 10g; **Dietary fiber:** 1g; **Protein:** 1g; **Sodium:** 265mg; **Potassium:** 109mg; **Calcium:** 11mg; **Iron:** trace; **Zinc:** trace; **Vitamin A:** 28IU.

Sweet Potato Pancakes

gluten milk soy egg corn nuts

A sweet and savory version of an old standby.

- 1 pound (455 g) sweet potatoes, peeled
- ½ cup (70 g) brown rice flour, or GF flour blend of choice
- 2 teaspoons (8 g) sugar or Sucanat
- 1 teaspoon brown sugar
- 1 teaspoon baking powder
- 1 teaspoon cinnamon
- ⅛ teaspoon cayenne (optional)
- 1 teaspoon curry powder
- ½ teaspoon cumin
- Salt and pepper to taste
- 2 large eggs, beaten
- ½ cup (120 ml) milk substitute
- 1 large onion, diced
- Oil for frying

Grate sweet potatoes coarsely. In a separate bowl, mix flour, sugars, baking powder, cinnamon, cayenne, curry powder, cumin, salt, and pepper. Add eggs and just enough milk substitute to make a stiff batter. Add potatoes and diced onion and mix. The batter should be moist but not runny. If too stiff, add milk substitute. Heat ¼ inch (0.6 cm) of oil in a frying pan until smoking. Drop batter by tablespoon and flatten. Fry over medium-high heat on each side until golden. Drain on paper towels.

YIELD: *16 pancakes*

Calories (kcal): 52; **Total fat:** trace; **Cholesterol:** 0mg; **Carbohydrate:** 12g; **Dietary fiber:** 1g; **Protein:** 1g; **Sodium:** 34mg; **Potassium:** 72mg; **Calcium:** 27mg; **Iron:** trace; **Zinc:** trace; **Vitamin A:** 4107IU.

Sautéed Cinnamon Carrots

     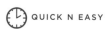

gluten   milk   soy   egg   corn   nuts

Sally Fallon notes in her book, Nourishing Traditions, that peeling carrots does not affect the nutrient content because nutrients are well distributed, unlike potatoes, which have the nutrients concentrated under the skin.

SCD Legal

- 1 pound (455 g) carrots
- $^1/_4$ cup (55 g) ghee or (60 ml) olive oil
- $^1/_4$ –$^1/_2$ teaspoon cinnamon (optional)
- $^1/_4$ teaspoon sea salt (optional)

Peel carrots and slice into rounds or cut into sticks about 3 inches (7.5 cm) long and $^1/_4$ inch (0.6 cm) wide. They may also be cut julienne-style (using a food processor).

Sauté in ghee or olive oil about 20 minutes, until golden but still slightly firm.

Add cinnamon and sea salt.

YIELD: *4 to 6 servings*

Calories (kcal): 109; **Total fat:** 9g; **Cholesterol:** 23mg; **Carbohydrate:** 7g; **Dietary fiber:** 2g; **Protein:** 1g; **Sodium:** 105mg; **Potassium:** 221 mg; **Calcium:** 21mg; **Iron:** 1mg; **Zinc:** trace; **Vitamin A:** 19284IU.

Zucchini Sticks

  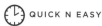

gluten   milk   soy   egg   corn   nuts

The "stick" form of the zucchini makes them less "vegetable-like" and more kid-friendly.

SCD Legal

- 2 small to medium size zucchini
- 1 tablespoon (15 ml) light olive oil (not extra virgin olive oil)
- 1 tablespoon (15 ml) lemon juice
- Pinch of salt
- Pinch of pepper

Cut zucchini in half lengthwise. Then, cut again lengthwise so they are quartered. Then, cut into sticks 2 to 3 inches (5 to 7.5 cm) long.

Mix oil, lemon juice, salt, and pepper. Either toss zucchini with mixture or brush zucchini with mixture using a pastry brush. Place on a cookie sheet, skin-side down.

Broil for 10–15 minutes or until starting to brown. Serve warm.

YIELD: *8 servings (4 sticks/serving)*

Calories (kcal): 20; **Total fat:** 2g; **Cholesterol:** 0mg; **Carbohydrate:** 1g; **Dietary fiber:** trace; **Protein:** 0g; **Sodium:** 20mg; **Potassium:** 76mg; **Calcium:** 5mg; **Iron:** 0mg; **Zinc:** 0mg; **Vitamin A:** 59IU.

QUICK N EASY

Simple Steamed Veggies

gluten milk soy egg corn nuts

This easy recipe lends itself to any variety of greens, depending on the likes and dislikes of your children.

- 2 cups (120 g) green vegetable (spinach, swiss chard, broccoli, kale, asparagus)
- 1 tablespoon (15 ml) olive oil
- $^1/_4$ teaspoon sea salt
- $^1/_8$ teaspoon white pepper
- $^1/_8$ teaspoon dried oregano
- $^1/_8$ teaspoon garlic powder
- $^1/_8$ teaspoon red chili flakes (optional)

Steam the green vegetable.

While steaming, combine the rest of the ingredients to taste in a large bowl. Add steamed vegetables. Stir and coat thoroughly and serve.

YIELD: *4 servings ($^1/_2$ cup [30 g] each)*

Calories (kcal): 40; **Total fat:** 4g; **Cholesterol:** 0mg; **Carbohydrate:** 2g; **Dietary fiber:** 1g; **Protein:** 1g; **Sodium:** 127mg; **Potassium:** 117mg; **Calcium:** 18mg; **Iron:** trace; **Zinc:** trace; **Vitamin A:** 1072IU.

Roasted Veggies

gluten milk soy egg corn nuts

A colorful crowd-pleaser.

- 2–3 sweet potatoes, cubed
- 1 butternut squash, cubed
- 1 red pepper, chopped
- 1 yellow pepper, chopped
- 1 zucchini, cubed
- 1 red onion, chopped
- $^1/_2$ cup (120 ml) balsamic vinegar
- 6 tablespoons (90 ml) olive oil
- 2 teaspoons (8 g) sugar or Sucanat
- 2 teaspoons fennel seed, crushed or whole, or dried rosemary
- 1 teaspoon salt
- $^1/_2$ teaspoon pepper

Lightly grease a roasting pan. Combine veggies. Mix remaining ingredients to make a sauce. Combine sauce with veggies. Bake uncovered for 45 minutes in a 450°F (230°C, or gas mark 8) oven, stirring twice during baking.

VARIATIONS: *Include turnips, parsnips, fennel bulbs, and/or new potatoes.*

YIELD: *10 to 12 servings*

Calories (kcal): 211; **Total fat:** 9g; **Cholesterol:** 0mg; **Carbohydrate:** 35g; **Dietary fiber:** 5g; **Protein:** 3g; **Sodium:** 227mg; **Potassium:** 820mg; **Calcium:** 106mg; **Iron:** 2mg; **Zinc:** trace; **Vitamin A:** 21878IU.

Butternut Squash Purée

gluten   milk   soy   egg   corn   nuts

This recipe, courtesy of Dr. Compart's sister-in-law, Lisa, is enjoyed by both children and adults. Once the purée has cooled a little, its consistency also makes this a good vehicle for hiding/mixing supplements.

- 1 medium to large butternut squash
- 2 teaspoons light olive oil (not extra virgin olive oil)
- 1 tablespoon (15 ml) maple syrup (*real* maple syrup, not pancake syrup)
- $^1/_4$ teaspoon salt

Preheat oven to 400°F (200°C, or gas mark 6). Pierce whole butternut squash in several places with a fork to allow air to escape. Place the butternut squash in a 9 x 13-inch (23 x 33 cm) baking dish.

Bake for approximately 1$^1/_2$ hours or until tender and easily pierced with fork. Let cool approximately 15 minutes. Cut squash open and scoop out the flesh.

Using a potato masher or an immersion blender, add oil, maple syrup, and salt and purée.

Serve warm.

YIELD: *4 servings*

Calories (kcal): 50; **Total fat:** 0g; **Cholesterol:** 0mg; **Carbohydrate:** 13g; **Dietary fiber:** 3g; **Protein:** 1g; **Sodium:** 150mg; **Potassium:** 264mg; **Calcium:** 42mg; **Iron:** 1mg; **Zinc:** 0mg; **Vitamin A:** 9956IU.

 QUICK N EASY

Butternut Squash "Fries"

gluten   milk   soy   egg   corn   nuts

Elaine Gotschall is the inspiration for this recipe. It is also good for those on the SCD eating plan.

- 1 butternut squash
- 2 tablespoons (28 g) GFCF butter substitute or ghee, melted
- Salt to taste

Preheat oven to 450°F (230°C, or gas mark 8).

Using only the neck of the squash, slice thinly ($^1/_4$ inch, or 6 mm).

Place the squash on a cookie sheet or pizza pan, dot with butter substitute or melted ghee, and sprinkle with salt. Bake until one side is brown. Turn over and brown the other side.

YIELD: *2 to 3 servings*

Calories (kcal): 335; **Total fat:** 10g; **Cholesterol:** 23mg; **Carbohydrate:** 66g; **Dietary fiber:** 10g; **Protein:** 6g; **Sodium:** 25mg; **Potassium:** 2,000mg; **Calcium:** 273mg; **Iron:** 4mg; **Zinc:** 1mg; **Vitamin A:** 44606IU.

Mashed Cauliflower—
The New Comfort Food
(Oven and Microwave Versions)

gluten milk soy egg corn nuts

Many children on the autism spectrum have strong aversions to vegetables, especially greens. They tend to focus on "the white diet." By substituting mashed cauliflower for mashed potato, the result is a healthy, high-fiber, nutrient-dense white food. To make the transition from mashed potatoes to cauliflower, combine both at the start. Depending on the type of milk substitute used, the recipe may or may not include non-GMO soy or nut (almond) milk.

Modified for SCD, Modified for Low Salicylate

- 1 head cauliflower, or 1 pound (455 g) frozen cauliflower florets
- $^1/_8$–$^1/_4$ cup (28–60 ml) rice milk (or non-GMO soy milk, coconut milk, almond milk) (For SCD, use coconut milk or almond milk; for low salicylate, use rice milk.)
- Salt and pepper to taste
- 1 tablespoon (15 g) ghee
- Optional seasoning: paprika, garlic

Boil, steam, or microwave (8–10 minutes) cauliflower until fork-tender. Drain thoroughly (squeeze excess water out, or it will be like soup).

Place cauliflower pieces in the blender, then add milk (rice, non-GMO soy, coconut, or almond), salt, pepper, and ghee. Whip until smooth.

Pour cauliflower into a small baking dish. If desired, sprinkle with seasonings. Bake in a hot oven until bubbly or heat quickly in the microwave.

VARIATION: *For those children who eat only white foods, white rice can be added as well as potato.*

YIELD: *4 servings*

Calories (kcal): 40; **Total fat:** 3g; **Cholesterol:** 9mg; **Carbohydrate:** 2g; **Dietary fiber:** 1g; **Protein:** 1g; **Sodium:** 9mg; **Potassium:** 78mg; **Calcium:** 6mg; **Iron:** trace; **Zinc:** trace; **Vitamin A:** 132IU.

Broccoli or "Little Tree" Purée

gluten milk soy egg corn nuts

According to Lisa Barnes in The Petit Appetit Cookbook, *no matter how old you are, everyone has referred to broccoli as "little trees." Look for compact heads that are dark green, sage green, or a purple-green color. The floret clusters should be firm, compact, and tightly closed. Avoid bunches that are wilted or shriveled and those with a pungent odor.*

SCD Legal

- 2 medium heads organic broccoli, stems removed, separated into equal-size florets, or 16 ounces (455 g) frozen broccoli florets
- Water
- Ghee, melted, if desired

Steamer Method:

Place broccoli in a steamer basket set in a pot filled with about 2 inches (5 cm) of lightly boiling water. Do not let water touch broccoli. Cover tightly for best nutrient retention and steam for 10 to 12 minutes or until broccoli is tender. Florets should pierce easily with a toothpick. Immediately transfer steamer basket to sink and run cold water over florets until completely cool, 2 to 3 minutes.

Purée broccoli in a food processor with a steel blade. Additional liquid is not usually needed.

Microwave Method:

Place broccoli florets in a microwave-safe dish. Add 1/2 cup (120 ml) water and cover tightly, lifting a corner to vent. Microwave on high for 4 minutes and stir broccoli. Re-cover and cook for 4 to 6 minutes or until tender. Check for doneness, cook, and proceed with directions above.

Top with melted ghee.

If the child has an aversion to green, mix the broccoli purée into spaghetti sauce or other food source in which the color will not be obvious.

NOTE: *The recipe is even more Quick N Easy when using the frozen organic broccoli florets.*

YIELD: *4 servings (1/2 cup [120 g] each)*

Calories (kcal): 79; **Total fat:** 7g; **Cholesterol:** 17mg; **Carbohydrate:** 4g; **Dietary fiber:** 2g; **Protein:** 2g; **Sodium:** 21mg; **Potassium:** 227mg; **Calcium:** 34mg; **Iron:** 1mg; **Zinc:** trace; **Vitamin A:** 2333IU.

Barb's Vegetable Combo

gluten milk soy egg corn nuts

- 3 tablespoons (45 g) ghee
- $^3/_4$ cup (175 ml) chicken broth
- 1 tablespoon (15 g) Dijon mustard
- 1 tablespoon (8 g) cornstarch
- Dash pepper
- $^1/_2$ teaspoon dried basil leaves, crushed
- $^1/_4$ teaspoon garlic powder
- 1 package (16 ounces, or 455 g) frozen Italian green beans
- 1 cup (50 g) cooked GFCF shell pasta or (165 g) cooked brown rice
- 1 small can (3 ounces, 85 g) button mushrooms, drained
- 1 small tomato, chopped
- $^1/_4$ cup (25 g) sliced black olives (optional)

Melt ghee in a large saucepan. Stir in broth, mustard, cornstarch, pepper, basil, and garlic. Cook until bubbling, stirring constantly. Add green beans, pasta shells or rice, and mushrooms. Stir until heated. The Italian green beans should be cooked to tender-crisp. Just before serving, stir in tomato and olives (optional). Heat to serving temperature.

YIELD: *4 servings*

Calories (kcal): 222; **Total fat:** 12g; **Cholesterol:** 26mg; **Carbohydrate:** 26g; **Dietary fiber:** 5g; **Protein:** 5g; **Sodium:** 275mg; **Potassium:** 435mg; **Calcium:** 73mg; **Iron:** 5mg; **Zinc:** 1mg; **Vitamin A:** 1171IU.

Fall Harvest Veggies

gluten milk soy egg corn nuts

Colorful, sweet, nutritious, and kid-friendly, this dish has it all.

- 2 jewel yams (or 1 jewel and 1 Japanese yam)
- 4 carrots
- 3 parsnips
- 2 tablespoons (30 ml) olive oil
- Fresh rosemary, to taste
- Dried oregano, to taste
- Salt
- Pepper

Preheat oven to 350°F (180°C, gas mark 4). Peel the vegetables and cut into small, thin pieces. Combine in a bowl. Add the remaining ingredients. Bake uncovered for 1 hour or until soft but not too mushy.

For those with sensory issues, this can be puréed.

VARIATION: *To sweeten the flavor, add 1 tablespoon (20 g) honey.*

YIELD: *4 to 6 servings*

Calories (kcal): 205; **Total fat:** 5g; **Cholesterol:** 0mg; **Carbohydrate:** 39g; **Dietary fiber:** 9g; **Protein:** 3g; **Sodium:** 33mg; **Potassium:** 989mg; **Calcium:** 62mg; **Iron:** 1mg; **Zinc:** 1mg; **Vitamin A:** 13502IU.

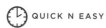

QUICK N EASY

Fried Summer Squash

gluten   milk   soy   egg   corn   nuts

This delicious summer squash recipe is good in any season.

- 1 egg
- 1 teaspoon (5 ml) water
- 2 medium summer squash
- Pecan meal or GFCF bread crumbs
- Olive oil

Beat egg and add 1 teaspoon (5 ml) water. Peel the squash and slice it about ¹/₄ inch (0.6 cm) thick. Drop squash slices into egg mixture to coat, then drop them into pecan meal or crushed bread crumbs, turning to coat evenly. Place on a plate until pan is ready.

A regular frying pan can be used, but be careful that it doesn't get too hot. Nut meal will brown quickly, so remember to cook below medium temperature. If using an electric frying pan, set the temperature to 250°F (120°C). Add a little oil to the pan (watch the amount of oil—just a little under each slice is sufficient) and add the squash slices. Cover the pan and cook 5 to 7 minutes on the first side. Flip the squash, add oil as necessary, and cover and cook for 3 to 4 minutes. Remove the cover and cook 2 to 3 minutes longer.

YIELD: *3 to 4 servings*

Calories (kcal): 147; **Total fat:** 8g; **Cholesterol:** 47mg; **Carbohydrate:** 12g; **Dietary fiber:** 3g; **Protein:** 8g; **Sodium:** 16mg; **Potassium:** 257mg; **Calcium:** 30mg; **Iron:** 1mg; **Zinc:** 1mg; **Vitamin A:** 281IU.

Pecan Meal

Pecan meal is sold in health food stores and online. Pecan "meal" refers to the flakes that occur as the result of chopping pecans. The meal is used in pie crusts, sprinkled on salads, and substituted as a breading for pan-fried foods.

QUICK N EASY

Glenda's Oven-Roasted Vegetables

gluten   milk   soy   egg   corn   nuts

This is an Ingham Family favorite. Vegetable choices can be changed to accommodate the people being served.

- 2–3 zucchini, sliced (medium thickness)
- 2 yellow squash, sliced (medium thickness)
- 3 peppers—one each of red, yellow, and green—sliced (medium thickness)
- 1 large onion, sliced (medium thickness)
- 3–4 cloves garlic, chopped
- 1 can (13.5 ounces, or 378 g) chopped tomatoes
- 1–2 tablespoons GFCF herbs de Provence (basil, oregano, rosemary, parsley, thyme)
- $1/8$ cup (8 g) fresh chopped cilantro (optional)
- $1/2$ cup (120 ml) olive oil

Place all vegetables in a 9 x 13-inch (23 x 33 cm) or other large pan. Sprinkle with herbs. Pour olive oil over top and mix well.

Cover with tin foil and roast in very hot (450°F [230°C, or gas mark 8]) oven for 7 to 10 minutes. Remove tin foil and roast for an additional 7 to 10 minutes.

VARIATIONS: *The vegetables can also be marinated in a GFCF marinade and then roasted in a grill pan. Leftovers can be served over brown rice for a quick, nutritious meal addition. (For SCD, use cauliflower rice.)*

With the addition of chicken broth or stock, this recipe also makes a good soup.

YIELD: *6 servings*

Calories (kcal): 223; **Total fat:** 19g; **Cholesterol:** 0mg; **Carbohydrate:** 14g; **Dietary fiber:** 4g; **Protein:** 3g; **Sodium:** 12mg; **Potassium:** 612mg; **Calcium:** 40mg; **Iron:** 1mg; **Zinc:** 1mg; **Vitamin A:** 1252IU.

Joyce's Versatile Vegetable Medley

gluten   milk   soy   egg   corn   nuts

Joyce Mulcahy's recipe is a family favorite and her standby when asked to bring a side dish to a party. Whether using the basic recipe or adding the optional vegetables, the dish is consistently delicious. Joyce provides two popular versions—Italian and Mexican—which depend on the herb combination used.

Basic Recipe

- $1/2$ onion, sliced or chopped
- 1 garlic clove, minced
- 1 red (or green) pepper
- 1 tablespoon (15 ml) olive oil

Basic vegetables

- 1 can (14.5 ounces, or 411 g) diced tomatoes with juice, or 1–2 fresh chopped tomatoes
- 2–3 sliced zucchini
- Salt and pepper to taste

Optional additions (one or more of the following):

- $1/2$ fennel bulb, chopped
- $2/3$ cup (100 g) white corn (frozen or fresh)
- 1 small eggplant, peeled and sliced

Herb Options:

Italian Herbs:

- 4–5 fresh basil leaves, minced, or $1/2$ –1 tablespoon (15 g) pesto
- $1/2$ teaspoon oregano

Mexican Herbs:

- 1 teaspoon cumin
- 1–2 tablespoons (4–8 g) chopped fresh cilantro

Sauté onion, garlic, and peppers in olive oil until the onions are translucent.

Add basic (and optional) vegetables and herbs and simmer on medium-low heat for 15 minutes, stirring occasionally.

VARIATIONS: *Purée the vegetable medley and serve it over GFCF pasta or rice. Add organic chicken broth and purée to make a delicious soup.*

YIELD: *4 to 6 servings*

Calories (kcal): 89; **Total fat:** 3g; **Cholesterol:** 0mg; **Carbohydrate:** 15g; **Dietary fiber:** 5g; **Protein:** 3g; **Sodium:** 24mg; **Potassium:** 662mg; **Calcium:** 35mg; **Iron:** 1mg; **Zinc:** trace; **Vitamin A:** 1006IU.

Sweet Potato Enchilada

gluten milk soy egg corn nuts

This hearty Mexican dish is easy to make, and its combination of sweet and spicy is something your whole family will love.

- 1 large onion, diced
- 1 teaspoon garlic, minced
- $1/4$ teaspoon cumin
- $1/4$ teaspoon coriander
- $1/8$ teaspoon chili powder
- Dash cayenne pepper
- $1/8$ teaspoon chipotle chili powder
- $1/8$ teaspoon garlic powder
- Approximately 3-4 cups (360–480 g) sweet potatoes, boiled and mashed
- $1/4$ cup (55 g) salsa
- 8 corn tortillas (cut in quarters)
- CF cheese (optional)

Sauté onion and garlic. Add spices to onion mixture and sauté until translucent. Add to mashed sweet potatoes. Adjust seasonings. Spray a baking pan with oil. Layer with half of the salsa, half of the tortillas, sweet potatoes, remaining salsa, and remaining corn tortillas. Top with CF cheese, if using. Bake at 350°F (180°C, gas mark 4) for 20 to 30 minutes, until done.

YIELD: *8 servings*

Calories (kcal): 193; **Total fat:** 1g; **Cholesterol:** 0mg; **Carbohydrate:** 43g; **Dietary fiber:** 4g; **Protein:** 4g; **Sodium:** 172mg; **Potassium:** 349mg; **Calcium:** 89mg; **Iron:** 22mg; **Zinc:** 1mg; **Vitamin A:** 19361IU.

Grandma Lillie's Sweet Potato Tzimmes Kugel

gluten milk soy egg corn nuts

Jody Cutler finds this unusual and delicious version of tzimmes perfect for any Jewish holiday.

- 1 cup (120 g) grated sweet potato
- 1 cup (120 g) grated carrots
- 1 cup (120 g) grated apples
- $1/2$ cup (70 g) chopped raisins
- $1/2$ cup (85 g) chopped prunes
- $1/2$ cup (100 g) sugar (may use honey, Sucanat, or agave nectar)
- $1/2$ cup (70 g) brown rice flour
- 2 tablespoons (30 ml) lemon juice
- $1/2$ teaspoon cinnamon
- $1/2$ teaspoon salt
- $1/2$ cup (112 g) butter substitute

In a large mixing bowl, mix all the ingredients together with a spoon. Pour into a greased 8 x 4-inch (20 x 10 cm) loaf pan and bake in a preheated 350°F (180°C, gas mark 4) oven for about 60 minutes or until brown.

YIELD: *6 to 8 servings*

Calories (kcal): 273; **Total fat:** 12g; **Cholesterol:** 0mg; **Carbohydrate:** 42g; **Dietary fiber:** 3g; **Protein:** 2g; **Sodium:** 276mg; **Potassium:** 288mg; **Calcium:** 27mg; **Iron:** 1mg; **Zinc:** trace; **Vitamin A:** 8340IU.

Purées

Purées are a great way to include vegetables in the diet. This approach is most helpful to those with sensory issues involving food choices, tastes, smells, and textures. One of the markers is a good appetite that becomes limited with the introduction of solids.

Please refer to detailed information in chapter 13. Purées are helpful for hiding vegetables within sauces, especially spaghetti sauce, and in muffins, cakes, brownies, pancakes, peanut butter, meatballs, smoothies, and anything chocolate. See also the main-dish recipes for adding meat purées to sauces to expand the protein content. Reminders:

- The secret is to add a very small amount (1 tablespoon [15 g] or less) blended well with a usual and well-liked food.

- Increase as tolerated to larger amounts, depending on the food in which it is mixed (e.g., 1/4 cup [60 g] or more in a recipe for spaghetti sauce or baked goods, less in a smoothie).

- Mix puréed/blended fruits with puréed/blended vegetables for flavor.

- Use lighter-colored vegetables in baked goods or smoothies:

Sweet potato	Cauliflower
Yellow squash	Turnips
Butternut squash	

- Darker colors work well in meatballs, spaghetti sauce, and chocolate items: (Do not use chocolate for SCD.)

Baby peas	Broccoli
Green beans	Beets
Asparagus	

Use 1 tablespoon to 1/4 cup (15–60 g) organic baby food vegetables or puréed vegetables, as suitable for the child.

Select single vegetables or combinations and use the amount appropriate for the recipes.

NOTE: This works well as long as the first introduction is a very small amount that is gradually increased according to tolerance. Eventually the child may begin to eat the new vegetables alone and may expand beyond the purées and hidden vegetables. The purées are listed first and are followed by more diverse family-friendly vegetable recipes.

Potato-Carrot Mash

gluten milk soy egg corn nuts

This recipe improves upon the standard mashed-potato recipe and is easy to make anytime. It can be made with leftover baked potatoes or leftover carrot purée for children. Russet potatoes work best in this recipe, as they have a high starch content and will become fluffy.

- 4 medium organic carrots, peeled and cut into chunks (about 2 cups, or 260 g)
- 3 medium organic baking potatoes, peeled and cut into chunks (about 3 cups, or 330 g)
- $^1/_2$ teaspoon sea salt
- $^1/_4$ cup (60 g) GMO non-GMO soy yogurt
- 1 tablespoon (15 g) ghee, melted
- 1$^1/_2$ teaspoons sweet GFCF mustard
- Sea salt and white pepper, to taste

Put carrots and potatoes in a large stockpot, cover with cold water, and sprinkle with the salt. Bring to a boil over medium-high heat, and boil until tender, about 10 minutes. Transfer potatoes and carrots to a food processor and purée. Stir in yogurt, ghee, and mustard. Season with salt and pepper.

VARIATION: *There are many colored and healthy mashed-potato variations that can be created by adding vegetables. How about asparagus for a green potato purée for St. Patrick's Day? Or maybe beets for red potato purée for Valentine's Day? Or make both, green and red, for the Christmas table.*

YIELD: *4 servings of 6 ounces (170 g) each*

Calories (kcal): 179; **Total fat:** 4g; **Cholesterol:** 9mg; **Carbohydrate:** 33g; **Dietary fiber:** 4g; **Protein:** 4g; **Sodium:** 293mg; **Potassium:** 985mg; **Calcium:** 31mg; **Iron:** 2mg; **Zinc:** 1mg; **Vitamin A:** 20381IU.

Yummy Mashed Carrots

gluten milk soy egg corn nuts

Children who dislike vegetables have difficulty tasting the natural flavors. Here is a way to bring more flavor to the food. Adding salt is not a problem. Most of the children have higher needs for salt (sodium chloride).

SCD Legal

- 1 pound (455 g) carrots
- 3 cups (710 ml) chicken stock (see page 294 or use chicken broth from the store)
- $^1/_4$ teaspoon sea salt

Optional ingredients

- 1 tablespoon (20 g) honey
- 2 tablespoons (30 g) applesauce (unsweetened)
- $^1/_4$ to $^1/_2$ teaspoon cinnamon

Peel carrots and slice into rounds or cut into sticks about 3 inches (7.5 cm) long and $^1/_4$ inch (0.6 cm) in width. They may also be cut julienne-style (using a food processor).

Combine carrots with chicken stock and cook in the microwave or simmer until soft enough to mash in a processor (medium speed) or in a mixer. Add salt.

Add one or more of the optional ingredients (honey, applesauce, cinnamon) to suit the child's taste.

YIELD: *4 servings*

Calories (kcal): 381; **Total fat:** 22g; **Cholesterol:** 127mg; **Carbohydrate:** 20g; **Dietary fiber:** 4g; **Protein:** 26g; **Sodium:** 295mg; **Potassium:** 737mg; **Calcium:** 72mg; **Iron:** 3mg; **Zinc:** 2mg; **Vitamin A:** 33714IU.

Carrot Soufflé

gluten   milk   soy   egg   corn   nuts

This is Welby Griffin's family's Thanksgiving favorite!

Low Phenol

For the Soufflé:

- 1 pound (455 g) carrots, peeled and cut into 2-inch (5 cm) pieces
- 3 large eggs
- $^1/_4$ cup (50 g) sugar
- 1 teaspoon baking powder
- $^1/_4$ teaspoon salt
- 1 teaspoon GF vanilla extract
- $^1/_3$ cup (80 ml) oil
- 3 tablespoons (26 g) GF flour blend or white rice flour

For the Topping:

- $^1/_4$ cup (7.5 g) GF corn flakes (or other similar cereal), crushed (Use buckwheat, rice, or millet for low phenol/low salicylate diet.)
- 1 tablespoon (14 g) melted ghee or GFCF spread
- 2 tablespoons (28 g) brown sugar

Preheat oven to 350°F (180°C, gas mark 4). Grease a 9-inch (23 cm) round casserole or soufflé dish. Boil carrots until tender, drain, and then mash them (they don't have to be perfectly smooth). Add remaining soufflé ingredients and beat well to combine. Pour mixture into the prepared dish. Blend topping ingredients together and sprinkle on top. Bake for 30 minutes or until lightly browned and bubbly.

NOTE: *This soufflé can be baked in small, individual ramekins or soufflé dishes, but be sure to reduce the baking time by 10 to 15 minutes.*

YIELD: *6 servings*

Calories (kcal): 270; **Total fat:** 17g; **Cholesterol:** 114mg; **Carbohydrate:** 25g; **Dietary fiber:** 3g; **Protein:** 5g; **Sodium:** 239mg; **Potassium:** 260mg; **Calcium:** 79mg; **Iron:** 1mg; **Zinc:** trace; **Vitamin A:** 19192IU.

Maple Mashed Sweet Potatoes

gluten   milk   soy   egg   corn   nuts

A sweet alternative to mashed potatoes.

Low Phenol

- 2 pounds (910 g) sweet potatoes
- $^1/_4$ cup (60 ml) maple syrup (preferably grade B)
- 2 tablespoons (28 g) ghee
- $^1/_2$ teaspoon ground nutmeg (optional)
- Salt and pepper

Peel and cut the sweet potatoes into large chunks. Place in a large pot with 1 teaspoon salt, cover with cold water, and bring to a boil. Reduce heat and simmer for 15 to 20 minutes, until tender. Drain and return to the pot. Add remaining ingredients, season with salt and pepper, and mash with a potato masher or fork. Serve.

YIELD: *6 servings*

Calories (kcal): 190; **Total fat:** 5g; **Cholesterol:** 12mg; **Carbohydrate:** 35g; **Dietary fiber:** 3g; **Protein:** 2g; **Sodium:** 17mg; **Potassium:** 251mg; **Calcium:** 38mg; **Iron:** 1mg; **Zinc:** trace; **Vitamin A:** 22031IU.

Grilled Zucchini "Parmesan"

gluten   milk   soy   egg   corn   nuts

Adapted from The Book of Yum
(http://www.bookofyum.com)

If your child likes eggplant, try it in place of the zucchini.

- $1/2$ cup (120 ml) extra virgin olive oil
- $1/4$ cup (60 ml) GFCF balsamic vinegar
- Salt and pepper, to taste
- 2 pounds (910 g) zucchini, washed and cut into $1/2$-inch (1.3 cm) slices lengthwise
- 2 cups (475 ml) GFCF marinara sauce of choice
- 4 ounces (115 g) Tofutti mozzarella cheese, cut into pieces
- 2 medium garlic cloves, minced

Preheat oven to 375°F (190°C, gas mark 5). Prepare grill for medium heat. Whisk oil, vinegar, salt, and pepper in a large shallow dish. Quickly dip each zucchini slice into the mixture and then place onto the grill. Cook until golden brown on both sides (flipping as necessary) but not mushy.

Grease a baking sheet. Arrange zucchini slices in an even layer on top. Spoon an equal portion of marinara sauce on top of each slice, and then sprinkle with cheese and a pinch of minced garlic. Bake until cheese is melted and lightly browned. Serve as is, or over your favorite GFCF pasta or polenta.

YIELD: *4 servings*

Calories (kcal): 384; **Total fat:** 32g; **Cholesterol:** 0mg; **Carbohydrate:** 21g; **Dietary fiber:** 4g; **Protein:** 7g; **Sodium:** 221mg; **Potassium:** 686mg; **Calcium:** 249mg; **Iron:** 2mg; **Zinc:** 1mg; **Vitamin A:** 1546IU.

Indian-Spiced Cauliflower and Potatoes

gluten   milk   soy   egg   corn   nuts

Low Phenol

- 4 tablespoons (60 ml) olive oil
- 2 medium onions, chopped
- 1 pound russet potatoes, peeled and cut into bite-size pieces
- 1 small head of cauliflower, cut into bite-size pieces
- 2 tomatoes, chopped
- $1/2$ teaspoon ground turmeric
- $1/2$ teaspoon chili powder
- 1 teaspoon cumin
- 1 teaspoon salt
- $1^1/2$ cups (200 g) frozen peas

Heat the oil in a large stock pot or Dutch oven over medium-high heat. Cook the onions for 3 to 4 minutes, until light brown. Add the potatoes, cauliflower, tomatoes, spices, and salt, and cook for another 3 minutes. Add the peas, cover, and reduce heat to medium-low and cook for 20 minutes, stirring occasionally to keep vegetables from sticking, until potatoes and cauliflower are tender. Serve.

NOTE: *For a smooth purée version, add 1 cup (235 ml) of water along with the peas, cook 20 minutes, and then mash everything together with a potato masher or food mill.*

YIELD: *6 servings*

Calories (kcal): 196; **Total fat:** 10g; **Cholesterol:** 0mg; **Carbohydrate:** 25g; **Dietary fiber:** 5g; **Protein:** 5g; **Sodium:** 413mg; **Potassium:** 678mg; **Calcium:** 33mg; **Iron:** 2mg; **Zinc:** 1mg; **Vitamin A:** 597IU.

Apple Butternut Squash Casserole

gluten   milk   soy   egg   corn   nuts

The apples add a nice twist to this vegetable casserole. For a nut-free version, simply omit the pecans and increase the cereal to 2 cups (80 g).

- 1¹⁄₂ cups (60 g) GF flaked cereal, crushed
- ¹⁄₂ cup (55 g) chopped pecans
- ¹⁄₂ cup (115 g) brown sugar, plus 1 tablespoon (15 g)
- ¹⁄₂ cup (112 g) ghee, melted and divided
- 1 small butternut squash, cooked and mashed (to yield 3 cups)
- ¹⁄₄ teaspoon salt
- 6 large or 8 small tart apples, peeled, cored, and sliced (to yield 6 cups)
- ¹⁄₄ cup (50 g) granulated sugar

Preheat oven to 350°F (180°C, gas mark 4). Combine the flaked cereal, pecans, ¹⁄₂ cup brown sugar, and 2 tablespoons (28 g) of the melted ghee in a medium bowl and set aside. In a separate bowl, mix the squash with ¹⁄₄ cup (56 g) ghee, 1 tablespoon brown sugar, and salt.

Heat 2 tablespoons (28 g) of ghee in a large skillet over medium-low heat. Add apples and granulated sugar, cover, and simmer for 5 to 8 minutes, until just tender. Spread apples in the bottom of a 3-quart (3 L) casserole dish. Top with squash mixture, and then sprinkle with cereal-nut topping. Bake for 15 to 20 minutes, until just beginning to bubble at the edges. Cool on wire rack 10 minutes and serve.

YIELD: *8 to 10 servings*

Calories (kcal): 359; **Total fat:** 16g; **Cholesterol:** 28mg; **Carbohydrate:** 58g; **Dietary fiber:** 7g; **Protein:** 3g; **Sodium:** 100mg; **Potassium:** 800mg; **Calcium:** 101mg; **Iron:** 2mg; **Zinc:** 1mg; **Vitamin A:** 13783IU.

CHAPTER 20

Salads

Incredible, Edible Gelatin

Gelatin is not just a fun food for kids, it is a healthy food. Gelatin in meat broths, desserts, and gelatin salads improves digestion by attracting digestive juices to the surface of cooked food particles. According to Sally Fallon in *Nourishing Traditions*, gelatin has been used throughout history in the treatment of many digestive and intestinal disorders. It is one of the "healing" ingredients in meat broths in chapter 21. Note that the vegetarian gelatin source, carrageenan, does not have the same healthy effect and can hinder the actions of digestive enzymes. The recipes here use only unflavored gelatin.

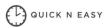

QUICK N EASY

Fruit Knox Blocks

gluten   milk   soy   egg   corn   nuts

This simple recipe is from the makers of Knox gelatin.

- 4 envelopes (1 tablespoon, or 7 g, each) unflavored gelatin
- 1 cup (235 ml) cold fruit juice (orange, grape, cranberry-apple, raspberry/cranberry)
- 3 cups (710 ml) fruit juice, heated to boiling
- 2 tablespoons (25 g) sugar or (40 g) honey (optional)

Sprinkle gelatin over cold juice in a large bowl and let stand 1 minute.

Add hot juice and stir with a metal spoon until gelatin completely dissolves (about 5 minutes). Stir in sugar or honey, if desired. Pour into 13 x 9 x 2-inch (33 x 22.5 x 5 cm) pan.

Refrigerate until firm, about 3 hours. To serve, cut into 1-inch (2.5 cm) squares.

YIELD: *9 dozen 1-inch (2.5-cm) squares*

Calories (kcal): 3; **Total fat:** 0g; **Cholesterol:** 0mg; **Carbohydrate:** 1g; **Dietary fiber:** 0g; **Protein:** trace; **Sodium:** 1mg; **Potassium:** trace; **Calcium:** trace; **Iron:** trace; **Zinc:** trace; **Vitamin A:** 0IU.

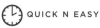

QUICK N EASY

Gelatin Fruit Purée

gluten   milk   soy   egg   corn   nuts

This is a great way for children to enjoy gelatin as part of a meal or dessert without the added sugars and preservatives of the boxed versions. The nutritional content of this real fruit version is far superior and tastier. This recipe is also a way to sneak in a few vegetables. Puréed carrots or sweet potato will mix nicely with the fruit. For a sick child, this is an easy way to increase liquids via the healing and soothing qualities of gelatin.

- 1 envelope (1 tablespoon, or 7 g) gelatin
- $1/3$ cup (80 ml) hot juice (apple, pear, or white grape)
- 1 cup (245 g) puréed fruit (apple, pear, peach) or applesauce or pear sauce
- If adding vegetables, reduce fruit to $3/4$ cup (185 g) and add $1/4$ cup (60 g) puréed carrots or sweet potato (Baby food may also be used.)

In a medium bowl, dissolve gelatin in hot juice, stirring continuously. Add purée and stir with a rubber spatula to combine. Pour mixture into an 8-inch (20 cm) square or round shallow glass dish, and chill in the refrigerator until firm, about 2 hours.

YIELD: *8 to 10 child-size servings*

Calories (kcal): 7; **Total fat:** 0g; **Cholesterol:** 0mg; **Carbohydrate:** 2g; **Dietary fiber:** 0g; **Protein:** trace; **Sodium:** 5mg; **Potassium:** trace; **Calcium:** trace; **Iron:** trace; **Zinc:** 0mg; **Vitamin A:** 0IU.

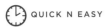
QUICK N EASY

Great Gelatin Fruit Salad

 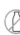
gluten   milk   soy   egg   corn   nuts

This fruit gelatin salad recipe can be adapted many ways, using a variety of fruits. Do not use fresh or frozen pineapple, guava, figs, kiwifruit, or gingerroot in molded salads. They contain bromelain, a protein-dissolving enzyme, which will break up the gelatin's protein bonds. The canned versions are fine because the heat used in canning denatures the bromelain enzymes. For those with sensitive digestive tracts, the fruits in this recipe may be partially cooked and puréed.

- 3 envelopes (1 tablespoon, or 7 g, each) unflavored gelatin
- 3 cups (710 ml) fruit juice (orange, grape, cranberry-apple, raspberry/cranberry, mixed fruit juices), divided as follows:
  - 1 cup (235 ml) cold
  - 2 cups (475 ml) heated to boiling
- 2 tablespoons (25 g) sugar or (40 g) honey (optional)
- 2 cups (300 g) assorted fresh fruits (sliced bananas or strawberries, chopped apples or melon, grapes or blueberries, cut-up peaches or pears)

Sprinkle gelatin over cold juice in a large bowl and let stand 1 minute.

Add hot juice and stir with a metal spoon until gelatin completely dissolves (about 5 minutes). Stir in sugar or honey, if desired.

Refrigerate gelatin mixture until partially chilled (about 1 hour). The gelatin will look like thick, unbeaten egg whites. This allows the added fruits to be evenly distributed. Fold in fruits.

Coat the inside of a 5-cup mold or individual dessert dishes with light oil (safflower) to prevent sticking, and turn the mixture into a mold or dishes. Refrigerate until completely set.

VARIATIONS: *Fruits can also be puréed to avoid lumps for those with oral sensory issues.*

This is another way to hide vegetables. If the puréed fruits work, then hide a few puréed vegetables with the fruits in the gelatin.

TIP: *Mix supplements into the gelatin solution once cooled and pour into ice-cube trays for full chilling so that 1 cube = 1 dose.*

YIELD: *8 servings*

Calories (kcal): 26; **Total fat:** 0g; **Cholesterol:** 0mg; **Carbohydrate:** 6g; **Dietary fiber:** 0g; **Protein:** trace; **Sodium:** 9mg; **Potassium:** trace; **Calcium:** trace; **Iron:** trace; **Zinc:** trace; **Vitamin A:** 0IU.

Dotty Lucey's Tangy Tomato Aspic

gluten milk soy egg corn nuts

Dana adapted this recipe from her mother's signature party dish. It is another way to sneak vegetables into children's diets. For those who have sensory issues with textures, try adding the vegetables as a purée.

- 3 envelopes (1 tablespoon, or 7 g, each) unflavored gelatin
- 3 cups (710 g) cold tomato juice, divided
- 2 cups (475 ml) tomato juice, heated to boiling
- 1/4 cup (60 ml) lemon juice
- 1/2 teaspoon vinegar
- 1 1/2 teaspoons GFCF Worcestershire sauce
- 1/2 teaspoon salt
- 2 tablespoons (25 g) sugar

Optional for Spicier Version:
- 1/2 teaspoon onion juice
- 1/8 teaspoon red pepper sauce
- Dash of cloves

Optional Additions:
- 1 cup (120 g) finely chopped celery
- 1 cup (180 g) cooked and cut-up asparagus

Sprinkle gelatin over 1 cup (235 ml) cold tomato juice in a large bowl; let stand 1 minute to soften gelatin. Add 2 cups (475 ml) hot tomato juice; stir 5 minutes or until gelatin is completely dissolved.

Add remaining 2 cups (475 ml) cold tomato juice, lemon juice, vinegar, Worcestershire sauce, salt, and sugar. For spicier version, add onion juice, red pepper sauce, and dash of cloves.

If adding celery and asparagus, chill for 1 hour until slightly thickened but not set.

Fold in finely chopped or puréed celery and asparagus and spoon into a lightly oiled ring gelatin mold.

Refrigerate for 3 to 4 hours or until firm. Unmold onto a serving platter. Place a dish of GFCF mayonnaise in the center of the ring.

YIELD: *Serves 8 to 12*

Calories (kcal): 49; **Total fat:** trace; **Cholesterol:** 0mg; **Carbohydrate:** 12g; **Dietary fiber:** 1g; **Protein:** 1g; **Sodium:** 566mg; **Potassium:** 283mg; **Calcium:** 13mg; **Iron:** 1mg; **Zinc:** trace; **Vitamin A:** 680IU.

Quick Pasta Salad

gluten　milk　soy　egg　corn　nuts

- 1 package (10–12 ounces, or 280–340 g) rice pasta
- 1 head garlic, baked in a 350°F (180°C, or gas mark 4) oven for 20 minutes or until soft
- 1/8 cup (30 ml) olive oil
- Salt
- Pepper
- Red chili flakes (optional)
- 1 jar (12–15 ounces, or 340–420 g) artichoke hearts, in water or oil, drained and diced
- 15 sundried tomatoes, diced
- 30 kalamata olives, sliced
- 1/4 cup (35 g) pine nuts

Cook pasta according to package directions. After garlic cools, push out the soft garlic from the outside casing. Combine garlic, oil, and spices and stir with a spoon. Combine all remaining ingredients.

YIELD: *4 to 6 servings*

Calories (kcal): 382; **Total fat:** 13g; **Cholesterol:** 0mg; **Carbohydrate:** 57g; **Dietary fiber:** 7g; **Protein:** 10g; **Sodium:** 471 mg; **Potassium:** 473mg; **Calcium:** 46mg; **Iron:** 2mg; **Zinc:** 1mg; **Vitamin A:** 171IU.

Wild Rice Fruit Salad

gluten　milk　soy　egg　corn　nuts

- 2 cups (330 g) cooked wild rice, cooled (For SCD, use cauliflower rice.)
- 1 cup (100 g) chopped celery
- 1/4 cup (35 g) golden raisins
- 1 cup (180 g) pineapple chunks, drained
- 1 cup (190 g) mandarin oranges, drained
- 1 cup (160 g) green seedless grapes
- 1 bunch scallions, sliced
- 1/2 cup (54 g) slivered almonds

Salad Dressing Options

- 1/2–3/4 cup (115–175 g) GFCF mayonnaise
- 1/2 cup (120 ml) Really Quick N Easy Raspberry Vinaigrette (page 173)

Combine all the ingredients. Add enough dressing to moisten the salad.

VARIATION: *Add 2 cups (280 g) chopped cooked chicken for a one-dish meal.*

YIELD: *6 servings*

Calories (kcal): 401; **Total fat:** 30g; **Cholesterol:** 10mg; **Carbohydrate:** 34g; **Dietary fiber:** 4g; **Protein:** 6g; **Sodium:** 181mg; **Potassium:** 410mg; **Calcium:** 64mg; **Iron:** 2mg; **Zinc:** 1mg; **Vitamin A:** 456IU.

QUICK N EASY

Apple Salad

gluten   milk   soy   egg   corn   nuts

Modified for SCD

- 2 large Red Delicious apples, unpeeled, cored and cut into 1-inch (2.5 cm) chunks
- $^2/_3$ cup (135 g) crushed pineapple, drained, or fresh pineapple, minced—reserve juice (For SCD, use 100% juice with no sugar added.)
- $^1/_3$ cup (40 g) celery, diced
- 2 tablespoons (18 g) raisins

Dressing

- 3 tablespoons (45 g) non-GMO soy yogurt (For SCD, use a non-soy homemade yogurt.)
- 2 teaspoons GFCF mayonnaise (For SCD, use homemade SCD legal mayonnaise.)
- 1 tablespoon (15 ml) pineapple juice (Avoid concentrate if on SCD and use 100% juice with no sugar added.)
- $^1/_8$ teaspoon cinnamon

In a medium bowl, combine the salad ingredients.

In a small bowl, combine the dressing ingredients. Pour the dressing over the fruit mixture and blend.

YIELD: *4 servings (1 cup [140 g] each)*

Calories (kcal): 105; **Total fat:** 3g; **Cholesterol:** 1mg; **Carbohydrate:** 22g; **Dietary fiber:** 3g; **Protein:** 1g; **Sodium:** 23mg; **Potassium:** 199mg; **Calcium:** 19mg; **Iron:** trace; **Zinc:** trace; **Vitamin A:** 73IU.

 QUICK N EASY

Apple Coleslaw

gluten   milk   soy   egg   corn   nuts

This great combination of fruit and vegetables in a sweet dressing is a definite favorite.

- 3 cups (270 g) chopped cabbage
- 1 unpeeled red Fuji or Gala apple, cored and chopped
- 1 unpeeled Granny Smith apple, cored and chopped
- 1 medium to large carrot, grated
- 1 scallion, finely chopped (optional)
- 1 cup (75 g) GFCF mayonnaise
- $^1/_3$ cup (75 g) GFCF brown sugar
- 1 teaspoon (5 ml) lemon juice
- Salt and pepper to taste

In a large bowl, combine cabbage, apples, carrot, and scallion. In a small bowl, mix together mayonnaise, brown sugar, and lemon juice. Whisk well and add more mayonnaise as needed. Season with salt and pepper to taste. Pour over salad.

YIELD: *6 to 8 servings*

Calories (kcal): 251; **Total fat:** 24g; **Cholesterol:** 10mg; **Carbohydrate:** 14g; **Dietary fiber:** 2g; **Protein:** 1g; **Sodium:** 167mg; **Potassium:** 170mg; **Calcium:** 29mg; **Iron:** 1mg; **Zinc:** trace; **Vitamin A:** 2669IU.

QUICK N EASY

Pasta Salad Supreme

     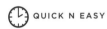

gluten　milk　soy　egg　corn　nuts

This dish can be made for all tastes in the family. The basic recipe should be acceptable to even the pickiest tastes. If only white foods are preferred, then adding the mashed cauliflower should be a good way to sneak in a vegetable. For a heartier dish, simply add the family's favorite protein, such as cooked shrimp or diced cooked chicken.

- 2 cups (210 g) GFCF pasta of choice, uncooked

Basic Version

- 1/4 cup (60 ml) red wine vinegar
- 2 tablespoons (30 ml) fresh lemon juice
- 1 teaspoon GFCF mustard
- 1/4 teaspoon salt
- 1/4 teaspoon white pepper
- 1/4 cup (60 ml) olive oil
- 1/2 cup (120 g) mashed cauliflower (page 267) (optional)

Expanded Version (add these ingredients as suitable to the family members)

- 1 tablespoon dried basil leaves
- 1 small garlic clove, minced
- 1 cup (63 g) snow peas, blanched
- 1 cup (70 g) broccoli florets, blanched
- 1 small red bell pepper
- 1/4 cup (25 g) black olives, halved
- 1/4 cup (35 g) pine nuts, toasted

Cook pasta in boiling, salted water to desired degree of doneness. Drain, chill.

For the basic version, whisk together vinegar, lemon juice, mustard, salt, pepper, olive oil, and optional mashed cauliflower. Add to pasta, toss, and chill.

For the expanded version, whisk together all of the dressing ingredients in a large bowl, then add desired optional ingredients. Toss with cooked pasta. Chill.

If making both versions of this salad to accommodate differing tastes, mix the pasta with the first set of ingredients and divide into 2 portions. Reserve the first portion as is (with or without the mashed cauliflower), and to the other portion add half of the listed rest of the ingredients: basil leaves, minced garlic, snow peas, broccoli florets, bell pepper, black olives, and pine nuts.

YIELD: *4 servings; 6 if child-size servings*

Calories (kcal): 85; **Total fat:** 9g; **Cholesterol:** 0mg; **Carbohydrate:** 2g; **Dietary fiber:** trace; **Protein:** trace; **Sodium:** 102mg; **Potassium:** 43mg; **Calcium:** 4mg; **Iron:** trace; **Zinc:** trace; **Vitamin A:** 3IU.

Cabbage Coleslaw

gluten   milk   soy   egg   corn   nuts

The mother of one of our patients passed this recipe on as a household favorite.

- 1 small cabbage, shredded
- 1 medium carrot, coarsely grated
- 2 celery stalks (cut into $^1/_4$-inch, or 6 mm, diagonals)
- 1 bunch scallions (cut into $^1/_4$-inch, or 6 mm, diagonals)

Dressing Ingredients

- 2 tablespoons (28 ml) apple cider vinegar
- 3 tablespoons (45 ml) fresh lemon juice
- 1 teaspoon honey
- $^1/_2$ tablespoon (8 g) GFCF mustard
- $^1/_3$ cup (80 ml) cooking oil (high oleic safflower, avocado, almond, extra virgin olive oil)
- $^1/_2$ teaspoon celery seed
- $^1/_2$ teaspoon salt
- $^1/_4$ teaspoon ground white pepper
- $^1/_4$ teaspoon paprika

In a large bowl, toss together cabbage, carrot, celery, and scallions. In a blender or food processor, blend the dressing ingredients, except paprika. Toss vegetables with dressing. Garnish with paprika. Serve chilled.

YIELD: *4 servings*

Calories (kcal): 190; **Total fat:** 18g; **Cholesterol:** 0mg; **Carbohydrate:** 7g; **Dietary fiber:** 2g; **Protein:** 1g; **Sodium:** 319mg; **Potassium:** 205mg; **Calcium:** 36mg; **Iron:** 1mg; **Zinc:** trace; **Vitamin A:** 5224IU.

Wonderful Waldorf Salad

gluten   milk   soy   egg   corn   nuts

There are numerous popular versions of this ageless salad. Contents can be adjusted according to individual tastes.

Modified for SCD

- 1 cup (155 g) pineapple chunks, fresh or unsweetened canned (For SCD, use 100% juice with no sugar added.)
- 3 cups (450 g) apples, cut in chunks or $^1/_2$-inch (1.25-cm) cubes, peeled or unpeeled
- $^1/_3$ cup (50 g) raisins
- 1 stalk celery, chopped
- 1 cup (120 g) carrots, thinly sliced
- $^1/_3$–$^1/_2$ cup (40–60 g) walnut pieces
- 1 cup (225 g) GFCF mayonnaise (For SCD, use homemade SCD legal mayonnaise.)
- $^1/_4$–$^1/_2$ cup (20–45 g) green pepper, thinly sliced (optional)

Combine all ingredients except mayonnaise. Blend with the mayonnaise.

Serve plain or on lettuce leaves.

YIELD: *4 to 6 servings*

Calories (kcal): 413; **Total fat:** 37g; **Cholesterol:** 13mg; **Carbohydrate:** 24g; **Dietary fiber:** 4g; **Protein:** 4g; **Sodium:** 223mg; **Potassium:** 358mg; **Calcium:** 36mg; **Iron:** 1mg; **Zinc:** 1mg; **Vitamin A:** 5980IU.

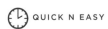

QUICK N EASY

Colleen's Fresh Salad Topped with Chicken and Pine Nuts

gluten milk soy egg corn nuts

Colleen Godbout offers this quick, healthy, and delicious salad, perfect for family and company.

- 1–2 tablespoons (15–30 ml) olive oil
- ¹/₂ cup (70 g) pine nuts
- 10 ounces (280 g) chicken breast strips (packaged or cut from baked or roasted chicken)
- 4 cups (120 g) organic baby spinach (well washed and dried)
- 4 cups (80 g) organic mixed greens (well washed and dried)
- 1 teaspoon sea salt, to taste

Splash the olive oil in a small frying pan on medium heat and toast the pine nuts until golden brown. Put the pine nuts/olive oil mixture in a dish and let cool.

Heat the chicken strips in the pan used for toasting the pine nuts.

Combine and mix spinach, mixed greens, and chicken or beef or shrimp. Top with pine nuts. Season with sea salt to taste.

VARIATIONS: *Add cranberries, raisins, or sliced strawberries. Substitute chicken with grilled steak tips or shrimp. (Do not use shellfish/shrimp for SCD.)*

YIELD: *4 servings*

Calories (kcal): 269; **Total fat:** 21g; **Cholesterol:** 36mg; **Carbohydrate:** 5g; **Dietary fiber:** 3g; **Protein:** 17g; **Sodium:** 583mg; **Potassium:** 426mg; **Calcium:** 72mg; **Iron:** 3mg; **Zinc:** 1mg Vitamin A: 3020IU.

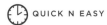

QUICK N EASY

Simple Egg Salad

     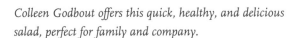
gluten milk soy egg corn nuts

This recipe is easy and a favorite among kids. They enjoy helping with boiling the eggs, peeling them, and "smashing" them.

Modified for Low Phenol, Modified for SCD

- 6 large eggs
- ³/₈ cup (85 g) GFCF mayonnaise (For SCD, use homemade SCD legal mayonnaise.)
- Salt to taste
- Pepper to taste (Omit for low phenol/low salicylate diet.)

Hard-boil eggs at least 15 minutes. Run under cold water and peel.

Place eggs in a bowl and smash with a fork until chopped up, or use an egg slicer to slice them one way first and then again at a 90-degree angle.

Add the mayonnaise and mix well. Add salt and pepper to taste.

Serve on GFCF bread as a sandwich, or simply on lettuce, or a sliced tomato, or garnish with a thin slice of avocado. (For low phenol, do not use tomato.)

YIELD: *4 servings*

Calories (kcal): 246; **Total fat:** 24g; **Cholesterol:** 288mg; **Carbohydrate:** 1g; **Dietary fiber:** 0g; **Protein:** 8g; **Sodium:** 200mg; **Potassium:** 87mg; **Calcium:** 36mg; **Iron:** 1mg; **Zinc:** 1mg; **Vitamin A:** 477IU.

Egg Salad with Zest

gluten milk soy egg corn nuts

This recipe is nice for sandwiches or for snacks and appetizers. Children enjoy helping, especially with peeling and slicing the eggs.

- 4 hard-boiled eggs
- 2 tablespoons (30 g) GFCF mayonnaise
- 1¹/₂ teaspoons GFCF mustard
- 2 teaspoons (10 ml) rice vinegar, cider vinegar, or pickle juice (Do not use rice vinegar for SCD. Use filtered apple cider vinegar as a substitute.)
- 1 teaspoon honey or real maple syrup (For SCD, use honey.)
- ¹/₄ teaspoon salt, or to taste
- 1 stalk celery, minced
- 2 teaspoons pickle relish
- Paprika, for garnish

Options:

- GFCF bread or crackers, lettuce leaves, sliced tomato

Place eggs in a bowl and smash with a fork until chopped up, or use an egg slicer to slice them one way first and then again at a 90-degree angle. Add all ingredients, except paprika, including salt to taste. Mix well, chill for at least 5 minutes, and spoon on bread, crackers, lettuce leaves, or tomato slices.

Sprinkle with paprika.

YIELD: *3 servings*

Calories (kcal): 185; **Total fat:** 15g; **Cholesterol:** 286mg; **Carbohydrate:** 5g; **Dietary fiber:** trace; **Protein:** 9g; **Sodium:** 383mg; **Potassium:** 134mg; **Calcium:** 44mg; **Iron:** 1mg; **Zinc:** 1mg; **Vitamin A:** 422IU.

 QUICK N EASY

Egg Salad

gluten milk soy egg corn nuts

Each version of egg salad has its own special flavor.

- 4 hard-boiled eggs
- 2 tablespoons (30 g) GFCF mayonnaise
- 1¹/₂ teaspoons GFCF mustard
- 2 teaspoons (10 ml) rice vinegar
- 1¹/₂ teaspoons granulated sugar
- ¹/₄ teaspoon salt, or to taste
- 1 stalk celery, minced
- 2 teaspoons pickle relish
- Paprika, for garnish

Place eggs in a bowl and smash with a fork until chopped up. Add all ingredients, except paprika, including salt to taste. Mix well, chill for at least 5 minutes, and spoon onto lettuce leaves or tomato slices. Sprinkle with paprika.

YIELD: *3 servings*

Calories (kcal): 186; **Total fat:** 15g; **Cholesterol:** 286mg; **Carbohydrate:** 5g; **Dietary fiber:** trace; **Protein:** 9g; **Sodium:** 383mg; **Potassium:** 133mg; **Calcium:** 44mg; **Iron:** 1mg; **Zinc:** 1mg; **Vitamin A:** 422IU.

Popular Potato Salad

gluten milk soy egg corn nuts

This is a popular recipe for an old standard.

- 3 cups (675 g) peeled and diced cooked potatoes
- 4 hard-boiled eggs, peeled and chopped
- ¹/₂ cup (60 g) celery, finely chopped
- ¹/₄ cup (25 g) scallions, finely chopped
- 2 tablespoons (30 g) sweet pickle relish
- ¹/₂ cup (115 g) GFCF mayonnaise
- 1 tablespoon (15 ml) vinegar
- 1 teaspoon sugar or honey
- ¹/₂ teaspoon celery salt
- ¹/₂ teaspoon celery seeds
- ¹/₄ teaspoon white pepper
- ¹/₂ teaspoon dry mustard
- Paprika, for garnish

Combine potatoes, eggs, celery, scallions, and relish in a large bowl. In a small bowl, whisk all remaining ingredients, except paprika, until smooth. Pour over potato mixture and toss until thoroughly coated. Turn into a serving bowl and sprinkle with paprika. Refrigerate until serving time.

YIELD: *6 servings*

Calories (kcal): 264; **Total fat:** 19g; **Cholesterol:** 148mg; **Carbohydrate:** 19g; **Dietary fiber:** 3g; **Protein:** 6g; **Sodium:** 659mg; **Potassium:** 403mg; **Calcium:** 90mg; **Iron:** 2mg; **Zinc:** 1mg; **Vitamin A:** 275IU.

Lady Di's Summertime Chicken Salad

gluten milk soy egg corn nuts

Diana Haan's family and friends love this recipe. It's a real child-pleaser.

- 4 organic chicken breasts, roasted and diced
- 2 celery stalks, diced
- 1 tablespoon (10 g) chopped red onion
- 1 cup (160 g) red grapes
- 1 cup (145 g) blueberries
- 1 can (10.5 ounces, or 294 g) mandarin oranges
- 1¹/₂ cups (340 g) GFCF mayonnaise
- 2 tablespoons (40 g) honey
- 1 tablespoon (15 ml) lemon juice
- 1 teaspoon sugar
- Salt to taste
- Pepper to taste
- 2 tomatoes, cut into wedges
- Mixed greens

Mix all ingredients except tomato wedges and stir. Add more mayonnaise for desired dressing consistency. Serve on mixed greens with tomato wedges.

YIELD: *4 to 6 servings*

Calories (kcal): 811; **Total fat:** 65g; **Cholesterol:** 143mg; **Carbohydrate:** 22g; **Dietary fiber:** 2g; **Protein:** 42g; **Sodium:** 454mg; **Potassium:** 718mg; **Calcium:** 50mg; **Iron:** 2mg; **Zinc:** 2mg; **Vitamin A:** 1042IU.

Bonnie's Easy Chicken Salad

gluten   milk   soy   egg   corn   nuts

Bonnie Gutman's version is without mayonnaise. It is perfect for summer meals.

- 5 cups (700 g) cubed cooked chicken
- 2 tablespoons (30 ml) oil (avocado, almond, safflower, light olive)
- 2 tablespoons (30 ml) orange juice
- 2 tablespoons (30 ml) vinegar
- 2 teaspoons salt
- 3 cups (495 g) cooked white rice, cooled (For SCD, use cauliflower rice.)
- 1¹/₂ cups (150 g) celery, sliced
- 1 can (15.75 ounces, or 440 g) pineapple chunks in juice, drained (For SCD, use 100% juice with no sugar added.)
- 1 can (10.5 ounces, or 294 g) mandarin oranges
- 1 cup (92 g) toasted sliced almonds (optional)

Combine chicken, oil, orange juice, vinegar, and salt. Let stand 30 minutes.

Add the remaining ingredients except the almonds and mix together well.

Sprinkle almonds over the top and serve.

YIELD: *12 servings*

Calories (kcal): 286; **Total fat:** 11g; **Cholesterol:** 50mg; **Carbohydrate:** 24g; **Dietary fiber:** 2g; **Protein:** 22g; **Sodium:** 416mg; **Potassium:** 376mg; **Calcium:** 60mg; **Iron:** 1mg; **Zinc:** 1mg; **Vitamin A:** 213IU.

Asian Cucumber Salad

gluten   milk   soy   egg   corn   nuts

If you can't find English cucumbers (sometimes sold as seedless cucumbers), substitute 2 medium regular cucumbers instead. Also, feel free to peel and seed the cucumbers if your child prefers them this way.

Low Phenol

- 2 tablespoons (30 ml) rice vinegar
- 2 tablespoons (26 g) sugar
- 1 English cucumber
- 2 teaspoons minced fresh ginger
- 1 teaspoon sesame oil

In a small saucepan, bring the sugar and vinegar to a boil; cook for 1 minute, until mixture has thickened slightly. Remove from heat and cool completely.

Cut cucumber in half lengthwise, and then cut each half into very thin slices. Toss with ginger and sesame oil and allow to marinate for 10 to 15 minutes.

Just before serving, pour the vinegar-sugar dressing over the cucumbers and toss to combine.

YIELD: *4 servings*

Calories (kcal): 46; **Total fat:** 1g; **Cholesterol:** 0mg; **Carbohydrate:** 9g; **Dietary fiber:** 1g; **Protein:** 1g; **Sodium:** trace; **Potassium:** 305mg; **Calcium:** 1mg; **Iron:** trace; **Zinc:** trace; **Vitamin A:** 200IU.

Sesame Green Bean Salad

gluten   milk   soy   egg   corn   nuts

- ¹/₂ pound (225 g) green beans, trimmed and cut into 2-inch (5 cm) pieces
- 1 medium red bell pepper, cored, seeded, and cut into 2-inch (5 cm) strips
- 1 tablespoon (6 g) minced fresh ginger
- 1¹/₂ teaspoons salt
- ¹/₂ teaspoon maple syrup
- 1 tablespoon (15 ml) sesame oil
- 1 tablespoon (8 g) toasted sesame seeds

Bring a pot of water to a boil; set up a bowl of ice water nearby. Boil the green beans until just tender, and then transfer them to the ice water until completely cool. Drain and transfer to a medium bowl. Add the remaining ingredients and toss well to combine and serve.

YIELD: *2 to 4 servings*

Calories (kcal): 68; Total fat: 4g; Cholesterol: 0mg; Carbohydrate: 7g; Dietary fiber: 3g; Protein: 2g; Sodium: 804mg; Potassium: 173mg; Calcium: 30mg; Iron: 1mg; Zinc: trace; Vitamin A: 512IU.

Chickpea Chicken Salad

gluten   milk   soy   egg   corn   nuts

This salad can be served as is with some GFCF crackers, or on top of a bed of salad greens.

- 1 can (14 ounces, or 400 g) chickpeas, drained and rinsed
- 2 cups (280 g) cooked, shredded chicken
- 4 scallions, thinly sliced
- 1 stick of celery, finely chopped
- ¹/₂ cup (120 ml) olive oil
- ¹/₄ cup (60 ml) lemon juice
- 1 teaspoon lemon zest
- 2 cloves garlic, minced
- 3 tablespoons (12 g) chopped parsley
- 1 tablespoon (4 g) chopped fresh dill
- ¹/₄ teaspoon mustard powder
- Salt and freshly ground black pepper

In a large bowl, combine the chickpeas, chicken, scallions, and celery. In a separate bowl, whisk together the oil, lemon juice, zest, garlic, parsley, dill, mustard powder, and salt and pepper to taste. Pour over the chickpea mixture, toss to combine, and then cover and chill for 2 hours to allow flavors to meld.

YIELD: *4 to 6 servings*

Calories (kcal): 328; Total fat: 21g; Cholesterol: 40mg; Carbohydrate: 17g; Dietary fiber: 3g; Protein: 18g; Sodium: 243mg; Potassium: 305mg; Calcium: 44mg; Iron: 2mg; Zinc: 1mg; Vitamin A: 184IU.

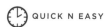

QUICK N EASY

Corn and Black Bean Salad

gluten milk soy egg corn nuts

This is great with sweet, summertime corn, but frozen corn can be substituted.

- 3 tablespoons (45 ml) fresh lime juice
- ¹/₄ teaspoon cumin
- ¹/₄ teaspoon chili powder
- ¹/₄ teaspoon salt
- 1 teaspoon agave nectar
- 3 tablespoons (45 ml) safflower oil
- 2 cups (450 g) cooked corn kernels
- 1 medium red bell pepper, seeded and chopped fine
- 1 can (15.5 ounces) black beans, rinsed
- 2 tablespoons (8 g) minced cilantro leaves

In a large bowl, whisk the lime juice, spices, and agave nectar together. Slowly add the oil while whisking vigorously, until the dressing is emulsified. Add the corn, pepper, beans, and cilantro and toss to combine. Serve.

YIELD: *4 servings*

Calories (kcal): 267; **Total fat:** 12g; **Cholesterol:** 0mg; **Carbohydrate:** 33g; **Dietary fiber:** 9g; **Protein:** 9g; **Sodium:** 486mg; **Potassium:** 283mg; **Calcium:** 8mg; **Iron:** 1mg; **Zinc:** trace; **Vitamin A:** 478IU.

"Julian is now ten years old. At age three, he was diagnosed with mild to moderate autism. At that time, my husband and I did not realize what a life-changing experience this would be. I thought that because we were both in the medical field, we had access to information and treatments that would cure him. As we started to gather information, we realized how sparse the options were. A visit to Dr. Compart yielded mixed feelings. She recommended blood and stool tests; supplements; and a GFCF diet. The tests and supplements were easy enough to comply with, but following the diet was too difficult. One morning, Julian's nanny fed him a large portion of chocolate cake and ice cream. For seven days, Julian was away somewhere. We were unable to get his attention. That was when we finally became serious about implementing the GFCF diet. Now he knows he eats only special food. We are still dealing with other issues, but I am convinced that his quality of life is much better by being on the diet."

—Maria Ribaya-Than, *MD*

CHAPTER 21

Soups and Stews

Stocks and Broths

The perfect beginning for this section is with the stocks that become the basis for many of the great soups. Whether homemade or purchased, these are an important part of healthy eating. The homemade versions of meat stocks contain natural gelatin, so important to digestion and healing. Unflavored gelatin can be added to store-bought versions to boost the healthy qualities of these broths. We have also included a vegetable broth; however, without the gelatin, the vegetable stocks are not as beneficial to digestion. Read the information on gelatin in chapter 9.

Chicken Stock

gluten   milk   soy   egg   corn   nuts

For those who prefer to make their own nutritious chicken stock, this recipe from Nourishing Traditions, *by Sally Fallon, is the best. It is nutritious and has healthy fatty acids and gelatin, which give chicken soup its healing reputation. See page 279 for a discussion of the health benefits of animal-source gelatin.*

Modified for Low Salicylate

- 1 whole organic chicken or 2–3 pounds (0.9–1.4 kg) bony chicken parts such as necks, backs, breastbones, and wings
- Gizzards from one chicken (optional)
- Chicken feet (optional)
- 4 quarts (3.8 L) cold filtered water
- 1 tablespoon (15 ml) vinegar (Use 50/50 lime and lemon juice for low salicylate diet.)
- 1 large onion, coarsely chopped
- 2 carrots, peeled and coarsely chopped
- 3 celery stalks, coarsely chopped
- 1 bunch parsley (Use basil for low salicylate diet.)

If using a whole chicken, remove the fat glands and the gizzards from the cavity. Chicken feet provide healthy, healing gelatin. Place chicken or chicken pieces, and gizzards and feet if using them, in a large stainless steel pot with the water, vinegar, onion, carrots, and celery. Bring to a boil and remove any scum that rises to the top. Cover and simmer for 12 to 24 hours. The longer the stock is cooked, the richer and more flavorful it will be. Add parsley 5 minutes before finishing the stock. (Parsley is a good source of minerals.)

Remove from heat and take out the chicken with a slotted spoon. Let it cool and remove chicken meat from the bones. Reserve the chicken meat for other uses such as chicken salads, enchiladas, sandwiches, or curries.

Strain the stock into a large bowl and reserve in your refrigerator until the fat rises to the top and congeals. Skim off this fat and reserve the stock in covered containers in your refrigerator or freezer.

VARIATIONS: Turkey Stock and Duck Stock

Prepare as chicken stock, using turkey wings and drumsticks or duck carcasses from which the breasts, legs, and thighs have been removed. These stocks will have a stronger flavor than chicken stock and will profit from the addition during cooking of several sprigs of fresh thyme tied together. The reserved duck fat is highly prized for cooking purposes.

YIELD: *2 quarts (1.9 L)*

Calories (kcal): 3361; **Total fat**: 234g; **Cholesterol**: 1358mg; **Carbohydrate**: 34g; **Dietary fiber**: 10g; **Protein**: 263g; **Sodium**: 1347mg; **Potassium**: 4287mg; **Calcium**: 419mg; **Iron**: 26mg; **Zinc**: 22mg; **Vitamin A**: 56507IU.

Clarified Stock

gluten milk soy egg corn nuts

If a perfectly clear stock is needed, the following will give the desired result.

- 2 egg whites, lightly beaten
- 2 quarts (1.9 L) defatted stock

Add egg whites to stock and bring to a boil, whisking with a wire whisk. When the stock begins to boil, stop whisking. Let it boil for 3 to 5 minutes. On the surface, a white foam will gradually form and become a spongy crust. Remove the pot from the heat, lift off the crust, and strain the stock through a strainer lined with several layers of cheesecloth.

YIELD: *2 quarts (1.9 L)*

Calories (kcal): 209; **Total fat:** 2g; **Cholesterol:** 0mg; **Carbohydrate**: 8g; **Dietary fiber:** 0g; **Protein:** 14g; **Sodium:** 17287mg; **Potassium:** 779mg; **Calcium:** 24mg; **Iron:** 12mg; **Zinc:** 0mg; **Vitamin A:** 0IU.

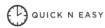 QUICK N EASY

Quick Chicken Stock

This lacks the flavor and nutritive properties of home-made stock, but it will do for a quick solution.

- 1 can (14 ounces, or 425 ml) chicken stock
- 1 tablespoon (7 g) unflavored gelatin

Mix stock with gelatin, bring to a boil.

YIELD: *Approximately 2 cups (475 ml) stock*

Calories (kcal): 92; **Total fat:** 2g; **Cholesterol:** 0mg; **Carbohydrate:** 15g; **Dietary fiber:** 0g; **Protein:** 3g; **Sodium:** 3530mg; **Potassium:** 140mg; **Calcium:** 4mg; **Iron:** 2mg; **Zinc:** 0mg; **Vitamin A:** 0IU.

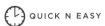 QUICK N EASY

Quick Beef Stock

gluten milk soy egg corn nuts

This lacks the flavor and nutritive properties of home-made stock, but will do for a quick solution.

- 1 can (14 ounces, or 425 ml) beef stock
- 1 tablespoon (7 g) unflavored gelatin

Mix stock with gelatin, bring to a boil.

YIELD: *Approximately 2 cups (475 ml) stock*

Calories (kcal): 92; **Total fat:** trace; **Cholesterol:** 0mg; **Carbohydrate:** 15g; **Dietary fiber:** 0g; **Protein:** 3g; **Sodium:** 3530mg; **Potassium:** 140mg; **Calcium:** 4mg; **Iron:** 2mg; **Zinc:** 0mg; **Vitamin A:** 4IU.

Beef Stock

gluten   milk   soy   egg   corn   nuts

Good beef stock must be made with several kinds of beef bones: knucklebones and feet impart large quantities of gelatin to the broth, marrow bones impart flavor and the particular nutrients of the bone marrow, and meaty rib or neck bones add color and flavor. In moving away from animal-source foods, we have lost many of the nutrients so common in human diets throughout the ages. Organic sources are important. See page 279 for a discussion of the health benefits of gelatin.

SCD Legal

- 6 pounds (2.7 kg) beef marrow and knuckle-bones
- 1 calf's foot, cut into pieces (optional)
- 4 quarts (3.8 L) or more cold filtered water, divided
- 5 pounds (2.3 kg) meaty rib or neck bones
- ¼ cup (60 ml) vinegar
- 3 onions, coarsely chopped
- 3 carrots, coarsely chopped
- 3 celery stalks, coarsely chopped
- 2 sprigs fresh thyme, tied together
- 1 teaspoon dried green peppercorns, crushed
- 1 bunch parsley

Place the beef marrow and knucklebones and optional calf's foot in a very large pot and cover with water.

Let stand for 1 hour.

Meanwhile, place the meaty bones in a roasting pan and brown at 350°F (180°C, gas mark 4) in the oven. When well browned, add to the pot along with vinegar and vegetables.

Pour fat out of the roasting pan, add cold water, set over a high flame and bring to a boil, stirring with a wooden spoon to deglaze. Add this liquid to the pot. Add more water if needed to cover the bones. The liquid should not be higher than within 1 inch (2.5 cm) of the rim of the pot since the volume expands during cooking. Bring to a boil.

Using a spoon, remove the scum that comes to the top. Reduce the heat and add thyme and crushed peppercorns.

Simmer stock for at least 12 and as long as 72 hours.

Before finishing, add parsley. Let it wilt, then remove from the stock.

At this point, the brown liquid with gelatinous fatty material is unattractive and smelly. But you are not finished yet! Clear, delicious broth is just ahead.

Remove bones with tongs or a slotted spoon. Strain the stock into a large bowl.

Let cool in the refrigerator and remove the congealed fat that rises to the top.

Reheat and transfer to storage containers.

This is now a wonderful stock for soups.

YIELD: *2 quarts (1.9 L)*

Calories (kcal): 306; Total fat: 2g; Cholesterol: 0mg; Carbohydrate: 71 g; Dietary fiber: 21 g; Protein: 10g; Sodium: 345mg; Potassium: 2097mg; Calcium: 523mg; Iron: 19mg; Zinc: 4mg; Vitamin A: 64377IU.

Anne Evans's Bone Marrow Stock

gluten   milk   soy   egg   corn   nuts

Anne's daughter Sarah, who has recovered from autism, wants to share this recipe because it made a huge difference in Sarah's health.

Beef marrow bones are a completely natural, easily digestible, and easy-to-assimilate source of all the amino acids. Amino acids improve immunity and are sources for the brain neurotransmitters. Stocks made the traditional way improve digestion and have a healing effect on the digestive tract.

<u>SCD Legal, Low Phenol, Low Salicylate, Low Oxalate</u>

- 8–10 pounds (3.6–4.5 kg) stew bones from (sliced 1–2 inches, or 2.5–5 cm, thick)
- Filtered water
- ¹/₂ teaspoon salt

In a large stockpot or Dutch oven, brown the bones and drain off the fat. Add enough filtered water to the pot to cover the bones. Add salt and bring to a boil.

Boil until the marrow falls out of the bones (approximately 45 minutes). Be sure to push all the marrow from all the bones back into the pot (this is essential).

Remove the bones from the pot. Let cool. Puree the stock plus marrow in small quantities in the blender. Store in the fridge—it keeps for a week.

Use this stock for sauces, gravies, soups, boiling rice pasta, moistening mashed potatoes, cooking vegetables, etc.

YIELD: *varies*

Calories (kcal): 0; **Total fat:** 0g; **Cholesterol:** 0mg; **Carbohydrate:** 0g; **Dietary fiber:** 0g; **Protein:** 0g; **Sodium:** 1066mg; **Potassium:** 0mg; **Calcium:** 7mg; **Iron:** 0mg; **Zinc:** 0 0mg; **Vitamin A:** 0IU.

Vegetable Potassium-Rich Broth

gluten   milk   soy   egg   corn   nuts

Recipe provided by Sara Keough, MS, CNS, LDN, who is an integrative nutritionist at Village Green Apothecary. This vegetarian potassium-rich broth is ideal for those who want a delicious healthy, vegetarian drink, warm or cold.

- 2 large handfuls of potato peelings (about 5 large potatoes)
- 1 large handful of carrot peelings (about 5 or 6 carrots)
- 4 celery stalks
- 3 medium beets AND their greens
- 1 large onion
- 3 bulbs of garlic
- 2 large handfuls of parsley
- A handful of sundried tomatoes
- 3 large handfuls of greens such as swiss chard, kale, spinach, collard greens, etc.
- Any extra "scraps" from veggies such as broccoli leaves, mushroom stems, etc.

Coarsely chop all vegetables and place into a large stockpot.

Fill pot with distilled or reverse-osmosis water until just covering all of the vegetables (almost to the top; you want to fill your stockpot with lots of veggies!). Bring to a boil and then simmer for 3 hours. Strain broth and compost remaining vegetables. Add a bit of salt and drink warm, or you can serve chilled for a revitalizing drink on a hot day.

YIELD: *Makes about 20+ cups (4.7 L) of broth depending on how large your stockpot is. There are loads of potassium in addition to many other minerals and vitamins.*

Calories (kcal): 15; **Total fat:** 0g; **Carbohydrate:** 1g; **Dietary fiber:** 1g; **Protein:** 0g; **Sodium:** 130mg; **Potassium:** 115mg; **Calcium:** 20mg; **Iron:** 0mg; **Zinc:** 0mg; **Vitamin A:** 1250IU.

Versatile Soup Template

gluten   milk   soy   egg   corn   nuts

Modified for GF, CF, and SF, Low Phenol, Low Salicylate, Low Oxalate, SCD, Anti-Yeast, Anti-Inflammatory, and FODMAPS

Vicki Kobliner, MS, RDN, provided this versatile recipe. She has this to say about it: "I love this recipe because it is extremely versatile—use any combination of vegetables, the flour, and 'cream' that works for your family. The same recipe can adapt to whatever you have on hand or whichever foods are best tolerated by your child. You can use the same base recipe every week, using different ingredients, and get a different result." This is a great meal starter that gets an additional veggie serving into the diet.

We also suggest adding fruit for a different flavor, and pastured-source poultry and meat for a protein boost. We have expanded on Vicki's excellent recipe by providing different diet-specific versions. In order to accommodate different texture preferences, the thickness of the soup can be varied by adjusting the amount of chicken broth included. This allows for a thin soup with vegetables and meats, a thick stew, and also a purée for those who want to avoid "lumps and bumps" in their food.

- 3¹/₂ cups (825 g) gluten-free organic chicken broth (see chicken stock recipe on page 294) (include the chicken fat)
- 3 tablespoons (45 g) organic ghee, safflower oil (works for most diets), or (45 ml) olive oil (not with low phenol, low salicylate, or low oxalate), or avocado oil (not with low salicylate).
- 3 tablespoons (23 to 30 g) of flour (See options under each diet in this recipe.)
- 1 minced garlic clove (not with Low FODMAP)
- 2 teaspoons salt, or to taste
- ¹/₂ diced medium onion (not with low phenol or low FODMAP)

- 1¹/₂ cups (355 g) organic half-and-half or other appropriate milk substitute. (Coconut milk/cream works well, but not for low salicylate.) See the suggestions under each diet.
- 3 cups (360 g) fresh vegetables*
- Fresh cracked white pepper (if tolerated)
- Celtic or Himalayan sea salt to taste
- Optional: poultry (pastured)—3 to 6 ounces (85 to 170 g)
- Optional: fruit to add flavor – ¹/₂ to 1 pear (peeled) or ¹/₄ to 1 mango (peeled) fits most of the diets. See the diet chapters for more diet-specific fruit choices.
- Optional for a creamy texture: avocado or coconut cream (suitable for all but the low salicylate diet)

*Use 3 cups (360 g) total of any combination of the appropriate diet-specific vegetables listed in this recipe:

- **Low Phenol Vegetable options:** asparagus (fresh only, not canned), beets, bean sprouts, cabbage (white), carrots, green beans, greens (chard, collard, kale *not curly*, watercress), mushrooms, peas (sugar snap peas, snow peas), squash (acorn, butternut, summer, winter), sweet potato, and white potato. Oil/fat options: ghee, safflower, or avocado. Milk substitutes: coconut milk/cream. GF flour options: amaranth, arrowroot, quinoa, white rice, and tapioca starch. Spice options: avoid most spices; include small amounts of chives, cilantro, coriander, dill, fennel, leeks, and Celtic or Himalayan sea salt.

- **Low Salicylate Vegetable options:** asparagus (fresh), beets, cabbage, carrots, cauliflower, greens (chard, collard, kale), lima beans, onions/shallots, peas (green, snow, snap) potato, and turnips. Oil/fat options: ghee, safflower, or flaxseed. Milk substitutes: non-GMO soy milk or tofu or cashew milk. GF flour options: amaranth, arrowroot, quinoa, rice, or tapioca starch. Spice options: avoid most; consider garlic, parsley, saffron, and Celtic or Himalayan sea salt to taste.

- **SCD and GAPS Vegetable options:** asparagus (fresh), avocado, beets, broccoli, carrots, cauliflower, celery, garlic, greens (chard, collard, endive, kale), lima beans, mushrooms, pumpkin (fresh), squash (acorn, butternut, summer, winter), tomatoes, watercress, and zucchini. Oil/fat options: ghee, safflower, almond, or coconut. Milk substitutes: coconut or almond milk. GF flour options: nut flours (almond, cashew, hazelnut, or pecan). Spice options: wide variety of individual spices permitted; avoid spice combinations. Consider black and white pepper, and Celtic or Himalayan sea salt to taste.

- **Anti-yeast Vegetable options:** asparagus, avocado, broccoli, cabbage, cauliflower, celery, greens (chard, collard, endive, kale, spinach, watercress), onions, parsley, spinach, tomatoes, turnips, and zucchini. Oil/fat options: ghee, almond, avocado, coconut, or olive. Milk substitutes: coconut, milk/cream. GF flour options: almond, coconut, or flax meal. Spice options: wide variety of spices and herbs, black and white pepper, and Celtic or Himalayan sea salt to taste.

- **Low Oxalate Vegetable options:** asparagus (fresh only), avocado, bean sprouts, cabbage, cauliflower, mushrooms, red sweet peppers, and squash (acorn, yellow). Oil/fat options: ghee, avocado, coconut, or safflower. Milk substitutes: coconut milk/cream. GF flour options: coconut flour and guar gum. Spice options: basil, cayenne, chives, cilantro, cloves, coriander, curry, dill, garlic powder, mustard seed, pepper (white), rosemary, saffron, tarragon, thyme, and Celtic or Himalayan sea salt to taste.

- **Anti-Inflammatory Non-Nightshade/Low Lectin Vegetable options:** asparagus (fresh), avocado, baby bok choy, broccoli, carrots, cauliflower, celery, greens (chard, collard, endive, kale, spinach, watercress), leeks, mushrooms, onions, pumpkin, scallions, sweet potatoes, turnips, and yams. Oil/fat options: ghee, avocado, coconut, or olive oil. Milk substitutes: coconut milk/cream. Flour options: arrowroot or sweet potato. Spice options: wide variety of non-nightshade, low-lectin spices: basil, bay leaf, chives, cilantro, cinnamon, cloves, onion, rosemary, saffron, thyme, turmeric, and Celtic or Himalayan sea salt.

- **FODMAP Vegetable options:** arugula, bean sprouts, bell peppers, cabbage, carrots, celery, chickpeas, chives, cucumbers, eggplant, green beans, greens (endive, kale), legumes, lima beans, parsnips, potatoes, pumpkin, scallions, (green portion), squash (acorn, zucchini, summer), sweet potatoes, turnips, and tomatoes. Oil/fat options: avocado, ghee, safflower, flaxseed oil, or coconut (MCT oil). Milk substitutes: almond milk, coconut milk/cream, hemp milk, and rice milk. GF flour options: arrowroot, buckwheat, quinoa, rice, or tapioca starch. Spice options: all spices except for onion and garlic; and sauces (soy, tomato, wasabi).

In a large stockpot, on medium heat, heat the fat until very hot and constantly whisk in flour to form a roux.

Add onion first (not with low phenol or low FODMAP) and continue to whisk. Then add the garlic (not with low FODMAP) and continue to whisk for about 1 minute until smooth and bubbly and the garlic is lightly cooked. (Adding the onion first prevents the garlic from burning.) Slowly add gluten-free chicken broth while whisking constantly, until mixture is smooth and creamy. Add fresh vegetables and fruit as suitable, and simmer until tender for stews, and until well-cooked for soups.

Add half-and-half, A2 milk if tolerated, or milk substitutes such as coconut cream (not if low salicylate diet). Add seasonings and stir until smooth. Be sure to add a small amount of hot liquid to the cold cream to bring the temperature down before adding it to the soup.

For a puréed soup, use an immersion or regular blender. Serve warm or cool completely and freeze.

YIELD: *5 to 6 servings*

Calories (kcal): 667; **Total fat:** 21g; **Cholesterol:** 0mg; **Carbohydrate:** 107g; **Dietary fiber:** 33g; **Protein:** 31g; **Sodium:** 1676mg; **Potassium:** 4850mg; **Calcium:** 247mg; **Iron:** 9mg; **Zinc:** 4mg; **Vitamin A:** 6144IU.

Vegetable Broth for the Whole Family

gluten   milk   soy   egg   corn   nuts

This recipe is perfect for use in a baby bottle or sippy cup. It is very nutritious and an easy way to hide nutritional supplements.

<u>SCD Legal</u>

- 4 cups (940 ml) cold water, or 3 cups (710 ml) cold water and 1 cup (235 ml) chicken broth
- 1 cup (150 g) cauliflower florets
- 1 cup (170 g) broccoli florets
- 1 cup (55 g) collard or dandelion greens, rinsed and roughly chopped
- 1 cup (130 g) carrots, cut into rounds

Place water (and chicken broth) in a medium pot with a lid. Add vegetables and bring to a boil over high heat. Reduce heat to a simmer and cover pot. Cook for 1 hour. Strain broth and reserve vegetables. These can be puréed or mashed. This broth freezes well in ice-cube trays for later use.

YIELD: *Makes about 3 cups (serving size ¹/₂ cup [120 ml])*

Calories (kcal): 85; **Total fat:** 1g; **Cholesterol:** 0mg; **Carbohydrate:** 18g; **Dietary fiber:** 7g; **Protein:** 4g; **Sodium:** 98mg; **Potassium:** 693mg; **Calcium:** 139mg; **Iron:** 1mg; **Zinc:** 1mg; **Vitamin A:** 37894IU.

Chicken Noodle Soup

gluten   milk   soy   egg   corn   nuts

Here's another tasty alternative to a childhood favorite. This GF version really satisfies a hungry tummy.

- 2 cups (475 ml) chicken broth
- 10 cups (2.4 L) water
- 2 medium onions, diced
- 3 large carrots, diced
- 2 medium potatoes, diced
- 1¹/₂ tablespoons parsley flakes
- 1 tablespoon (18 g) salt
- 1 teaspoon pepper
- ¹/₂ teaspoon garlic
- 16–20 ounces (455–560 g) brown rice spaghetti
- 1 cooked chicken, diced

Put all ingredients except spaghetti and chicken in a stockpot. Simmer 1 hour. Break spaghetti into 1-inch (2.5 cm) lengths and boil in a separate pot (rice pasta is very starchy). Add chicken to stockpot and simmer 15 additional minutes. Add noodles and serve.

YIELD: *12 servings*

Calories (kcal): 443; **Total fat:** 20g; **Cholesterol:** 113mg; **Carbohydrate:** 36g; **Dietary fiber:** 3g; **Protein:** 27g; **Sodium:** 761 mg; **Potassium:** 481 mg; **Calcium:** 33mg; **Iron:** 2mg; **Zinc:** 2mg; **Vitamin A:** 6125IU.

> All soups and stews can be puréed to achieve a texture that is best suited to your child's sensory development.

Jane's Lentil Vegetable Soup

gluten   milk   soy   egg   corn   nuts

This recipe is quick to put together and can be a meal in itself.

- 2 cups (400 g) lentils
- 6 cups (1.4 L) water
- 2 cups (475 ml) beef broth
- 2 slices bacon, diced (optional)
- $^1/_2$ cup (80 g) chopped onion
- $^1/_2$ cup (50 g) chopped celery
- $^1/_4$ cup (35 g) chopped carrot
- 3 tablespoons (12 g) parsley
- 1 clove garlic, minced
- 2 teaspoons salt
- $^1/_4$ teaspoon pepper
- $^1/_2$ teaspoon oregano
- 1 tablespoon (15 ml) GFCF Worcestershire sauce
- 1 can (14.5 ounces, or 411 g) diced tomatoes
- 2 tablespoons (30 ml) apple cider vinegar

Rinse lentils and place in a large soup kettle. Add water and beef broth and the remaining ingredients except tomatoes and vinegar. Cover and simmer for $1^1/_2$ hours.

Add tomatoes and vinegar and simmer for $^1/_2$ hour more.

YIELD: *8 servings*

Calories (kcal): 207; **Total fat:** 1g; **Cholesterol:** 1mg; **Carbohydrate:** 33g; **Dietary fiber:** 16g; **Protein:** 17g; **Sodium:** 920mg; **Potassium:** 714mg; **Calcium:** 51mg; **Iron:** 5mg; **Zinc:** 2mg; **Vitamin A:** 1561IU.

Turkey Noodle Soup

gluten   milk   soy   egg   corn   nuts

Turkey is not just for Thanksgiving, although turkey soup is one of the most popular ways to serve leftovers from Thanksgiving. Perfect as a meal or part of a meal, like chicken noodle soup, it is soothing to digestion and healing. If using ready-to-eat chicken broth, add gelatin to enhance the quality.

- 4 cups (940 ml) homemade Chicken Stock (see page 294) or ready-to-eat chicken broth with 1 envelope (1 tablespoon, or 7 g) plain gelatin added
- $^1/_2$ cup (80 g) yellow onion, chopped
- $^1/_2$ cup (65 g) carrot, chopped
- 1 tablespoon (4 g) minced fresh parsley
- $^1/_2$ teaspoon minced fresh thyme
- 1 bay leaf
- $^1/_2$ teaspoon black pepper
- 4 ounces (115 g) uncooked GF macaroni or small pasta shells
- 2 cups (about $^3/_4$ pound, or 340 g) cubed cooked turkey
- 1 cup (180 g) chopped tomatoes

In a large sauce pot over medium heat, combine broth, onion, carrot, parsley, thyme, bay leaf, and pepper. Bring to a boil. Stir in macaroni, cover, and reduce heat. Simmer for about 6 minutes. Stir in turkey and tomatoes. Cook until heated through and macaroni is tender. Discard bay leaf before serving.

YIELD: *Makes 8 servings of 1 cup (215 ml) each*

Calories (kcal): 336; **Total fat:** 17g; **Cholesterol:** 111mg; **Carbohydrate:** 16g; **Dietary fiber:** 2g; **Protein:** 28g; **Sodium:** 115mg; **Potassium:** 478mg; **Calcium:** 43mg; **Iron:** 3mg; **Zinc:** 3mg; **Vitamin A:** 6232IU.

Joyce's Versatile Vegetable Medley Soup

 gluten milk soy egg corn nuts

Joyce Mulcahy uses her vegetable medley as the basis for a delicious puréed soup with the addition of organic chicken broth.

Modified for SCD

- $1/2$ onion, sliced or chopped
- 1 garlic clove, minced
- 1 red or green bell pepper, chopped
- 1 tablespoon (15 ml) olive oil

Basic vegetables

- 1 can (14.5 ounces, or 411 g) diced tomatoes with juice, or 1-2 fresh chopped tomatoes
- 2-3 sliced zucchini
- Salt and pepper to taste

Optional additions (one or more of the following):

- $1/2$ fennel bulb, chopped
- $2/3$ cup (105 g) white corn, frozen or fresh (Do not use corn for SCD.)
- 1 small eggplant, peeled and sliced

Herb Options:

Italian Herbs:

- 4-5 minced basil leaves or $1/2$-1 tablespoon (15 g) pesto
- $1/2$ teaspoon oregano

Mexican Herbs:

- 1 teaspoon cumin
- 1-2 tablespoons (8 g) chopped cilantro (fresh)
- 1-2 cups (235-475 ml) chicken broth, depending on desired consistency of soup

Sauté onion, garlic, and bell pepper in olive oil until the onions are translucent.

Add basic (and optional) vegetables and herbs and simmer on medium-low heat for 15 minutes, stirring occasionally.

Place the ingredients in a blender. Add $1/2$ cup (120 ml) chicken broth and begin blending. Continue to add chicken broth and blend until the desired consistency is reached.

YIELD: *5 to 6 servings*

Calories (kcal): 667; **Total fat:** 21g; **Cholesterol:** 0mg; **Carbohydrate:** 107g; **Dietary fiber:** 33g; **Protein:** 31g; **Sodium:** 1676mg; **Potassium:** 4850mg; **Calcium:** 247mg; **Iron:** 9mg; **Zinc:** 4mg; **Vitamin A:** 6144IU.

Greek Lemon Chicken Soup

gluten milk soy egg corn nuts

Modified for Low Salicylate

- 2 chicken breasts
- 6 cups (1.4 L) broth or water
- 3 celery ribs
- 1 onion
- 5 garlic cloves
- Salt to taste
- 1/2 cup (90 g) long-grain rice
- 3 eggs, room temperature
- 1/4 cup (60 ml) lemon juice
- 1/2 teaspoon xanthan gum
- 1 teaspoon dill
- Salt to taste

Boil chicken in broth with celery ribs, onion, garlic, and salt for 30 minutes or longer. Pour mixture through a sieve. Put broth back into pot. Add rice.

Beat eggs in a blender. Add lemon juice. Add xanthan gum.

When rice is cooked, add lemon juice/egg mixture slowly, stirring constantly. Add dill and cut-up chicken. Adjust seasonings and salt to taste.

YIELD: *6 to 8 servings*

Calories (kcal): 311; **Total fat:** 13g; **Cholesterol:** 155mg; **Carbohydrate:** 18g; **Dietary fiber:** 1g; **Protein:** 29g; **Sodium:** 871 mg; **Potassium:** 578mg; **Calcium:** 55mg; **Iron:** 2mg; **Zinc:** 2mg; **Vitamin A:** 259IU.

Peter's Beef Stew

gluten milk soy egg corn nuts

- 2 pounds (910 g) cubed beef
- 1 bag (1 pound, or 455 g) baby carrots
- 1/2 celery head, cubed
- 1 teaspoon oregano
- 2 teaspoons salt
- 3 tablespoons Sofrito (45 g) (page 179)
- 1/2 cup (130 g) tomato paste
- 1 1/2 cups (355 ml) water
- 1 teaspoon (5 ml) apple cider vinegar
- 4 medium potatoes, cubed
- 1 teaspoon xanthan gum

Put all ingredients in a slow cooker except potatoes and xanthan gum. Cook on low for 6 hours. One hour before it's finished cooking, add potatoes. When fully cooked, take out 1 cup (235 ml) of liquid and blend it with xanthan gum in the blender. Pour into slow cooker and mix gently.

Serve with rice or quinoa.

YIELD: *8 servings*

Calories (kcal): 373; **Total fat:** 22g; **Cholesterol:** 76mg; **Carbohydrate:** 20g; **Dietary fiber:** 3g; **Protein:** 23g; **Sodium:** 753mg; **Potassium:** 1007mg; **Calcium:** 41mg; **Iron:** 3mg; **Zinc:** 5mg; **Vitamin A:** 8951IU.

Best Beef Soup Ever

gluten   milk   soy   egg   corn   nuts

This hearty and yummy winter soup is good any time of the year.

- 8–10 cups (1.9–2.4 L) water
- 2 large onions, quartered
- 5 pounds (2.3 kg) short ribs with bone cut into 1-inch (2.5 cm) chunks (results in 2$\frac{1}{2}$ pounds, or 1.1 kg, beef chunks)
- 1 tablespoon (18 g) kosher salt
- 1 tablespoon (6 g) ground black pepper
- 4 medium potatoes, quartered
- 1 small head cabbage, cut into bite-size pieces
- 1 large carrot, sliced into thick coins
- 1–2 tablespoons (15–30 ml) GFCFSF fish sauce

Combine the first 5 ingredients in a large saucepan or stockpot. Cooked (uncovered) on medium-high heat until beef is tender.

Simmer (covered) for about 3 hours. Add potatoes for the last 30 minutes. Add cabbage and carrot for the last 15 to 20 minutes. Add fish sauce to taste (this is quite salty but does add to the taste).

NOTE: *When buying fish sauce, check the ingredient list. Some have hydrolyzed wheat protein added. Thai Kitchen fish sauce is GFCFSF (www.thaikitchen.com).*

YIELD: *8 to 10 servings*

Calories (kcal): 117; **Total fat:** 104g; **Cholesterol:** 216mg; **Carbohydrate:** 16g; **Dietary fiber:** 2g; **Protein:** 43g; **Sodium:** 861 mg; **Potassium:** 1095mg; **Calcium:** 50mg; **Iron:** 5mg; **Zinc:** 9mg; **Vitamin A:** 2545IU.

Vegetable Purée Soup

gluten   milk   soy   egg   corn   nuts

This is a tasty way to expand on vegetables in a way that is acceptable with most who have sensory issues.

- 12 cups (2.8 L) water
- $\frac{1}{4}$ cup (35 g) yellow split peas
- $\frac{1}{4}$ cup (35 g) green split peas
- 4–6 medium carrots
- 2 sweet potatoes
- 2 medium zucchini
- 2 medium parsnips
- 1 large onion
- 1 teaspoon salt
- 1 teaspoon dried dill

Bring water to a boil. Lower heat and add yellow and green peas. Cover and simmer for 1 hour. Peel and cut remaining vegetables into large chunks. Add vegetables, salt, and dill. Bring to a boil, then lower heat and simmer, covered, for 1 more hour. Purée with an immersion blender in the pot or in batches in a blender (at low/medium speed) or a food processor.

YIELD: *8 to 12 servings*

Calories (kcal): 120; **Total fat:** trace; **Cholesterol:** 0mg; **Carbohydrate:** 26g; **Dietary fiber:** 7g; **Protein:** 4g; **Sodium:** 245mg; **Potassium:** 554mg; **Calcium:** 54mg; **Iron:** 1mg; **Zinc:** 1mg; **Vitamin A:** 15497IU.

Mary Lou's North African Vegetable Stew

gluten   milk   soy   egg   corn   nuts

This tasty stew is perfect for a cold winter day. It warms you from the inside.

- 2 teaspoons vegetable oil
- 1 medium onion, sliced
- $^1/_2$ teaspoon ground coriander
- $^1/_4$ teaspoon turmeric
- $^1/_2$ teaspoon cinnamon
- $^1/_2$ teaspoon ground ginger
- $^1/_4$ teaspoon ground cumin
- 2 medium tomatoes, chopped
- 1 medium sweet potato, peeled and cut
- $^1/_4$ cup (60 ml) water
- 2 tablespoons (30 ml) lemon juice
- 1 can (15 ounces, or 420 g) garbanzo beans, drained and rinsed
- 1 small zucchini, cut into 1-inch (2.5 cm) chunks
- $^1/_2$ cup (30 g) chopped fresh parsley
- $^1/_4$ cup (35 g) raisins
- Hot pepper sauce to taste (optional)

Heat oil. Add onion and spices, cooking until onion is limp, about 10 minutes, stirring frequently. Add tomatoes, sweet potato, water, and lemon juice. Bring to a boil, reduce heat, cover, and simmer approximately 30 minutes. Add beans, zucchini, parsley, and raisins. Cover and simmer another 10 minutes, until zucchini is tender. Season with hot pepper sauce to taste, if desired.

VARIATION: *Add sautéed boneless chicken to stew.*

YIELD: *4 to 6 servings*

Calories (kcal): 506; **Total fat:** 9g; **Cholesterol:** 0mg; **Carbohydrate:** 88g; **Dietary fiber:** 22g; **Protein:** 23g; **Sodium:** 44mg; **Potassium:** 1430mg; **Calcium:** 157mg; **Iron:** 8mg; **Zinc:** 4mg; **Vitamin A:** 7536IU.

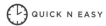 QUICK N EASY

Doug's Potato Leek Soup

gluten   milk   soy   egg   corn   nuts

Doug and Jeannette DeLawter enjoy sharing this recipe. It is a delicious light soup that is also easy on the digestive system and a good addition to any meal. As with all soups, this soup can be puréed as needed for those children with sensory food-texture issues.

- 3 medium leeks
- 1 medium onion
- 4 carrots, peeled or scrubbed
- 2 stalks celery
- 3 medium white potatoes, peeled
- Salt and pepper to taste
- $1/4$ teaspoon garlic powder
- 2 bay leaves
- 3 cans (14.5 ounces, or 411 g, each) chicken broth
- 3 chicken broth cans water

Under cool running water, clean dirt from leeks. Split leeks lengthwise into 4 sections, and chop into small pieces up to and including part of the green stalk.

Chop onion, carrots, and celery into small pieces. Cut potatoes into $1/4$-inch (6 mm) cubes.

Place leeks, onion, carrots, and celery into a large dry pot and simmer until ingredients soften.

Wash potato cubes in colander to rinse off starch and dry with paper towel before adding to vegetables. Add seasonings. Stir all ingredients frequently, not allowing them to stick to bottom of pot. When vegetables are softened, add broth and water. Bring the soup to a boil and then simmer until potatoes are cooked. Remove bay leaves before serving.

YIELD: *8 to 10 servings*

Calories (kcal): 105; **Total fat:** 1g; **Cholesterol:** 0mg; **Carbohydrate:** 19g; **Dietary fiber:** 3g; **Protein:** 5g; **Sodium:** 543mg; **Potassium:** 613mg; **Calcium:** 49mg; **Iron:** 2mg; **Zinc:** 1mg; **Vitamin A:** 10173IU.

QUICK N EASY

Carrot Veggie Stew

     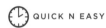

gluten   milk   soy   egg   corn   nuts

*From the Lambert Hill Farm, originally from Marilyn Lammers, with quite a
bit of revising along the way, as it has been passed down through generations!
This nutrient-rich stew has a good amount of beta-carotene. This is a good stew
for adding more vegetables into the diet, easily mixed in with the others. It can also
be puréed in a blender for those who do not tolerate "lumps and bumps" in foods.*

- 1 large onion, chopped (Vidalia recommended)
- 2 cloves garlic, diced
- 1 tablespoon (15 ml) olive oil
- 2 cans (12 ounces, or 355 ml, each) carrot juice
- 1/2 cup (120 ml) chicken broth
- 1 tablespoon (8 g) chili powder (This is very conservative; use more or use cayenne for a spicier stew.)
- 1 tablespoon (15 ml) vinegar
- 20 ounces (570 ml) water
- 3 cups (360 g) chopped fresh vegetables (carrots or cook's choice of vegetables)
- 1 can (19 ounces, or 530 g) red kidney beans

Sauté onion and garlic in olive oil until transparent, about 5 minutes. Add
juice (reserve empty cans), broth, chili powder, and vinegar. Bring to a
boil. Pour water into empty carrot-juice cans and swish around; add to
soup. Add veggies. Cover and simmer slowly (so the veggies keep their
texture) until veggies are tender, about 15 minutes. Add beans and simmer for another couple of minutes to heat through.

YIELD: *12 servings*

Calories (kcal): 192; **Total fat:** 2g; **Cholesterol:** 0mg; **Carbohydrate:** 34g; **Dietary fiber:** 8g; **Protein:** 11g;
Sodium: 62mg; **Potassium:** 814mg; **Calcium:** 57mg; **Iron:** 3mg; **Zinc:** 1mg; **Vitamin A:** 14823IU.

Super Carrot Soup

gluten milk soy egg corn nuts

- 1 small onion, chopped
- 2 tablespoons (30 g) ghee, divided
- 5–6 medium carrots, peeled and chopped
- 1 large potato, peeled and cubed
- 1 can (14.5 ounces, or 406 ml) chicken broth
- 1^1/$_2$ cups (105 g) chopped fresh mushrooms
- 1 stalk celery, chopped
- 1 clove garlic, minced
- ^{1}/$_2$ teaspoon sugar
- ^{1}/$_2$ teaspoon salt
- ^{1}/$_2$ teaspoon dried thyme
- ^{1}/$_4$ teaspoon GFCF hot pepper sauce
- ^{1}/$_2$ cup (120 ml) milk substitute (rice, non-GMO soy, coconut)
- Salt and pepper to taste

In a large saucepan, sauté onion in 1 tablespoon (15 g) ghee until tender. Add carrots and potato and cook for 2 minutes. Add broth, mushrooms, celery, garlic, sugar, salt, thyme, and pepper sauce. Bring to a boil and reduce heat. Cover and simmer for 50 minutes.

Let mixture cool slightly, then transfer to a blender and blend on medium until smooth.

Return to saucepan. Stir in milk substitute and remaining ghee and heat.

Season with salt and pepper.

YIELD: *6 to 8 servings*

Calories (kcal): 88; **Total fat:** 4g; **Cholesterol:** 9mg; **Carbohydrate:** 12g; **Dietary fiber:** 2g; **Protein:** 2g; **Sodium:** 327mg; **Potassium:** 390mg; **Calcium:** 27mg; **Iron:** 1mg; **Zinc:** trace; **Vitamin A:** 15328IU.

 QUICK N EASY

Corn Chowder

gluten milk soy egg corn nuts

This is a good way to add in a few more vegetables in order to expand variety.

- 2 tablespoons (30 ml) oil
- 1 large yellow onion, diced
- 5 medium Yukon Gold potatoes, peeled and chopped
- Salt to taste
- Pepper to taste
- 3 cups (710 ml) water
- 1 bag (16 ounces, or 455 g) frozen corn, defrosted and drained
- 1 cup (235 ml) rice milk

Heat oil over medium-high heat in a large pot or stockpot. Sauté onion until translucent and soft. Add potatoes and mix to coat with oil; sauté 1 to 2 minutes. Add salt and pepper. Add water and corn. Cook until potatoes are soft. Add rice milk and purée until smooth.

VARIATIONS: *Add some squash, carrots, or yams in place of some of the potatoes.*

YIELD: *8 servings*

Calories (kcal): 153; **Total fat:** 4g; **Cholesterol:** 0mg; **Carbohydrate:** 28g; **Dietary fiber:** 3g; **Protein:** 4g; **Sodium:** 10mg; **Potassium:** 557mg; **Calcium:** 13mg; **Iron:** 1mg; **Zinc:** 1mg; **Vitamin A:** 74IU.

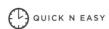 QUICK N EASY

Dana's Really Quick N Easy Vegetable Soup or Purée

gluten   milk   soy   egg   corn   nuts

This soup can be made as a soup or puréed for those with sensory issues who do not tolerate the "lumps and bumps" in soups or stews. Adding organic beef gelatin provides a better food that helps digestion. The addition of apple juice adds natural sweetness and enhances the flavor.

- 1 tablespoon (15 ml) olive oil
- 3 tablespoons (30 g) frozen minced onion
- ¼ teaspoon minced garlic (optional)
- 4 cups (940 ml) store-bought or homemade GFCF chicken broth (page 294)
- 1 cup (235 ml) apple juice (or apple cider)
- 1 tablespoon (7 g) organic unflavored gelatin
- 1 bag (16 ounces, or 455 g) frozen mixed organic vegetables (peas, non-GMO corn, carrots)
- Pepper to taste
- Salt, or GFCF fish sauce, to taste

Heat oil over medium-high heat in a 3- to 4-quart (2.8 to 3.8 L) pot or stockpot. Sauté onion (and optional garlic) until translucent and soft. Add chicken broth and apple juice (or cider). Add in gelatin and stir until it dissolves. Add in vegetables. Cook (covered) on medium heat for 15 to 20 minutes.

Add pepper to taste and salt or fish sauce to taste.

Serve as a soup, or purée in blender (medium/high speed) until smooth. Add more liquid if needed.

VARIATION: *Add chicken, turkey, or beef to this for a hearty soup/stew or purée.*

YIELD: *Serves 6 to 8*

Calories (kcal): 94; **Total fat:** 3g; **Cholesterol:** 0mg; **Carbohydrate:** 14g; **Dietary fiber:** 2g; **Protein:** 5g; **Sodium:** 414mg; **Potassium:** 267mg; **Calcium:** 22mg; **Iron:** 1mg; **Zinc:** trace; **Vitamin A:** 2880IU.

"To feel safe and warm on a cold wet night, all you really need is soup."

—Laurie Colwin

Thai-Style Pumpkin Soup

gluten　milk　soy　egg　corn　nuts

Here is another excellent recipe by Jody Cutler. This is a wonderful blend of colors and flavors. Guaranteed to warm you!

- 1 quart (940 ml) vegetable or chicken broth
- 1 can (15 ounces, or 420 g) pumpkin purée
- 1 can (12 ounces, or 355 ml) mango nectar
- ¼ cup (65 g) chunky GFCF peanut butter
- 2 tablespoons (30 ml) rice vinegar
- 1½ tablespoons (9 g) minced scallion
- 1 teaspoon grated peeled fresh ginger
- ½ teaspoon grated orange rind
- ¼ teaspoon crushed red pepper
- 1 clove garlic, crushed
- Chopped fresh cilantro (optional)

Combine first 3 ingredients in a large Dutch oven and bring to a boil. Cover, reduce heat, and simmer 10 minutes. Combine 1 cup (235 ml) pumpkin mixture and peanut butter in a blender or food processor; process until smooth. Return mixture to pan. Stir in vinegar and next 5 ingredients (through garlic); cook 3 minutes or until thoroughly heated. Ladle into soup bowls. Sprinkle with cilantro, if using.

YIELD: *6 servings (1 cup [235 ml] each)*

Calories (kcal): 121; **Total fat:** 6g; **Cholesterol:** 0mg; **Carbohydrate:** 11g; **Dietary fiber:** 2g; **Protein:** 6g; **Sodium:** 567mg; **Potassium:** 322mg; **Calcium:** 25mg; **Iron:** 2mg; **Zinc:** 1mg; **Vitamin A:** 9017IU.

White Bean Stew with Swiss Chard

gluten　milk　soy　egg　corn　nuts

This is a nice, hearty soup for those cold weather months.

Modified for SCD

- 2 ounces (55 g) nitrate-free bacon, chopped fine
- 1 small onion, chopped fine
- 1 carrot, chopped fine
- 2 cloves garlic
- 1 bay leaf
- 1 sprig rosemary
- 3 cups (710 ml) GFCF chicken broth
- 2 cans (15.5 ounces, or 450 g each) cannellini beans, rinsed (For SCD, use haricot beans.)
- 3 cups (165 g) chopped Swiss chard (from about 1 bunch)
- 2 tablespoons (8 g) chopped parsley
- Salt and ground black pepper
- Extra virgin olive oil for drizzling (optional)

Cook bacon in a large pot or Dutch oven over medium-high heat for 3 to 5 minutes, until golden and most of the fat has rendered. Add onion and carrot and cook until softened, 5 minutes. Stir in the garlic, bay leaf, and rosemary and cook for a few seconds, until fragrant. Pour in broth, beans, and chard, and bring to a boil. Reduce heat and simmer for 15 minutes. Remove bay leaf and rosemary, add parsley, and season to taste with salt and pepper. Serve with a drizzle of olive oil if desired.

TIP: *You can use curly leaf spinach in place of the chard.*

YIELD: *4 servings*

Calories (kcal): 427; **Total fat:** 10g; **Cholesterol:** 13mg; **Carbohydrate:** 61g; **Dietary fiber:** 21g; **Protein:** 26g; **Sodium:** 642mg; **Potassium:** 1458mg; **Calcium:** 238mg; **Iron:** 9mg; **Zinc:** 3mg; **Vitamin A:** 6079IU.

Black Bean Soup

gluten   milk   soy   egg   corn   nuts

- 1 tablespoon (15 ml) extra virgin olive oil
- 1 medium onion, diced
- 1 tablespoon (7.5 g) chili powder
- 1 teaspoon ground cumin
- 1 teaspoon dried oregano
- 1/2 teaspoon salt
- 3 cups (710 ml) GFCF chicken broth
- 2 cans (15 ounces, or 420 g, each) black beans, drained and rinsed
- 2 garlic cloves, minced
- 1 can (15 ounces, or 420 g) pumpkin purée
- 1/4 cup (15 g) minced fresh cilantro
- 1 tablespoon (15 ml) lime juice

Heat olive oil in large pot over medium-high heat and cook onion, chili powder, cumin, oregano, and salt for 2 minutes, stirring frequently. Add the garlic and cook for 30 seconds. Add the broth and black beans and bring to a boil over high heat; reduce heat and simmer for 3 minutes. Off heat, stir in the cilantro and lime juice and serve.

YIELD: *4 to 6 servings*

Calories (kcal): 197; **Total fat:** 5g; **Cholesterol:** 3mg; **Carbohydrate:** 27g; **Dietary fiber:** 11g; **Protein:** 10g; **Sodium:** 921mg; **Potassium:** 216mg; **Calcium:** 36mg; **Iron:** 2mg; **Zinc:** trace; **Vitamin A:** 16093IU.

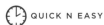 QUICK N EASY

Special Ingredient Noodles

gluten   milk   soy   egg   corn   nuts

Inspired by a certain blockbuster Panda, Ellen Demattia came up with this tasty dinner for her family. Their favorite part about this dish is using a special noodle spoon—the flat, ceramic kind offered in Chinese restaurants.

- 1 quart (940 ml) GFCF chicken broth
- 8 ounces (225 g) dried Pad Thai–style Rice Noodles
- 2 cups (280 g) chopped precooked chicken
- 2 cups (about 400 g) chopped cooked mixed vegetables of your choice

Bring the broth to a boil in a large pot. Off heat, add noodles and let sit for 10 to 15 minutes, until noodles are tender. Add chicken and vegetables and cook over medium heat, about 3 minutes. Serve.

YIELD: *4 servings*

Calories (kcal): 462; **Total fat:** 16g; **Cholesterol:** 83mg; **Carbohydrate:** 58g; **Dietary fiber:** 5g; **Protein:** 19g; **Sodium:** 920mg; **Potassium:** 344mg; **Calcium:** 49mg; **Iron:** 3mg; **Zinc:** 2mg; **Vitamin A:** 6952IU.

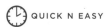

QUICK N EASY

Simple Egg Drop Soup

gluten   milk   soy   egg   corn   nuts

- 1 large egg
- Salt and ground black pepper
- 4 cups (940 ml) GFCF chicken broth
- 1 clove garlic, minced
- 1 tablespoon (8 g) chopped fresh ginger
- 3 scallions, chopped fine
- 1 teaspoon sesame oil

In a small bowl, lightly beat the egg with a pinch of salt and pepper.

In a large saucepan, bring the chicken broth, garlic, ginger, and 1 teaspoon salt to a boil over high heat; reduce heat and simmer for 3 minutes. Pour the egg in a very thin stream along the prongs of a fork over the surface of the soup. When the egg has set, add the scallions and sesame oil and serve.

YIELD: *4 servings*

Calories (kcal): 69; **Total fat:** 5g; **Cholesterol:** 59mg; **Carbohydrate:** 1g; **Dietary fiber:** trace; **Protein:** 4g; **Sodium:** 598mg; **Potassium:** 55mg; **Calcium:** 16mg; **Iron:** trace; **Zinc:** trace; **Vitamin A:** 123IU.

Tomato Rice Soup

gluten   milk   soy   egg   corn   nuts

- 2 tablespoons (30 ml) olive oil
- 1 small onion, chopped
- 1 clove garlic, minced
- 2 teaspoons tomato paste (For SCD, use fresh tomatoes that have been puréed in the blender and squeezed to remove the juice.)
- 1 large can (28 ounces, or 800 g) whole tomatoes
- 2 teaspoons agave syrup (For SCD, use honey.)
- $^1/_2$ teaspoon salt
- $^1/_4$ teaspoon coarsely ground pepper
- $1^1/_2$ cups (355 ml) GFCF chicken broth
- 1 cup (165 g) cooked rice (For SCD, use cauliflower rice.)

Heat oil in large pot over medium heat; cook onion, garlic, and tomato paste 5 minutes, or until onion is soft. Add the tomatoes and their juices, agave syrup, salt and pepper and cook another 5 minutes. Carefully purée mixture in a blender or a food processor until smooth, and then return to the pot. Add the broth and cooked rice and return soup to a boil. Serve.

NOTE: *If you are using white rice, the rice can be puréed along with the tomato mixture for a completely smooth and creamy soup.*

YIELD: *4 servings*

Calories (kcal): 188; **Total fat:** 8g; **Cholesterol:** 2mg; **Carbohydrate:** 26g; **Dietary fiber:** 3g; **Protein:** 4g; **Sodium:** 801mg; **Potassium:** 508mg; **Calcium:** 72mg; **Iron:** 1mg; **Zinc:** 1mg; **Vitamin A:** 1248IU.

Cream of Cauliflower Soup

gluten milk soy egg corn nuts

Coconut milk is the secret to this "creamy" soup, and is healthy for the GI tract. See the discussion about the health benefits of this fabulous food on page 69.

- 1 medium head (about 2 pounds, or 910 g) cauliflower
- 4 tablespoons (60 ml) olive oil, divided
- 2 to 3 teaspoons mild GFCF curry powder
- Salt and ground black pepper
- 1 medium onion, chopped fine
- 2 cups (475 ml) GFCF chicken broth
- 1 can (14 ounces, or 425 ml) unsweetened coconut milk

Preheat oven to 450°F (230°C, gas mark 8). Cut the cauliflower into 1-inch (2.5 cm) florets, and toss with 3 tablespoons (45 ml) of the oil, curry powder, and $\frac{1}{2}$ teaspoon salt in a large bowl. Transfer to a baking sheet and roast for 15 to 20 minutes, until cauliflower is golden brown on the edges, stirring once halfway through.

In a large pot, heat remaining oil over medium heat. Add onion and cook until softened, 5 minutes. Add roasted cauliflower and stock and bring to a boil; reduce heat and simmer, covered, until cauliflower is very soft. Carefully purée soup in a blender with the coconut milk until smooth; season to taste with salt and pepper. Serve, or return to pot to gently reheat if necessary, but do not boil.

YIELD: *6 servings*

Calories (kcal): 265; **Total fat:** 25g; **Cholesterol:** 2mg; **Carbohydrate:** 10g; **Dietary fiber:** 3g; **Protein:** 4g; **Sodium:** 241mg; **Potassium:** 95mg; **Calcium:** 12mg; **Iron:** trace; **Zinc:** trace; **Vitamin A:** 14IU.

Erika's Chicken Noodle Soup

gluten milk soy egg corn nuts

SCD Legal

- 3 large boneless skinless chicken breasts
- Water
- 8 cups (1.9 L) GFCF organic chicken broth
- 1 pound (455 g) celery, cut into bite-sized pieces
- 1 pound (455 g) carrots, peeled and cut into bite-size pieces
- 1 large onion, chopped fine
- 2 tablespoons (8 g) chopped parsley
- Salt and ground black pepper to taste
- 1 pound (455 g) GF noodles (For SCD, use cauliflower rice.)

Add chicken and broth to a large stockpot and bring to boil. Skim off brown foam and yellow patches. Add celery, carrots, onion, and parsley, cover, reduce heat to low and simmer for at least 1 hour, stirring occasionally to break chicken up into pieces (or you can remove breasts after 20 minutes and shred with a fork, and then return to the pot).

Meanwhile, boil another large pot of water and cook the noodles according to package directions. Drain and rinse noodles.

When soup is done, add noodles, and season to taste with salt and pepper. Serve.

YIELD: *6 to 8 servings*

Calories (kcal): 373; **Total fat:** 4g; **Cholesterol:** 56mg; **Carbohydrate:** 51g; **Dietary fiber:** 6g; **Protein:** 28g; **Sodium:** 701mg; **Potassium:** 569mg; **Calcium:** 59mg; **Iron:** 2mg; **Zinc:** 1mg; **Vitamin A:** 14380IU.

CHAPTER 22

Fruits, Sweets, and Treats

FRUITS CAN BE SERVED A VARIETY OF WAYS, and fresh is always the healthiest. Fresh fruit cut up is easy to handle for most children. For those with sensory issues, use puréed fruits and fruit sauces such as applesauce and pear sauce. Baby foods are readily available and easy to use.

For an easy, tasty, and healthy "syrup" topping, blend frozen raspberries or strawberries (organic is the best choice). Spoon on top of any mix of cut-up fruit.

QUICK N EASY

Baked Honey Apple Slices

gluten   milk   soy   egg   corn   nuts

This is very appealing to little ones, and another quick and easy recipe.

- ¹/₄ cup (85 g) honey
- Juice of 1 lemon (fresh or bottled)
- 3 large cooking apples
- ¹/₂ teaspoon cinnamon
- 2 teaspoons ghee

Mix honey and lemon juice in a shallow baking dish or pie pan.

Peel and core apples. Cut apples in quarters, then slices.

Place apples in honey-juice mixture, coating well. Sprinkle with cinnamon.

Melt ghee and pour over the mix.

Bake in a moderate oven, 350°F (180°C, gas mark 4), for 30 to 40 minutes or until tender.

Baste with pan liquid twice during baking.

YIELD: *4 to 6 servings*

Calories (kcal): 149; **Total fat:** 3g; **Cholesterol:** 6mg; **Carbohydrate:** 35g; **Dietary fiber:** 3g; **Protein:** trace; **Sodium:** 2mg; **Potassium:** 153mg; **Calcium:** 16mg; **Iron:** 1mg; **Zinc:** trace; **Vitamin A:** 145IU.

Poached Pears

gluten   milk   soy   egg   corn   nuts

Poached fruit is an easy, but elegant dessert for a festive occasion. Serve pears alone or with poaching liquid, warm or chilled, spooned over ice cream, yogurt, or angel-food cake. (For SCD, use almond- or cashew-based ice cream or non-soy homemade yogurt.)

Modified for SCD

- 4 medium pears (about 1¹/₄ pounds, or 560 g), peeled, cored, and quartered
- 2 cups (475 ml) cranberry juice (For SCD, use 100% juice without added sugar.)
- 2 cinnamon sticks
- 3 whole cloves
- Zest of ¹/₂ orange, in strips

Put all ingredients into a large saucepan. Be sure that pan is not too large, so that the juice completely covers the pears. If the juice does not cover the pears and the fruit floats, place a small plate upside down in pot, to weight pears down in liquid. Bring to a simmer over medium heat and cook for 7 (for ripe fruit) to 10 minutes (for less ripe fruit). Pears should pierce easily with a fork.

To make syrup, transfer pears to a bowl. Simmer the poaching liquid until it is reduced by one-third and thickened to desired consistency, 30 to 40 minutes. Store in poaching liquid in a covered container in the refrigerator for up to 3 days.

This recipe works well with fruit of the same firmness and ripeness. Try combining apples with pears. Softer fruits such as peaches and plums are also a good option, but you'll need to reduce the cooking time so the fruit does not become mushy.

YIELD: *Makes 4 servings of 4 quarters each*

Calories (kcal): 204; **Total fat:** 2g; **Cholesterol:** 0mg; **Carbohydrate:** 52g; **Dietary fiber:** 9g; **Protein:** 1g; **Sodium:** 16mg; **Potassium:** 320mg; **Calcium:** 138mg; **Iron:** 4mg; **Zinc:** trace; **Vitamin A:** 84IU.

QUICK N EASY

Warm Stewed Fruit

gluten   milk   soy   egg   corn   nuts

This recipe title says it all—a warm, tasty comfort food. It is especially good for those with oral motor difficulties who do not handle raw fruit well and prefer softer textures.

- 6 medium apples (can use different varieties), peeled and chopped
- 1/2 teaspoon cinnamon
- 1/4 teaspoon dried ginger
- 1/4 cup (60 ml) apple juice or white grape juice
- 1/4 cup (60 ml) water
- 1 teaspoon sugar-free mixed berry jam (optional)

Combine all ingredients in a saucepan. Bring to a boil. Reduce heat and simmer, uncovered, until apples are soft.

VARIATION: *Use apples and pears or apples and cranberries. This recipe can also be made with 6 cups (660 g) of fresh strawberries instead of apples—just omit the cinnamon, ginger, and water.*

YIELD: *4 to 6 servings*

Calories (kcal): 87; **Total fat:** 1g; **Cholesterol:** 0mg; **Carbohydrate:** 22g; **Dietary fiber:** 4g; **Protein:** trace; **Sodium:** 1mg; **Potassium:** 173mg; **Calcium:** 13mg; **Iron:** trace; **Zinc:** trace; **Vitamin A:** 74IU.

Fruit Clafouti

gluten   milk   soy   egg   corn   nuts

This is a classic French dessert. It falls somewhere between a pancake and a custard, and is surprisingly simple to make. Traditionally, sour cherries are used, but you can use any fresh fruit in season you like (although softer fruits work better than crunchy ones like apples, which require more baking time).

- 1 pound (455 g) fruit (either cherries, berries, or chopped fruit such as peaches, apricots, or plums)
- 1 cup (235 ml) rice milk
- 1/2 cup (100 g) sugar
- 3 large eggs
- 1/2 cup (70 g) GF flour blend
- 2 teaspoons GFCF vanilla extract
- 1 teaspoon lemon zest
- 1/4 teaspoon salt

Preheat the oven to 350°F (180°C, gas mark 4). Distribute the fruit evenly on the bottom of a greased baking dish or large pie plate. Combine the rice milk, sugar, eggs, flour blend, vanilla extract, zest, and salt in a blender for 1 minute. Pour over the fruit and bake for 45 to 50 minutes, until edges have puffed and top is lightly browned (center should be set and should not look liquid-y when jiggled). Cool for 5 to 10 minutes, then cut into wedges and serve.

YIELD: *6 servings*

Calories (kcal): 225; **Total fat:** 3g; **Cholesterol:** 112mg; **Carbohydrate:** 44g; **Dietary fiber:** 3g; **Protein:** 6g; **Sodium:** 142mg; **Potassium:** 179mg; **Calcium:** 23mg; **Iron:** 1mg; **Zinc:** trace; **Vitamin A:** 918IU.

Fried Bananas

gluten   milk   soy   egg   corn   nuts

Small bananas, called baby, finger, or apple bananas, are best for this dish, but slightly green, regular bananas can be used. Just cut them in half lengthwise, and then in half again crosswise.

- 1³/₄ cups (175 g) rice flour
- ¹/₄ cup (20 g) unsweetened shredded coconut
- 1 tablespoon (13 g) sugar
- 1 tablespoon (8 g) sesame seeds
- 1 teaspoon baking powder
- ¹/₄ teaspoon salt
- ¹/₂ cup (120 ml) water
- 3 cups (710 ml) canola oil (or other oil suitable for frying)
- ¹/₂ pound (225 g) slightly green baby bananas, peeled and cut in half lengthwise
- Honey, for drizzling

Mix the rice flour, coconut, sugar, sesame seeds, baking powder, and salt together in a medium bowl. Whisk in the water until the batter is smooth and free of lumps. Heat the oil in a wok or deep pan to 350°F (180°C).

Dip the banana pieces into the batter and then carefully slide them into the hot oil. Cook for 3 minutes, then flip over and cook another 2 minutes, until golden brown all over. Remove with a slotted spoon and drain on a plate lined with paper towels. Drizzle with honey and serve immediately.

YIELD: *2 to 4 servings*

Calories (kcal): 181; **Total fat:** 10g; **Cholesterol:** 30mg; **Carbohydrate:** 19g; **Dietary fiber:** 2g; **Protein:** 3g; **Sodium:** 99mg; **Potassium:** 237mg; **Calcium:** 101mg; **Iron:** 1mg; **Zinc:** 1mg; **Vitamin A:** 30IU.

Cashew Cookies

gluten   milk   soy   egg   corn   nuts

Every child loves cookies and these protein-packed cookies are sure to win them over.

Low Phenol

- 16 ounces (455 g) cashews
- 1 cup (235 ml) sunflower oil plus 2 tablespoons (30 ml) for making cashew butter
- ³/₄ cup (170 g) brown sugar
- ³/₄ cup (150 g) sugar
- 4 eggs
- ¹/₂ cup (120 ml) water
- 1 tablespoon (14 g) baking soda
- 1 tablespoon (8 g) xanthan gum
- ³/₄ teaspoon salt
- 2¹/₄ cups (315 g) brown rice flour
- 1¹/₂ cups (180 g) quinoa flour
- 1¹/₂ cups (180 g) tapioca starch

Grind cashews in a food processor and add enough sunflower oil to make a smooth nut butter. Mix additional 1 cup (235 ml) sunflower oil and all remaining ingredients. Chill dough at least 1 hour.

Place dough in a cookie press or roll out between 2 sheets of wax paper and shape with cutters. Bake pressed cookies at 375°F (190°C, or gas mark 5) for 12 to 15 minutes, cut-out cookies for 10 to 12 minutes. This dough can also be rolled into balls and crisscrossed with a fork.

YIELD: *18 to 24 cookies*

Calories (kcal): 480; **Total fat:** 27g; **Cholesterol:** 42mg; **Carbohydrate:** 55g; **Dietary fiber:** 3g; **Protein:** 9g; **Sodium:** 322mg; **Potassium:** 328mg; **Calcium:** 32mg; **Iron:** 3mg; **Zinc:** 2mg; **Vitamin A:** 62IU.

Chocolate Chip Cookies

gluten   milk   soy   egg   corn   nuts

Almost every child wants to be able to eat a chocolate chip cookie, so we are giving you a recipe for a GFCF version of this favorite treat.

- 1 cup (225 g) ghee, softened
- 2 cups (450 g) Sucanat
- 2 large eggs
- $^1/_2$ teaspoon salt
- 2 tablespoons (30 ml) vanilla
- 1 cup (120 g) almond flour
- 1 cup (140 g) garbanzo bean flour
- 1 teaspoon baking soda
- 2 cups (350 g) GFCF semisweet chocolate chips
- 2 cups (190 g) ground almonds or walnuts (You can substitute with the above almond flour.)

Place a rack in the center of the oven. Preheat oven to 375°F (190°C, or gas mark 5). Line several baking sheets with Silpat sheets or parchment paper. With an electric mixer, beat the ghee with the Sucanat until very fluffy. In a separate small bowl, mix together the eggs, salt, and vanilla until well blended. Add to the ghee/Sucanat mixture. Stir until well blended. In a separate large bowl, mix together the almond flour, garbanzo bean flour, and baking soda. Add to the ghee/Sucanat mixture. Stir until well blended. Stir in chocolate chips and the ground almonds or walnuts. If the dough is too stiff to work, add more ghee. Drop onto the baking sheets, spacing the cookies 2 inches (5 cm) apart.

Bake until the cookies are just slightly colored on top and rimmed with brown at the edges (8 to 10 minutes). Be sure to rotate the sheets halfway through the baking time (front to back). Be careful: Since the recipe does not use regular flour, the cookies can burn more quickly than usual. Watch them closely. Remove the sheets to a rack. Let the cookies cool for a few minutes before transferring them to a rack to finish cooling. You can freeze them when completely cool. Place wax paper between layers of cookies before freezing them.

YIELD: *48 cookies*

Calories (kcal): 157; **Total fat:** 10g; **Cholesterol:** 19mg; **Carbohydrate:** 15g; **Dietary fiber:** 1g; **Protein:** 3g; **Sodium:** 55mg; **Potassium:** 100mg; **Calcium:** 23mg; **Iron:** 1mg; **Zinc:** trace; **Vitamin A:** 197IU.

Maya's Cookies

gluten   milk   soy   egg   corn   nuts

Extra protein has been added to these cookies, reducing the negative effect on blood sugar. This is also a way to sneak protein into the picky eater.

Low Phenol

- $^7/_8$ cup (105 g) almond meal flour
- $^7/_8$ cup (88 g) GF oat flour
- $^7/_8$ cup (125 g) garbanzo and fava bean flour
- $1^1/_2$ cups (210 g) GF flour
- 1 teaspoon baking soda
- $^1/_2$ teaspoon salt
- 1 cup (200 g) sugar
- $^1/_2$ teaspoon cinnamon
- $1^1/_4$ cups (295 ml) safflower oil
- $^1/_4$ cup (85 g) molasses
- 5 eggs, or 3 eggs and 3 egg whites
- 2 teaspoons vanilla

Preheat oven to 350°F (180°C, gas mark 4).

Combine all dry ingredients in a bowl.

In a large bowl, beat the liquid ingredients on medium speed until smooth. Add dry ingredients and mix thoroughly with a wooden spoon.

Drop by rounded teaspoons on an ungreased cookie sheet. Flatten with bottom of a glass that has been dipped in sugar.

Bake 8 minutes, until edges are lightly browned. Transfer to a wire rack to cool. These cookies can be stored in a covered container for up to 3 days or in a sealed freezer bag in the freezer for up to 6 months.

YIELD: *44 cookies*

Calories (kcal): 135; Total fat: 8g; Cholesterol: 21mg; Carbohydrate: 14g; Dietary fiber: 1g; Protein: 3g; Sodium: 61mg; Potassium: 105mg; Calcium: 21mg; Iron: 1mg; Zinc: trace; Vitamin A: 33IU.

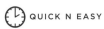 QUICK N EASY

Peanut Butter Truffle Cookies

gluten   milk   soy   egg   corn   nuts

The yummy taste of this recipe, which has been modified from a Skippy peanut butter recipe, is excellent for hiding nutritional supplements.

Low Phenol

- 1 cup (260 g) creamy GFCF peanut butter
- 1 cup (225 g) light brown sugar
- 1 large egg
- 1 teaspoon baking soda
- $^1/_2$ cup (90 g) GFCF semisweet chocolate chips

Preheat oven to 350°F (180°C, gas mark 4). Cream together all the ingredients, except for the chocolate chips, with a wooden spoon. Add chocolate chips. Drop by rounded teaspoonfuls onto a greased cookie sheet. Bake 9 minutes. Allow to cool for 5 minutes on the sheet before removing to cool completely.

NOTE: *Be sure to read the peanut butter label, some brands contain soy.*

YIELD: *36 cookies*

Calories (kcal): 71; Total fat: 4g; Cholesterol: 5mg; Carbohydrate: 7g; Dietary fiber: 1g; Protein: 2g; Sodium: 72mg; Potassium: 72mg; Calcium: 7mg; Iron: trace; Zinc: trace; Vitamin A: 13IU.

Welby's 3-in-1 Cookie Recipe

gluten milk soy egg corn nuts

Using one standard dry mix, we present Welby Griffin's 3 cookie variations. The addition of almond meal and sorghum also makes these cookies high in protein.

Dry Mix

- 1/2 cup (60 g) tapioca flour
- 1/2 cup (70 g) sorghum flour
- 1/2 cup (60 g) almond meal
- 1/4 cup (40 g) potato starch
- 1 teaspoon baking powder
- 1/2 teaspoon baking soda
- 1/4 teaspoon salt
- 1/4 teaspoon xanthan gum

For the Chocolate Chip Cookies

- 1/2 cup (120 g) GFCF Spread (such as Earth Balance)
- 3/4 cup (170 g) brown sugar
- 1/4 cup (50 g) granulated sugar
- 1 large egg
- 1 1/2 teaspoons GF vanilla
- 6 ounces (170 g) GFCF chocolate chips

For the Peanut Butter Cookies

- 1/3 cup (80 g) GFCF Spread
- 1/3 cup (87 g) peanut butter
- 3/4 cup (150 g) granulated sugar
- 1 large egg
- 1 teaspoon honey
- 1 teaspoon GF vanilla extract
- 1/2 cup (72.5 g) chopped peanuts (optional)

For the Sugar Cookies

- 1/2 cup (120 g) GFCF Spread
- 1 cup (200 g) granulated sugar
- 1 large egg
- 1 1/2 teaspoons GF vanilla extract
- Dash of nutmeg

To make dry mix: Blend all dry mix ingredients in a bowl and set aside.

To make all cookies: Preheat oven to 350°F (180°C, gas mark 4). Spray a baking sheet with cooking spray or line with parchment paper and set aside.

In a large bowl, cream together the GFCF spread and sugar(s). (For the peanut cookie variation, also add in the peanut butter.) Then add the remaining ingredients for your chosen recipe, except for any chocolate chip or nut additions. Stir in the dry mix, and then gently fold in the nuts or chips. Chill dough until firm.

Roll dough into 1-inch (2.5 cm) balls and place 2 to 3 inches (5 to 7.5 cm) apart on the prepared cookie sheet (if dough becomes too warm, place cookie sheet in refrigerator for 10 minutes to firm it up). Bake cookies for 10 to 15 minutes (depending on whether you like your cookies chewy or crispy). Allow cookies to cool on sheet for 5 minutes before moving to a cooling rack.

NOTE: To achieve classic look, flatten peanut butter with a fork or slotted spatula halfway through baking.

TIP: *Make several batches of dry mix at once, and store them in separate, labeled, freezer bags.*

VARIATION: Sugar cookie variations: Roll balls of cookie dough in cinnamon sugar to make Snickerdoodles or in colored sugar for a holiday look.

YIELD: 3¹/₂ dozen cookies

Dry Mix: Calories (kcal): 20; **Total fat:** trace; **Cholesterol:** 0mg; **Carbohydrate:** 4g; **Dietary fiber:** trace; **Protein:** 1g; **Sodium:** 39mg; **Potassium:** 23mg; **Calcium:** 13mg; **Iron:** trace; **Zinc:** trace; **Vitamin A:** 0IU.

Chocolate Chip Cookies: Calories (kcal): 76; **Total fat:** 4g; **Cholesterol:** 5mg; **Carbohydrate:** 10g; **Dietary fiber:** trace; **Protein:** 1g; **Sodium:** 42mg; **Potassium:** 34mg; **Calcium:** 22mg; **Iron:** 1mg; **Zinc:** trace; **Vitamin A:** 8IU.

Peanut Butter Cookies: Calories (kcal): 62; **Total fat:** 4g; **Cholesterol:** 5mg; **Carbohydrate:** 6g; **Dietary fiber:** trace; **Protein:** 2g; **Sodium:** 51mg; **Potassium:** 51mg; **Calcium:** 16mg; **Iron:** trace; **Zinc:** trace; **Vitamin A:** 8IU.

Sugar Cookies: Calories (kcal): 60; **Total fat:** 3g; **Cholesterol:** 5mg; **Carbohydrate:** 8g; **Dietary fiber:** trace; **Protein:** 1g; **Sodium:** 41mg; **Potassium:** 25mg; **Calcium:** 14mg; **Iron:** trace; **Zinc:** trace; **Vitamin A:** 8IU.

QUICK N EASY

Chocolate Date Balls

gluten   milk   soy   egg   corn   nuts

From Susan Lyttek, Springfield, VA

- 1¹/₂ cups (267 g) pitted, chopped dates
- 1¹/₂ cups (180 g) chopped walnuts, toasted
- ¹/₂ cup (40 g) GFCF unsweetened cocoa powder
- 1 teaspoon cinnamon
- ¹/₄ cup (60 ml) coconut milk

Pulse dates, walnuts, cocoa powder, and cinnamon in food processor until finely ground. Add coconut milk and process until combined. Form into 1-inch balls and freeze.

YIELD: 3¹/₂ dozen balls

Calories (kcal): 51; **Total fat:** 3g; **Cholesterol:** 0mg; **Carbohydrate:** 6g; **Dietary fiber:** 1g; **Protein:** 1g; **Sodium:** 7mg; **Potassium:** 69mg; **Calcium:** 6mg; **Iron:** trace; **Zinc:** trace; **Vitamin A:** 17IU.

QUICK N EASY

Apple Pie Cake

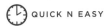
gluten   milk   soy   egg   corn   nuts

This recipe combines the better of two family favorites into one really fantastic dessert.

- ¹/₃ cup (40 g) quinoa flour
- ¹/₃ cup (45 g) brown rice flour
- ¹/₃ cup (40 g) tapioca starch
- ²/₃ cup (135 g) sugar
- 1 teaspoon baking soda
- 1 teaspoon xanthan gum
- ¹/₂ teaspoon cinnamon
- Pinch of salt
- 2 tablespoons (30 ml) oil
- 1 egg
- 1 tablespoon (15 ml) hot water
- 4 apples, sliced thin
- ¹/₄ cup (35 g) crushed nuts (optional)

Mix all ingredients except crushed nuts, adding apples last. Pour into ungreased 9-inch (23 cm) pie pan. Sprinkle with nuts (optional). Bake in a 350°F (180°C, gas mark 4) oven for 35 minutes.

YIELD: 8 servings

Calories (kcal): 238; **Total fat:** 7g; **Cholesterol:** 23mg; **Carbohydrate:** 43g; **Dietary fiber:** 3g; **Protein:** 3g; **Sodium:** 184mg; **Potassium:** 184mg; **Calcium:** 19mg; **Iron:** 1mg; **Zinc:** 1mg; **Vitamin A:** 73IU.

Meringue Cookies

gluten milk soy egg corn nuts

These cookies are lighter than air, chewy on the inside, and crunchy on the outside. They are portable and a favorite for many. A protein treat that will please the kids who love something crunchy.

- 4 egg whites, at room temperature
- $^1/_4$ teaspoon salt
- $^1/_4$ teaspoon cream of tartar
- $1^1/_2$ cups (300 g) sugar
- $1^1/_2$ teaspoons vanilla extract

Basics

Use a clean, dry bowl that is absolutely grease-free. Glass, ceramic, stainless steel are best. Avoid copper. Plastic bowls should be avoided because they can have trace amounts of oil.

Cold eggs separate easily, but eggs whip to a higher volume when at room temperature. Separate the cold eggs, and then set them aside for 10 or 15 minutes. There can be absolutely no yolk mixed in the whites. Save the yolks for another dish.

Superfine sugar is best. Simply process granulated sugar in the food processor.

Beat egg whites with salt and cream of tartar until stiff. Add sugar 1 tablespoon (13 g) at a time, beating well after each addition. Add vanilla extract.

Adding sugar early in the beating process results in a firmer, finer-textured meringue. When the mixture becomes stiff and shiny like satin, stop mixing, the meringue is ready.

If making a variation, add extra ingredient.

Line large baking sheets with parchment paper. Drop meringue by tablespoonful $1^1/_2$ inches (3.75 cm) apart onto prepared baking sheets.

Bake at 250°F (120°C, or gas mark $^1/_2$) for 30 to 40 minutes (until they crack). Turn off oven and let them cool down (15 minutes).

VARIATIONS:

- **ALMOND MERINGUES:** *1 teaspoon GFCF almond extract*
- **CINNAMON MERINGUES:** *$^1/_8$ teaspoon ground cinnamon*
- **CHOCOLATE CHIP:** *1 cup (85 g) GFCF chocolate chips*
- **CHOCOLATE MERINGUES:** *1 cup (85 g) GFCF chocolate chips, melted*

YIELD: *2 dozen*

Calories (kcal): 52; **Total fat:** 0g; **Cholesterol:** 0mg; **Carbohydrate:** 13g; **Dietary fiber:** 0g; **Protein:** 1g; **Sodium:** 31 mg; **Potassium:** 13mg; **Calcium:** 1mg; **Iron:** trace; **Zinc:** trace; **Vitamin A:** 0IU.

Carrot Cake

gluten   milk   soy   egg   corn   nuts

- 1 package (10.5 ounces, or 294 g) extra-firm silken tofu
- 1¹/₂ ounces (42 ml) canola oil
- 2¹/₄ cups (450 g) sugar
- 1¹/₂ cups (355 ml) canola oil
- 6 cups (720 g) shredded carrots
- 1¹/₂ cups (180 g) tapioca flour
- 1¹/₂ cups (180 g) arrowroot flour
- 1 cup (140 g) garbanzo and fava bean flour
- ¹/₂ cup (70 g) sorghum flour
- 1 teaspoon xanthan gum
- 1 tablespoon (14 g) baking powder
- 1 tablespoon (14 g) baking soda
- 1 tablespoon (7 g) ground cinnamon
- ³/₄ teaspoon ground nutmeg
- ³/₄ teaspoon ground clove
- 1 teaspoon salt
- Frosting, recipe follows
- 3 cups (315 g) toasted, finely chopped walnuts

Preheat oven to 350°F (180°C, gas mark 4). Spray two 9-inch (23 cm) cake pans with canola oil, line bottom with parchment paper, and spray again. Lightly flour the pans with white rice flour. In a food processor, purée the tofu and 1¹/₂ ounces (42 ml) canola oil until very smooth and set aside. Beat together in a mixer with the paddle attachment (or by hand) the sugar and the tofu mixture for about 3 minutes; add in the shredded carrot. While the oil and sugar are mixing, combine together with a whisk in a separate bowl the flours, xanthan gum, baking powder, baking soda, spices, and salt. Add this mixture to the carrot mixture and mix until combined. Do not overmix, as it will result in a dense, unleavened cake. Divide mixture between prepared cake pans and bake for about 50 to 60 minutes or until a toothpick comes out clean.

After the cake is completely cool, you can cut each cake into 2 layers to make a 4-layer cake (or do not cut the cakes, to make a 2-layer cake). Frost the top of the first layer and lightly sprinkle with walnuts. Place the second layer on top of the first, frost, and sprinkle with walnuts. Do this for all 4 layers, omitting the walnuts on the top layer. Frost the sides of the cake and then press the remainder of the nuts onto the sides and top of the frosting.

YIELD: *8 to 16 servings*

Calories (kcal): 835; **Total fat:** 55g; **Cholesterol:** 0mg; **Carbohydrate:** 81g; **Dietary fiber:** 4g; **Protein:** 11g; **Sodium:** 735mg; **Potassium:** 321 mg; **Calcium:** 109mg; **Iron:** 2mg; **Zinc:** 1mg; **Vitamin A:** 12956IU.

Frosting

gluten   milk   soy   egg   corn   nuts

- 2¹/₄ pounds (1 kg) vegan cream cheese
- 1 tablespoon (1 ml) vanilla extract
- 1¹/₂ tablespoons (23 ml) lemon juice
- 9 ounces (255 g) confectioners' sugar, sifted

In a mixer, soften cream cheese by beating with the paddle attachment. Add the vanilla extract and lemon juice until combined. Add the confectioners' sugar and mix until there are no lumps.

Travis Martin's Favorite Flourless Chocolate Mousse Cake

gluten   milk   soy   egg   corn   nuts

Using bittersweet chocolate avoids the dairy-based milk chocolate and lessens the glucose effect without sacrificing taste. Serve sweet things in small half portions and do so after a meal of protein and fiber. This will slow the entry of sugar into the bloodstream and avoid the glucose rise and fall that can trigger behavior and attention problems.

- 8 ounces (225 g) GFCF bittersweet chocolate, finely chopped
- 6 tablespoons (90 g) nondairy spread (non-hydrogenated)
- 6 large eggs, separated
- ½ cup (100 g) sugar

Preheat oven to 275°F (140°C, or gas mark 1) and place rack in center of oven. Grease a 9-inch (23 cm) springform pan.

Place chopped chocolate and spread in a large, microwave-safe bowl and microwave on high in 30-second increments. Stir after each increment, continuing until the chocolate is completely melted. Allow to cool slightly, then whisk in the egg yolks.

Beat egg whites to soft peaks. Gradually add sugar, beating until stiff and glossy.

Whisk one-fourth of the egg whites into the chocolate mixture to lighten it.

Using a rubber spatula, gently fold the chocolate mixture into the rest of the egg whites.

Pour mixture into the prepared pan and smooth the top.

Bake 40 to 50 minutes. The thin mousse cake will have pulled away from the pan side.

Allow to cool.

To serve, dust the top of the cake with confectioners' sugar or spread with raspberry fruit spread.

YIELD: *8 servings*

Calories (kcal): 322; **Total fat:** 27g; **Cholesterol:** 140mg; **Carbohydrate:** 21g; **Dietary fiber:** 4g; **Protein:** 7g; **Sodium:** 146mg; **Potassium:** 281 mg; **Calcium:** 40mg; **Iron:** 2mg; **Zinc:** 1mg; **Vitamin A:** 616IU.

Hot Chocolate Pudding Cake

gluten milk soy egg corn nuts

This is a great rustic treat for a cold winter's night, and delicious served with GFCF vanilla ice cream.

- $^2/_3$ cup (54 g) GFCF unsweetened cocoa powder, divided
- $^1/_3$ cup (75 g) brown sugar
- $^1/_4$ cup (22 g) GFCF chocolate chips
- $^3/_4$ cup (105 g) GF flour blend
- 1 teaspoon baking powder
- $^1/_4$ teaspoon salt
- 6 tablespoons (85 g) ghee, melted
- 1 large egg yolk
- 1 cup (200 g) granulated sugar
- $^1/_3$ cup (80 ml) rice milk
- 2 teaspoons GFCF vanilla extract
- $1^1/_2$ cups (355 ml) hot water

Preheat oven to 325°F (170°C, gas mark 3), and grease an 8-inch (20 cm) square baking dish. In a small bowl, combine $^1/_3$ cup (27 g) cocoa powder, brown sugar, and chocolate chips and set aside. In another bowl, whisk together flour, baking powder, and salt, and set aside.

In a medium bowl, whisk together the ghee and remaining cocoa powder until smooth. Add yolk, granulated sugar, rice milk, and vanilla extract and whisk to combine. Stir in flour mixture until just combined. Spread batter evenly into baking dish, and then sprinkle with reserved cocoa-brown sugar mixture. Pour hot water evenly over batter and bake for 40 to 45 minutes, until edges have puffed up and begun to pull away from the sides of the pan (center will still jiggle slightly). Cool on wire rack 20 minutes; serve warm.

YIELD: *6 to 8 servings*

Calories (kcal): 347; **Total fat:** 14g; **Cholesterol:** 54mg; **Carbohydrate:** 55g; **Dietary fiber:** 4g; **Protein:** 3g; **Sodium:** 192mg; **Potassium:** 31mg; **Calcium:** 52mg; **Iron:** 1mg; **Zinc:** trace; **Vitamin A:** 424IU.

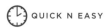 QUICK N EASY

Pie Crust

gluten   milk   soy   egg   corn   nuts

- 1 package (6 ounces, or 170 g) Snickerdoodle cookies
- 3 tablespoons (45 g) nondairy margarine, melted
- 1 teaspoon (5 ml) vanilla extract
- $1/4$ teaspoon cinnamon
- $1/3$ cup (75 g) brown sugar
- $1/2$ cup (35 g) coconut or (60 g) chopped nuts (optional)

Process all ingredients in a food processor until well combined.

Place in a 9-inch (23 cm) pie shell. Press down and smooth crumbs up the sides.

Bake at 350°F (180°C, gas mark 4) for 8 minutes. Let cool.

Fill as desired—works great for pumpkin or pecan pies!

YIELD: *One 9-inch (23 cm) pie shell*

Calories (kcal): 120 9; **Total fat:** 65g; **Cholesterol:** 0mg; **Carbohydrate:** 146g; **Dietary fiber:** 15g; **Protein:** 13g; **Sodium:** 427mg; **Potassium:** 330mg; **Calcium:** 180mg; **Iron:** 66mg; **Zinc:** 1mg; **Vitamin A:** 2649IU.

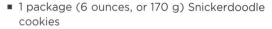

These pie and crumble dessert recipes include ready-to-eat GFCF cookies as a quick and delicious substitute for flours.

Banana Cake or Muffins

gluten   milk   soy   egg   corn   nuts

Besides being downright delicious, this versatile treat can be made as a cake or muffins.

- 1 cup (120 g) quinoa flour
- $2/3$ cup (90 g) brown rice flour
- $1/3$ cup (40 g) tapioca starch
- 1 cup (200 g) sugar
- 1 teaspoon xanthan gum
- $1/2$ tablespoon (7 g) baking soda
- 2 teaspoons baking powder
- $3/4$ teaspoon salt
- 2 eggs + 1 egg white
- 1 cup (225 g) mashed banana
- $1/2$ cup (120 ml) oil (safflower, almond, sunflower, or canola)
- $1/2$ cup (120 ml) rice milk

Combine dry ingredients in a mixing bowl. Add remaining ingredients and mix with electric mixer on low speed until blended. Mix on medium-high speed for 2 minutes. Oil a 9 x 13-inch (23 x 33 cm) pan and cover with parchment paper or use cupcake papers. Bake in a 350°F (180°C, gas mark 4) oven; cake bakes for 45 minutes, muffins for 20 minutes.

NOTE: *Nut butter makes a great, healthy frosting for this recipe.*

YIELD: *8 cake servings or 12 medium muffins*

Calories (kcal): 393; **Total fat:** 16g; **Cholesterol:** 47mg; **Carbohydrate:** 58g; **Dietary fiber:** 3g; **Protein:** 6g; **Sodium:** 585mg; **Potassium:** 328mg; **Calcium:** 91mg; **Iron:** 33mg; **Zinc:** 1mg; **Vitamin A:** 93IU.

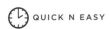

QUICK N EASY

Baked Apple Crumble

gluten　milk　soy　egg　corn　nuts

- 5 large apples, peeled and cut into chunks
- 3 tablespoons (45 ml) lemon juice
- $^1/_2$ cup (100 g) granulated sugar
- $^1/_2$ teaspoon cinnamon
- $^1/_4$ teaspoon nutmeg
- 1 package (6 ounces, or 170 g) No-oats "Oatmeal" cookies
- $^1/_2$ cup (115 g) brown sugar
- 6 tablespoons (90 g) nondairy spread
- $^1/_4$ teaspoon vanilla extract
- Pinch of salt

Put apples in a bowl with the lemon juice. Combine apples with the granulated sugar, cinnamon, and nutmeg. Toss to coat.

Spray an 8 x 8-inch (20 x 20 cm) pan with GFCF cooking spray. Spread apples in the bottom of the pan. Place the cookies, brown sugar, margarine, vanilla extract, and salt in a food processor and process until well combined. Spread the cookie mixture over the apples and bake in a 350°F (180°C, gas mark 4) oven for 40 minutes.

Can be served warm or at room temperature.

NOTE: *Read the label on the margarine—some brands may contain soy or corn.*

YIELD: *12 servings of $^1/_2$ cup (125 g) each*

Calories (kcal): 189; **Total fat:** 7g; **Cholesterol:** 0mg; **Carbohydrate:** 31g; **Dietary fiber:** 3g; **Protein:** 1g; **Sodium:** 80mg; **Potassium:** 96mg; **Calcium:** 22mg; **Iron:** 1mg; **Zinc:** trace; **Vitamin A:** 378IU.

American Apple Pie

gluten　milk　soy　egg　corn　nuts

This is adapted from www.gfutah.org recipes online.

- 1 teaspoon ground cinnamon
- 3 tablespoons (24 g) cornstarch
- $^3/_4$ cup (150 g) granulated sugar
- 5 cups (750 g) peeled, cored, and sliced baking apples
- Unbaked 8-inch (20 cm) double Pie Crust (page 326)

Mix cinnamon, cornstarch, and sugar together in a medium bowl and stir in apples.

Spread apple mixture in an unbaked pie shell.

Cover with top crust and crimp edges with your fingers to seal. Cut slits in top.

Bake in preheated 400°F (200°C, or gas mark 6) for 10 minutes. Turn oven to 350°F (180°C, gas mark 4) and continue cooking for 30 to 40 minutes or until crust is lightly brown.

VARIATION: *Omit top crust and sprinkle pie with Walnut Streusel (recipe follows).*

NOTE: *This recipe can also be made with peaches or pears.*

YIELD: *8 servings*

Calories (kcal): 287; **Total fat:** 8g; **Cholesterol:** 0mg; **Carbohydrate:** 53g; **Dietary fiber:** 4g; **Protein:** 2g; **Sodium:** 54mg; **Potassium:** 142mg; **Calcium:** 32mg; **Iron:** 1mg; **Zinc:** trace; **Vitamin A:** 378IU.

Walnut Streusel

gluten   milk   soy   egg   corn   nuts

Modified for Low Phenol

- $^1/_2$ cup (80 g) rice flour
- $^1/_4$ cup (50 g) granulated sugar
- $^1/_4$ cup (60 g) brown sugar
- $^1/_4$ teaspoon ground cinnamon
- $^1/_4$ teaspoon ground nutmeg
- $^1/_4$ cup (55 g) nondairy spread
- $^1/_2$ cup (65 g) walnuts, chopped fine (Use cashews or sunflower seeds for low phenol diet.)

Combine flour, sugars, and spices.

Cut in cold spread with knives or pastry blender until coarse and crumbly. Add in walnuts. Sprinkle over pie; bake until topping is golden brown.

YIELD: *1$^1/_2$ cups (310 g)*

Calories (kcal): 140; **Total fat:** 82g; **Cholesterol:** 0mg; **Carbohydrate:** 157g; **Dietary fiber:** 5g; **Protein:** 20g; **Sodium:** 549mg; **Potassium:** 543mg; **Calcium:** 100mg; **Iron:** 3mg; **Zinc:** 3mg; **Vitamin A:** 2205IU.

Tracey's Pie Crust

gluten   milk   soy   egg   corn   nuts

- $^1/_2$ cup (70 g) brown rice flour
- $^1/_2$ cup (60 g) quinoa flour
- $^1/_2$ cup (60 g) tapioca starch
- $^1/_2$ cup (80 g) sweet rice flour
- $^1/_4$ cup (35 g) garbanzo bean flour
- 2 teaspoons xanthan gum
- 1 teaspoon salt
- $^1/_2$ cup (120 ml) + 2 tablespoons (30 ml) oil (sunflower, almond, safflower, or canola)
- $^1/_4$ cup (60 ml) milk substitute
- $^1/_2$ cup (120 ml) water

Stir together dry ingredients. Add oil, milk substitute, and water and mix thoroughly. Divide dough in half and roll out bottom crust between two pieces of floured parchment paper. Lift parchment paper and dough and place both in bottom of an ungreased pie pan. Roll out second pie crust. Loosely roll together crust with parchment paper and unroll carefully over filled pie crust. Bake per pie's instructions.

TIP: *A small, one-handled roller works well.*

VARIATION: *For pot pies, replace flours with the following mixture: $^3/_4$ cup (105 g) brown rice flour, $^1/_2$ cup (60 g) quinoa flour, $^1/_2$ cup (60 g) tapioca starch, $^1/_2$ cup (70 g) garbanzo bean flour.*

YIELD: *1 double pie crust or 2 single pie crusts*

Calories (kcal): 119 9; **Total fat:** 73g; **Cholesterol:** 0mg; **Carbohydrate:** 125g; **Dietary fiber:** 7g; **Protein:** 14g; **Sodium:** 1088mg; **Potassium:** 558mg **Calcium:** 48mg; **Iron:** 5mg; **Zinc:** 3mg; **Vitamin A:** 5IU.

Pumpkin Pie (Pareve)

gluten   milk   soy   egg   corn   nuts

This is Travis Martin's favorite Kosher recipe, and it is as good as the usual version. Enjoy!

- 3 cups (675 g) canned pumpkin
- 1 cup (225 g) brown sugar
- 1 cup (200 g) granulated sugar
- 1 teaspoon salt
- 1 teaspoon nutmeg
- 1 teaspoon cinnamon
- 1 teaspoon ginger
- $^1/_4$ teaspoon cloves
- $^1/_4$ teaspoon allspice
- 4 eggs, beaten
- $^1/_4$ cup (55 g) margarine, ghee, or nondairy shortening, melted
- 1 unbaked (10-inch, or 25 cm) pie shell

In a large bowl, mix together pumpkin, sugars, salt, and spices.

In a small bowl, mix together eggs and margarine or ghee. Add to pumpkin mixture.

Pour mixture into a pie shell. Bake for 10 minutes in a preheated 450°F (230°C, or gas mark 8) oven.

Reduce heat to 350°F (180°C, gas mark 4) and bake 40 minutes longer or until a knife inserted into center comes out clean.

YIELD: *8 servings*

Calories (kcal): 443; **Total fat:** 17g; **Cholesterol:** 111mg; **Carbohydrate:** 69g; **Dietary fiber:** 5g; **Protein:** 5g; **Sodium:** 362mg; **Potassium:** 329mg; **Calcium:** 80mg; **Iron:** 3mg; **Zinc:** 1mg; **Vitamin A:** 20992IU.

Blender Pecan Pie

gluten   milk   soy   egg   corn   nuts

This is a simple way to make a holiday favorite.

- 2 cups (200 g) pecan halves, divided
- 2 large eggs
- $^2/_3$ cup (135 g) sugar
- $^1/_2$ teaspoon salt
- $^1/_2$ cup (170 g) agave nectar
- 2 tablespoons (28 g) ghee, melted
- 1 teaspoon GFCF vanilla extract
- 1 9-inch (23 cm) prebaked GFCF pie crust

Preheat oven to 425°F (220°C, gas mark 7). Select 1 cup (100 g) of the best-looking pecan halves and reserve for top. Combine the remaining filling ingredients in a blender and purée until smooth. Pour into prebaked crust, top with reserved pecan halves and bake for 15 minutes. Reduce oven temperature to 350°F (180°C, gas mark 4) and bake for another 30 minutes, until center of pie is set. Cool completely on a wire rack, 2 to 3 hours. Serve.

YIELD: *8 servings*

Calories (kcal): 398; **Total fat:** 26g; **Cholesterol:** 70mg; **Carbohydrate:** 42g; **Dietary fiber:** 3g; **Protein:** 4g; **Sodium:** 43mg; **Potassium:** 123mg; **Calcium:** 16mg; **Iron:** 1mg; **Zinc:** 2mg; **Vitamin A:** 242IU.

Apple, Pear, and Cranberry Crisp

gluten   milk   soy   egg   corn   nuts

This is a great, simple-to-make, holiday dessert. If you can't find fresh cranberries, frozen ones can be thawed and used instead. Or, if cranberries are too tart for your taste, try substituting an equal amount of raspberries or blueberries.

For Topping

- $^1/_2$ cup (70 g) GF flour blend
- $^1/_2$ cup (55 g) chopped pecans
- $^1/_2$ cup (120 g) brown sugar
- 1 teaspoon ground ginger
- $^1/_2$ teaspoon ground cinnamon
- $^1/_8$ teaspoon salt
- 4 tablespoons (56 g) Spectrum Palm Shortening, chilled

For Filling

- 3 medium tart apples, peeled, cored, and cut into $^1/_2$-inch (1.3 cm) pieces
- 3 semi-firm pears, such as Bosc or Bartlett, peeled, cored, and cut into $^1/_2$-inch (1.3 cm) pieces
- 1 cup (100 g) fresh cranberries
- $^1/_2$ cup (100 g) granulated sugar
- $^1/_2$ teaspoon lemon zest
- Pinch of salt

TO MAKE THE TOPPING: In food processor, pulse dry ingredients until combined. Add shortening and continue pulsing until small clumps form and mixture appears sandy. Set aside in the refrigerator until ready to use.

TO MAKE THE FILLING: Preheat oven to 350°F (180°C, gas mark 4). In large bowl, toss apples, pears, and cranberries with sugar, salt, and lemon zest until evenly coated. Transfer mixture to an 8- or 9-inch square baking dish and sprinkle evenly with chilled topping. Bake for 40 to 45 minutes, until fruit is bubbling and topping is golden brown.

YIELD: *6 servings*

Calories (kcal): 414; **Total fat:** 16g; **Cholesterol:** 0mg; **Carbohydrate:** 70g; **Dietary fiber:** 7g; **Protein:** 3g; **Sodium:** 56mg; **Potassium:** 281mg; **Calcium:** 32mg; **Iron:** 1mg; **Zinc:** 1mg; **Vitamin A:** 74IU.

Apricot Almond Torte

gluten   milk   soy   egg   corn   nuts

Substitute sliced peaches/plums in place of the apricots.

- $^1/_3$ cup (37 g) slivered almonds
- $^3/_4$ cup (150 g) sugar, plus 2 tablespoons (26 g) for sprinkling
- $^3/_4$ cup (105 g) GF flour blend, plus more for dusting pan
- $^1/_2$ teaspoon baking powder
- $^1/_4$ teaspoon xanthan gum
- $^1/_4$ teaspoon salt
- 6 tablespoons (83 g) Spectrum Palm Shortening, plus more for greasing pan
- 1 large egg
- 1 large egg yolk
- 1 teaspoon GFCF vanilla extract
- $^1/_4$ teaspoon GFCF almond extract
- 1 pound (455 g) fresh apricots, halved and pitted

Preheat oven to 350°F (180°C, gas mark 4). Grease and flour a 9-inch (23 cm) springform pan. In the bowl of a food processor, grind nuts and $^3/_4$ cup sugar together until fine. Add flour blend, baking powder, xanthan gum and salt and continue processing until combined. Add shortening and pulse until all the nut mixture is coated. Add the egg, yolk, and extracts and process until smooth, scraping sides if necessary. Spread batter evenly in the prepared pan, and then arrange apricots cut-side up on top. Sprinkle apricots with the remaining sugar and bake for 55 to 60 minutes. Cool for 30 minutes on wire rack; serve warm or at room temperature.

YIELD: *6 to 8 servings*

Calories (kcal): 321; **Total fat:** 14g; **Cholesterol:** 54mg; **Carbohydrate:** 45g; **Dietary fiber:** 4g; **Protein:** 5g; **Sodium:** 115mg; **Potassium:** 212mg; **Calcium:** 46mg; **Iron:** 1mg; **Zinc:** trace; **Vitamin A:** 1459IU.

Chocolaty Pumpkin Bars

gluten   milk   soy   egg   corn   nuts

These bars are for those who love chocolate! Calcium and magnesium powders can be hidden in this recipe.

- 2 cups (280 g) GF flour blend
- $^1/_2$ teaspoon xanthan gum
- $^3/_4$ cup (150 g) sugar
- 1 cup (125 g) finely chopped pecans (optional)
- 2 teaspoons baking powder
- 1 teaspoon ground cinnamon
- $^1/_2$ teaspoon baking soda
- $^1/_2$ teaspoon salt
- 4 large eggs, beaten
- 1 can (15 ounces, or 420 g) pumpkin purée
- $^1/_2$ cup (120 ml) canola oil
- $^1/_4$ cup (60 ml) milk substitute
- $^1/_2$ cup (80 g) GFCF mini chocolate chips

Preheat oven to 350°F (180°C, gas mark 4). Whisk together the flour, xanthan gum, sugar, pecans, baking powder, cinnamon, baking soda, and salt in a large bowl. In a separate bowl, combine the eggs, pumpkin, oil, and milk substitute. Stir the wet and dry mixtures together, then add chocolate chips. Spread the batter evenly into a greased 15 x 10 x 1-inch (37.5 x 25 x 2.5 cm) pan (a jellyroll pan with an edge) that has been sprayed with nonstick spray.

Bake 25 minutes. Check with a toothpick in the middle—bars are done when the toothpick comes out clean. Cool completely on a wire rack in the pan before cutting and serving.

YIELD: *2 dozen bars*

Calories (kcal): 186; **Total fat:** 10g; **Cholesterol:** 31mg; **Carbohydrate:** 22g; **Dietary fiber:** 2g; **Protein:** 2g; **Sodium:** 122mg; **Potassium:** 93mg; **Calcium:** 37mg; **Iron:** 1mg; **Zinc:** 1mg; **Vitamin A:** 3962IU.

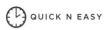
Chocolate Mousse

gluten   milk   soy   egg   corn   nuts

It doesn't get easier than this! A sweet source of protein and a terrific way to hide supplements.

- 1 bag (12 ounces, or 340 g) or 2 cups GFCF chocolate chips
- 1 package (12 ounces, or 340 g) silken tofu

Melt the chocolate chips. Drain the tofu of its water. Combine chocolate and tofu in food processor. Blend until smooth (this may take several minutes). Chill in the refrigerator for at least a few hours.

YIELD: *4 to 6 servings*

Calories (kcal): 599; **Total fat:** 37g; **Cholesterol:** 0mg; **Carbohydrate:** 73g; **Dietary fiber:** 8g; **Protein:** 12g; **Sodium:** 18mg; **Potassium:** 512mg; **Calcium:** 125mg; **Iron:** 8mg; **Zinc:** 2mg; **Vitamin A:** 96IU.

Chocolate-Almond Truffles

gluten   milk   soy   egg   corn   nuts

The better-quality chocolate used, the richer and more delectable these simple, not-too-sweet truffles will taste. This is also a good way to hide supplements.

- 1 cup (235 ml) vanilla non-GMO soy milk
- 16 ounces (455 g) GFCF semisweet chocolate, chips or chopped
- 6 ounces (170 g) GFCF unsweetened chocolate, chopped
- $1/2$ teaspoon almond extract (optional)
- 1 cup (145 g) raw almonds
- Pinch of salt

Heat soy milk in a saucepan until hot but not boiling. Remove from heat and whisk in chocolates until smooth. Add almond extract, if desired, and whisk. Place in refrigerator and cool for 2 hours or until firm.

Preheat oven to 300°F (150°C, or gas mark 2). Toast almonds for 10 minutes or until lightly browned and fragrant. Cool. Transfer almonds to a food processor and add a pinch of salt. Grind until fine.

When chocolate is firm, scoop out portions and roll quickly between the palms, forming walnut-size balls. Roll each ball in crushed almonds, pressing into sides. Transfer to a parchment-lined baking sheet and keep cool until ready to serve.

YIELD: *36 truffles*

Calories (kcal): 111; **Total fat:** 9g; **Cholesterol:** 0mg; **Carbohydrate:** 10g; **Dietary fiber:** 2g; **Protein:** 2g; **Sodium:** 7mg; **Potassium:** 124mg; **Calcium:** 18mg; **Iron:** 1mg; **Zinc:** 1mg; **Vitamin A:** 33IU.

QUICK N EASY

Healthy Truffles

gluten milk soy egg corn nuts

A tasty, high-protein snack and a good way to hide supplements.

- 1¹/₃ cups (230 g) pitted dates
- ¹/₂ cup (85 g) flaxseed
- ¹/₂ cup (70 g) peanuts
- ¹/₂ cup (60 g) dried cranberries
- ¹/₄ teaspoon cinnamon
- ¹/₂–³/₄ cup (130–195 g) GFCF peanut butter
- 1–2 tablespoons (15–30 ml) flaxseed oil (optional)
- Cinnamon or unsweetened shredded coconut (optional)

Mash dates in a bowl with the back of a spoon (or chop dates if too hard to mash). Grind flaxseed, and then add peanuts, to form a fine meal (use short bursts in the food processor to avoid an oily paste). Add to the dates and combine with a spoon or fingers. Add cranberries and cinnamon and combine. Add peanut butter and flax oil and mix well.

Shape the mixture into small balls. Roll in cinnamon or coconut, if desired. Place in an airtight container and refrigerate or freeze immediately. Eat at room temperature, cold, or frozen.

YIELD: *12 to 24 (depending on the size)*

Calories (kcal): 216; **Total fat:** 13g; **Cholesterol:** 0mg; **Carbohydrate:** 21g; **Dietary fiber:** 5g; **Protein:** 7g; **Sodium:** 79mg; **Potassium:** 323mg; **Calcium:** 31mg; **Iron:** 1mg; **Zinc:** 1mg; **Vitamin A:** 10IU.

QUICK N EASY

Lemon Pudding

gluten milk soy egg corn nuts

This is another good food for hiding mild-tasting supplement powders.

- 6 egg yolks
- ¹/₂ cup (65 g) cornstarch
- 1¹/₂ cups (300 g) sugar
- 2 cans (14 ounces, or 425 ml, each) coconut milk
- 3 cups (710 ml) dairy-free milk substitute
- Rind from 1 lemon
- 2 cinnamon sticks
- Juice from 1¹/₂ lemons

Beat egg yolks. Mix all ingredients together. Heat on medium to a boil. Continue cooking on low, stirring constantly, until thickened. Refrigerate for at least 2 hours or until firm.

YIELD: *6 servings*

Calories (kcal): 644; **Total fat:** 37g; **Cholesterol:** 213mg; **Carbohydrate:** 79g; **Dietary fiber:** 6g; **Protein:** 7g; **Sodium:** 34mg; **Potassium:** 411mg; **Calcium:** 107mg; **Iron:** 5mg; **Zinc:** 2mg; **Vitamin A:** 337IU.

QUICK N EASY

Banana Mango "Pudding"

gluten milk soy egg corn nuts

This recipe is not just tasty, it is a good way to hide supplements.

- 1¹⁄₃ cups (315 ml) water
- ¹⁄₄ cup (50 g) basmati or white rice
- 2 juicy ripe mangoes
- 2 large bananas
- 1 teaspoon (5 ml) vanilla
- ¹⁄₈ teaspoon cinnamon, to taste (optional)

Bring the water to a boil in a small pan. Add the rice and cover. Simmer gently for 10 minutes, stirring occasionally to prevent sticking. Remove from the heat and set aside to cool to just above room temperature.

Purée the mangoes, bananas, and rice in the blender. Add vanilla and cinnamon to taste.

YIELD: *2¹⁄₂ cups (500 g)*

Calories (kcal): 668; **Total fat:** 3g; **Cholesterol:** 0mg; **Carbohydrate:** 164g; **Dietary fiber:** 16g; **Protein:** 8g; **Sodium:** 23mg; **Potassium:** 1635mg; **Calcium:** 78mg; **Iron:** 3mg; **Zinc:** 1mg; **Vitamin A:** 16313IU.

Apple Coconut Milk Pudding

gluten milk soy egg corn nuts

This sweet treat is enjoyable as a dessert. It also can be used for hiding supplements for children who are unable to swallow pills and capsules; the richness of the coconut milk and sweetness of the honey is good for masking the taste and texture of supplement powders.

- 1 13.5 ounce (400 ml) can unsweetened, full-fat coconut milk (without guar gum)
- 2 apples (peeled and chopped)
- 1 teaspoon vanilla extract
- ¹⁄₂ teaspoon ground cinnamon
- 2 tablespoons (40 g) honey (Adjust to taste.)
- 1 teaspoon unflavored organic gelatin

Add coconut milk, apples, vanilla, cinnamon, and honey to a saucepan and cook over medium heat until apples are soft. Transfer ingredients to a blender and add gelatin while blending at high speed. Refrigerate until pudding is set.

YIELD: *6 servings*

Calories (kcal): 180; **Total fat:** 14g; **Cholesterol:** 0mg; **Carbohydrate:** 15g; **Dietary fiber:** 1g; **Protein:** 2g; **Sodium:** 10mg; **Potassium:** 194mg; **Calcium:** 17mg; **Iron:** 2mg; **Zinc:** trace; **Vitamin A:** 21IU.

Autumn Sweet Cake

gluten   milk   soy   egg   corn   nuts

This is a "must" at our house for every Thanksgiving. Everyone loves it. There is no pumpkin in this pudding!

- 2 pounds (910 g) sweet potatoes (garnet or white Japanese)
- 2 pounds (910 g) butternut squash
- 3 quarts (2.8 L) + ¹/₂ cup (120 ml) water
- 1 teaspoon salt, plus ¹/₄ teaspoon
- 1 thin slice fresh ginger, peeled
- 1 cinnamon stick
- 5 cloves
- 1 cup (235 ml) Thai coconut milk
- ¹/₄ cup (40 g) rice flour
- 1 teaspoon xanthan gum
- 2 ounces (55 g) GFCF buttery sticks, room temperature
- 3 eggs
- 1³/₄ cups (350 g) sugar
- ¹/₄ teaspoon salt

Peel, seed, and cut squash into large chunks. Peel sweet potatoes and cut into chunks. In a very large pot, bring 3 quarts (2.8 L) water to a boil. Add salt. Add squash and sweet potato chunks. Cook until soft.

In a separate small saucepan, add spices to ¹/₂ cup (120 ml) water. Bring to a boil. Cook on medium for 5 minutes.

Meanwhile, preheat oven to 400°F (200°C, or gas mark 6) and grease a 9-inch (23 cm) round cake pan.

Mix coconut milk with flour and xanthan gum.

Mash squash and sweet potatoes after draining, while still hot. (Tip: Save some of the liquid to drink warm as a vegetable broth. It is delicious and packed with vitamins.)

Add buttery sticks, eggs, coconut milk mixture, sugar, salt, and the liquid in which the spices were boiled. This liquid should have been significantly reduced.

Mix everything. Pour mixture into a greased pan. Bake for 1¹/₂ hours or until a knife inserted in the center comes out clean. Let cool before turning over. This can also be served warm out of the baking dish.

YIELD: *8 servings*

Calories (kcal): 490; **Total fat:** 17g; **Cholesterol:** 88mg; **Carbohydrate:** 84g; **Dietary fiber:** 7g; **Protein:** 6g; **Sodium:** 397mg; **Potassium:** 662mg; **Calcium:** 135mg; **Iron:** 3mg; **Zinc:** 1mg; **Vitamin A:** 24229IU.

QUICK N EASY

Rice Cream

gluten milk soy egg corn nuts

"I scream, you scream, we all scream for rice cream."

- 2 cups (475 ml) rice milk
- ¼ cup (50 g) sugar
- 1 tablespoon (8 g) powdered egg whites
- 1 tablespoon (15 ml) oil
- ¼ teaspoon salt
- ½ cup (75 g) fruit, optional

Put all ingredients in a blender. Add additional rice milk to 4-cup (940 ml) mark and blend. Pour into an ice cream maker and mix.

This has a texture like ice milk.

YIELD: *4 servings*

Calories (kcal): 112; **Total fat:** 3g; **Cholesterol:** 0mg; **Carbohydrate:** 19g; **Dietary fiber:** trace; **Protein:** 1g; **Sodium:** 144mg; **Potassium:** 15mg; **Calcium:** 6mg; **Iron:** trace; **Zinc:** trace; **Vitamin A:** 0IU.

 QUICK N EASY

Aidan's Avocado Fruit Surprise

   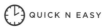
gluten milk soy egg corn nuts

Carla and Aidan provide this dessert, which is like a creamy mousse. The raspberries add a nice tang; however, if lumps are a problem, they can be eliminated.

- 1 ripe avocado (soft but not discolored)
- 1 cup (155 g) frozen blueberries
- 1 cup (135 g) frozen raspberries
- 1 teaspoon (5 ml) lemon juice

Peel and pit the avocado and place in a food processor or blender along with the berries and lemon juice. Blend until smooth.

Store in the freezer in one container or separately in ¼-cup (125 g) servings.

NOTE: *If omitting raspberries because they are too "lumpy," double the amount of blueberries for a total of 2 cups (310 g) frozen berries.*

YIELD: *1 cup (4 servings, ¼ cup [125 g] each)*

Calories (kcal): 165; **Total fat:** 8g; **Cholesterol:** 0mg; **Carbohydrate:** 25g; **Dietary fiber:** 5g; **Protein:** 2g; **Sodium:** 6mg; **Potassium:** 395mg; **Calcium:** 18mg; **Iron:** 1mg; **Zinc:** trace; **Vitamin A:** 377IU.

Creamy Fruit Ice Cream

gluten   milk   soy   egg   corn   nuts

The basics of these ice cream recipes are listed first, and the additions are listed last. There are directions for making the recipes without an ice cream machine. If making these using an ice cream machine, follow the manufacturer's instructions. This is also a good source for hiding some supplements.

AUTHORS' NOTE: *Palm shortening has no trans-fatty acids. Palm and coconut oils are excellent for baking and for making ice cream. The taste is mild. If you want an ice cream that is as tasty as the "real thing"—the palm oil shortening will work well.*

Ice cream machines are the easiest way to achieve a good, smooth ice cream.

Basics

- 1 cup (125 g) potato milk powder
- 1 cup (100 g) confectioners' sugar (pure)
- 1 cup (235 ml) very hot water
- 2 tablespoons (28 g) palm shortening
- $1/2$ tablespoon guar gum
- $1/4$ teaspoon vanilla

Fruit choices

- $1^1/2$ cups (165 g) fresh strawberries
- 4 ripe medium bananas

Combination of fruits:

- $3/4$ cup (85 g) fresh strawberries
- 2 ripe medium bananas

Combine the basic ingredients and the fruit choice(s). Blend all ingredients thoroughly in a blender (medium to medium-high speed). Place into a tightly lidded plastic container. Place in freezer until frozen.

If using an ice cream maker, follow the manufacturer's instructions.

YIELD: *6 servings*

Calories (kcal): 230; **Total fat:** 4g; **Cholesterol:** 0mg; **Carbohydrate:** 51g; **Dietary fiber:** 0g; **Protein:** 0g; **Sodium:** 108mg; **Potassium:** 45mg; **Calcium:** 1mg; **Iron:** trace; **Zinc:** trace; **Vitamin A:** 0IU.

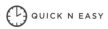

Banana Peanut Butter Mush

gluten   milk   soy   egg   corn   nuts

This guilt-free nutritious ice-cream alternative is also a superior food for hiding nutritional supplements, even those that have a stronger taste.

Modified for SCD

- 2 ripe bananas, sliced and frozen
- $^1/_2$ cup (130 g) GFCF peanut butter
- $^1/_4$ cup (60 ml) milk substitute (For SCD, use coconut or almond milk.)
- Dash of cinnamon
- $^1/_4$ teaspoon vanilla extract

Blend in a food processor until smooth. Eat immediately or put in freezer for 10 minutes to set.

VARIATION: *Use almond butter and almond extract instead of GFCF peanut butter and vanilla extract.*

YIELD: *2 cups (about 450 g)*

Calories (kcal): 250; **Total fat:** 17g; **Cholesterol:** 0mg; **Carbohydrate:** 21g; **Dietary fiber:** 3g; **Protein:** 9g; **Sodium:** 152mg; **Potassium:** 451 mg; **Calcium:** 17mg; **Iron:** 1mg; **Zinc:** 1mg; **Vitamin A:** 48IU.

Lemon Strawberry Ice

gluten   milk   soy   egg   corn   nuts

Try adding $^1/_4$ cup (30 g) non-GMO rice protein powder to this recipe. Adding some protein is both nutritious and helps to reduce the glucose-raising effect of foods that are glycemic.

- 1 cup (170 g) sliced strawberries
- $^3/_4$ cup (180 ml) fresh-squeezed lemon juice
- $^3/_4$ cup (255 g) agave nectar
- 2 cups (475 ml) water
- Pinch of salt

Purée all ingredients in a blender or food processor. Pour mixture into 2 ice cube trays and freeze completely, at least 3 hours. Process one tray of ice cubes in the food processor at a time, transferring slush to a container in the freezer before proceeding with the remaining cubes. Serve immediately. Alternatively, freeze mixture using an ice cream machine.

TIP: *Try substituting fresh raspberries or blackberries for the strawberries, or lime juice for lemon juice (you may want to reduce the agave nectar to taste).*

YIELD: *6 servings*

Calories (kcal): 127; **Total fat:** trace; **Cholesterol:** 0mg; **Carbohydrate:** 34g; **Dietary fiber:** 3g; **Protein:** trace; **Sodium:** 3mg; **Potassium:** 84mg; **Calcium:** 8mg; **Iron:** trace; **Zinc:** trace; **Vitamin A:** 14IU.

Honey Peach Sorbet

gluten milk soy egg corn nuts

Nectarines can be substituted for the peaches.

- 2 pounds (910 g) ripe peaches
- ³/₄ cup (255 g) mild honey
- 2 tablespoons (30 ml) lemon juice
- 1¹/₂ cups (355 ml) water, divided
- Pinch of salt

Preheat oven to 375°F (190°C, gas mark 5). Halve and pit peaches, but leave skins on. Place cut-side down in a roasting pan or baking dish, drizzle with honey, and add ¹/₂ cup (120 ml) water. Cover with foil, bake for 20 minutes, flip peaches over, and continue baking uncovered for 20–40 minutes, until peaches are very tender. Let peaches sit until cool enough to handle, and then slip off their skins and discard. Purée peaches, their roasting juices, lemon juice, salt, and remaining water until smooth. Freeze in an ice cream machine according to the manufacturer's instructions.

YIELD: *8 servings*

Calories (kcal): 135; **Total fat:** trace; **Cholesterol:** 0mg; **Carbohydrate:** 36g; **Dietary fiber:** 2g; **Protein:** 1g; **Sodium:** 3mg; **Potassium:** 191mg; **Calcium:** 7mg; **Iron:** trace; **Zinc:** trace; **Vitamin A:** 462IU.

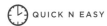 QUICK N EASY

Frozen Melon-Ball Pops

gluten milk soy egg corn nuts

Modified for Low Phenol

- 1 cantaloupe or honeydew melon, or ¹/₂ seedless watermelon (For low phenol, use cantaloupe or watermelon.)

Make small balls of the melon of your choice with a melon baller (or make a medley of different melons). Arrange them on a baking sheet or large plate, skewer them with a fun toothpick, and then freeze. Serve.

YIELD: *8 servings*

Calories (kcal): 24; **Total fat:** trace; **Cholesterol:** 0mg; **Carbohydrate:** 6g; **Dietary fiber:** 1g; **Protein:** 1g; **Sodium:** 6mg; **Potassium:** 213mg; **Calcium:** 8mg; **Iron:** trace; **Zinc:** trace; **Vitamin A:** 2225IU.

Appendix: Resources

BOOKS

Baker, Sidney MacDonald
Detoxification and Healing: The Key to Optimal Health
www.yourmedicaldetective.com

Barkley, Russell A.
Taking Charge of ADHD: The Complete, Authoritative Guide for Parents

Bock, Kenneth, and Stauth, Cameron
Healing the New Childhood Epidemics: Autism, ADHD, Asthma and Allergies. The Groundbreaking Program for the 4-A Disorders

Campbell-McBride, Natasha
Gut and Psychology Syndrome (GAPS)

Crook, William
Tired—So Tired! and the Yeast Connection

Dorfman, Kelly
Cure Your Child with Food
www.kellydorfman.com

Edelson, Stephen M., and Rimland, Bernard
Treating Autism: Parent Stories of Hope and Success
Recovering Autistic Children

Fallon, Sally, and Enig, Mary G.
Nourishing Traditions
www.nourishingtraditions.com

Fenster, Carol
Gluten-Free Quick & Easy: From Prep to Plate Without the Fuss

Gates, Donna
The Body Ecology Diet

Gottschall, Elaine
Breaking the Vicious Cycle: Intestinal Health Through Diet

Grandin, Temple
Emergence: Labeled Autistic
Thinking in Pictures: And Other Reports from My Life with Autism

Hagman, Bette
The Gluten-Free Gourmet series of cookbooks

Hallowell, Edward M., and Ratey, John J.
Delivered from Distraction: Getting the Most out of Life with Attention Deficit Disorder

Herbert, Martha
The Autism Revolution
Autism and EMF: Plausibility of a pathophysiological link (with Cindy Sage)

Jepson, Bryan, Wright Katie, and Johnson, Jane
Changing the Course of Autism: A Scientific Approach for Parents and Physicians

Hyman, Mark
The Blood Sugar Solution
Food: What the Heck Should I Eat?

Kranowitz, Carol
The Out-of-Sync Child

Lemer, Patricia S.
Envisioning a Bright Future: Interventions That Work for Children and Adults with Autism Spectrum Disorders

Lewis, Lisa
The Encyclopedia of Dietary Interventions for the Treatment of Autism and Related Disorders (with Karyn Seroussi)
Special Diets for Special Kids Two

Lipski, Elizabeth
Digestive Wellness
Digestion Connection
Digestive Wellness for Children
Leaky Gut Syndrome

Matthews, Julie
Nourishing Hope for Autism
www.nourishinghope.com
Cooking to Heal

Pangborn, Jon, and Baker, Sidney
Autism: Effective Biomedical Treatments and 2007 Supplement

Pizzorno, Joseph
The Toxin Solution
Clinical Environmental Medicine (with Walter J. Crinnion)

Price, Weston A.
Nutrition and Physical Degeneration

Rapp, Doris J.
32 Tips That Could Save Your Life.

Rimland, Bernard
Infantile Autism
Dyslogic Syndrome

Segersten, Alissa, and Malterre, Tom
The Whole Life Nutrition Cookbook, 2nd edition

Semon, Bruce, and Kornblum, Lori
Feast Without Yeast: 4 Stages to Better Health

Seroussi, Karyn
Unraveling the Mystery of Autism and Pervasive Developmental Disorder
The Encyclopedia of Dietary Interventions for the Treatment of Autism and Related Disorders (with Lisa Lewis)

Shaw, William
Biological Treatments for Autism and PDD

Vess, Sueson
Special Eats: Simple, Delicious Solutions for Gluten-Free & Dairy-Free Cooking

OTHER RESOURCES

ADDitude Magazine
www.additudemag.com
Information on ADD symptoms, medication, treatment, diagnosis, and parenting

The Autism Exchange
www.theautismexchange.com
Information on therapies, biomedical, diet, daily living, education, AEX Blog Discount products, interactive tools, library, and consumer corner

Autism Hope Alliance
www.autismhopealliance.org

Autism Research Institute
www.autism.com
Resources, webinars, research, newsletter, diet information, education

Autism Society of America (ASA)
www.autism-society.org

Autism Speaks USA
www.autismspeaks.org

Barnhill, Kelly
The Johnson Center for Child Health & Development
www.johnson-center.org

Celiac Disease Foundation
https://celiac.org

Children and Adults with Attention-Deficit/Hyperactivity Disorder (CHADD)
www.chadd.org

Environmental Working Group (EWG)
www.ewg.org

Food-Medication Interactions
www.foodmedinteractions.com
The foremost handbooks and software on food/herb/medication reactions

Feingold Association
www.feingold.org

The GFCF Diet
www.gfcfdiet.com
Includes the GFCF Kids Forum (http://health.groups.yahoo.com/group/GFCFKids/)

The Johnson Center for Child Health and Development
www.johnson-center.org/

Kobliner, Vicki
Holcare Nutrition
https://holcarenutrition.com

Medical Academy for Pediatric Special Needs
medmaps.org

The Neurological Health Foundation (NHF)
https://neurologicalhealth.org
The Healthy Child Guide, preconception/prenatal information

Nourishing Hope
www.nourishinghope.com
Julie Matthews, CNC

Talk About Curing Autism (TACA)
www.tacanow.org

The US Davis MIND Institute (Medical Investigation of Neurodevelopmental Disorders)
http://www.ucdmc.ucdavis.edu/mind-institute/

Weston A. Price Foundation
www.westonaprice.org

PRODUCT SOURCES

Applegate Farms, LLC
https://applegate.com

Arrowhead Mills
www.arrowheadmills.com

Ener-G Foods, INC
www.ener-g.com

Enjoy Life Foods
https://enjoylifefoods.com

Gluten Free Mall
www.glutenfreemall.com

Glutino
www.glutino.com

Kinnikinnick Foods Inc.
www.kinnikinnick.com

Lundberg Family Farms
www.lundberg.com

Pacific Foods
www.pacificfoods.com

Pamela's Products
www.pamelasproducts.com

Udi's Gluten Free
www.udisglutenfree.com

Vance's Foods
www.gfcf-foods.com

Wellshire Farms Inc.
www.wellshirefarms.com

Acknowledgments

PAMELA J. COMPART, MD

This book could not have been written without the input and support of so many people; in many ways, this was a community effort.

My deep gratitude and thanks go out to:

All my friends who nourished me, with both food and emotional support, through my medical training and residency and beyond, and who are likely stunned that my name is on a cookbook;

My incredible former colleagues at HeartLight Healing Arts who inspired me daily with their clinical astuteness, the bigness of their hearts, and the brightness of their lights;

All the friends, colleagues, and patients who contributed recipes and testimonials; and all the teachers and healers who came before, whose shoulders I stand on.

Special thanks and abiding gratitude go to Jennifer Sima, RN, who labored above and beyond the call of duty, who collected, collated, and taste-tested innumerable recipes, and who provided me with unflagging faith and support during the writing of this book.

This book would not have been possible without the incredible knowledge and creativity of my colleague and coauthor, Dana Laake, whose brilliance and dedication to her work are unparalleled.

Thanks beyond measure and words go to my parents, who gave me unwavering support through all the various changes in my career till I landed at this place, which gives me such joy.

I thank my brothers, who, after they stopped laughing and realized I wasn't kidding about being asked to write a cookbook, supported me 110 percent.

Last, but certainly not least, I give thanks to my patients and their families, who inspire me daily to be better and do better. I get so much more from them than they do from me.

Pamela J. Compart, MD

"If you have knowledge, let others light their candles at it."

—M. Fuller

DANA GODBOUT LAAKE, RDH, MS, LDN

As a college freshman, I chose the path less traveled and began a journey that has given me far more sunny days than bumps along the way. More than the journey itself, it is the traveling companions I joined who have made the trip extraordinary.

The pioneers and mentors who left their legacy, lit the way for so many of us, endured much opposition, and with noble humility, prevailed: Emanuel Cheraskin, Linus Pauling, Hans Selye, Carl Pfeiffer, Mildred Seelig, William (Billy) Crook, Bernard Rimland, Candace Pert, and Mary Enig.

I am thankful for the pioneers who continue to devote their lives to the biomedical interventions: Sidney MacDonald Baker, Jon Pangborn, Jeffrey Bland, Leo Galland, Doris Rapp, Martha Herbert, Robert Naviaux, Temple Grandin, and the exceptional professionals in the Autism Research Institute under Steve Edelson's guidance.

To the brilliant nutrition colleagues—thank you for your wisdom and generosity in sharing your knowledge: Kelly Dorfman, Julie Matthews, Victoria Wood, Kelly Barnhill, Vicki Kobliner, Sally Fallon, Steven Nadell, Lisa Lewis, and Karyn Seroussi.

Special thanks to Samantha Tucker, Susan Drescher, and Joyce Mulcahy for contributions to this edition. And always—gratitude to the children and their families

To my resourceful, precise, and wise coauthor, Pamela Compart, thank you for being my companion along this journey through our books on ADHD and autism. To my parents for love, wisdom, and believing that their daughters could do anything! Friends and family are the people who do not lead or follow—they walk beside us: Judy Eisenacher, the Pam Foster Friends and family; Mary Kay Almy, Glenda Ingham, Bev Bailey, and the Garrett Park friends; Bonnie Gutman; Linda Schmidt; Susan Polydoroff, and Pam Wilson.

Our blended family is a village, made strong by love and humor: the Clarks—Susie, Tim, Rachel and Bill; the ever-expanding Godbout clan; our sons and daughters-in-law: Pete Jr. and Carron Laake; Steve and Marisa Laake; Rich and Julie Godbout; and Greg and Colleen Godbout; and always the Grands: Peter Laake III, Ella Godbout, Kit Laake, Sammi Laake, Skylar Laake, Brody Godbout, and Melody Laake. With love and genuine appreciation for the one who makes my work possible and keeps me laughing, Pete Laake, Sr.—thank you for asking me to dance!

With gratitude times infinity,

Dana Godbout Laake, RDH, MS, LDN

About the Authors

PAMELA J. COMPART, MD

Pamela J. Compart, MD, is a developmental pediatrician in Columbia, Maryland. She completed a pediatric residency at Children's National Medical Center in Washington, DC, and fellowship training in Behavioral and Developmental Pediatrics at the University of Maryland School of Medicine. She combines traditional and complementary medicine approaches to the treatment of ADHD, autism, and other behavioral and developmental disorders. Dietary changes and use of nutritional supplements complement traditional treatments such as appropriate educational placement and speech therapy, occupational therapy, and other therapies. She founded and directed HeartLight Healing Arts, a multi-disciplinary integrated holistic health care practice providing services for children, adults, and families for 15 years. She is currently in solo practice, focusing on her passions of patient care, teaching, and writing. She is also coauthor of *The ADHD and Autism Nutritional Supplement Handbook.*

DANA LAAKE, RDH, MS, LDN

Dana Laake is a licensed nutritionist in Kensington, Maryland. Within her practice, Dana Laake Nutrition, she provides preventive and therapeutic medical nutrition therapy to adults and children. An honors graduate from Temple University (health sciences, dental hygiene), she received her master's degree in nutrition from the University of Maryland. A recipient of the Temple University 50th Anniversary Outstanding Alumnus award, Ms. Laake has served as a Maryland legislative assistant on health issues, was coauthor of the legislation that established licensure boards for dietetics and nutrition in both Maryland and Washington, DC, and has served four gubernatorial appointments on two health care regulatory boards (dentistry and dietetics). She has been a partner in three functional medicine practices and provides local and national continuing education courses. In addition to writing and hosting a radio show, *The Essentials of Healthy Living* 1500 AM, Dana is a scientific advisor and content contributor for the Autism Exchange and for the Neurological Health Foundation Healthy Child Guide. She is also an autism treatment researcher and coauthor of *The ADHD and Autism Nutritional Supplement Handbook.*

Index